MYOTHERAPY

Books by Bonnie Prudden

MYOTHERAPY
Bonnie Prudden's Complete Guide to Pain-Free Living

by
Bonnie Prudden

THE DIAL PRESS
DOUBLEDAY & COMPANY, INC., GARDEN CITY, NEW YORK

Myotherapy^{sm} is a service mark of Bonnie Prudden, Inc.

Illustrations by Debbie Schmalbach/*Elbow Room Graphics*
Photographs by Bob Curtis

Library of Congress Cataloging in Publication Data
Prudden, Bonnie, 1914–
   Myotherapy.
   Includes index.
   1. Pain—Treatment. 2. Exercise therapy. I. Title.
RB127.P778 1984   616′.0472   83-10062
ISBN 0-385-27755-5

Published by *The Dial Press*
DESIGN BY M FRANKLIN-PLYMPTON
MANUFACTURED IN THE UNITED STATES OF AMERICA
9 8 7 6 5 4 3

For "Beanie" Whittaker, who
made this book a reality.

Contents

Foreword

This book was written for *you*, a human being, to help keep yourself free from pain. It is geared for the executive in the front office, the shop foreman, the salesman on the road, the lady of the house . . . children, oldsters . . . *people*.

For your protection and your family's health and safety, you should purchase a medical dictionary. Should any of you be injured or fall ill, you *must* know what the doctor is talking about when he says your son has cervical radiculitis or you have spondylosis. If someone suggests an operation, you *must* know the facts insofar as the doctor does. You have no right to lay the whole responsibility on him or her. There are many names for pain, and most of them merely tell you *where* the pain is and what type of pain it is, not the cause of the pain. This is particularly true in chronic pain. You must know well that medicine is not an exact science, but that *you* are exactly in the middle when any decisions about your pain are made.

Also, for your protection and peace of mind, you need a book on anatomy. You already have a dictionary and probably a thesaurus to guide you in the world of words. You have an atlas, which provides you with information about the countries of the world, and in your car a road map, so you won't get lost in your own country. Can you afford to be ignorant about that most valuable country of all, your body?

The world is full of people, but each of us is really alone. We would *like* to have others take the responsibility for our well-being, our education and our happiness for several reasons—the main one being lack of self-confidence. Since time began, there have been people telling other people that *they* knew better and even best. The only edge those leaders had was that they believed in themselves or at least in their own ability to sway others. They could read what others said; they could also communicate. It seems that was enough for thousands of years. But now you too can communicate and read. More important than either, you can think and ask questions, and it's time.

For centuries, parents believed that being able to read and write made teachers superior people, so they placed the minds and bodies of their helpless children during their most creative years in the hands of those teachers. Look around you and see what this "education" has accomplished, both mentally and physically.

Health too has been made the responsibility of others, and that hasn't worked either. America has one of the highest infant-mortality rates in the civilized world. Failure due to abdication of responsibility is everywhere: obesity, alcoholism, drug addiction, mental crack-ups, crippled hearts, sports injuries and millions in chronic pain.

We can look everywhere for someone else to blame, but in the end we must look to ourselves. Then we must change.

When you have finished this book you will be wiser than you were. You will also have new weapons for your protection and a start on a new and different kind of education, one for which you will have instant and endless use. You will be different from the person you are now. You will have some control over your own body. And you will be needed.

MYOTHERAPY

The Future Depends on Today

This is the best of all possible times in which to take out a new lease on life. Just about all the things we used to believe in, take for granted or expect have gone, or gone askew. We don't believe in them anymore. We don't trust in them anymore. And we are right. Even our children, coming along behind us, look at the world with cynical eyes. They have no faith in school or teachers, and they are right. When we turn to the law, the lawyers win and *we* lose. When we go to church, nobody's there. We have been horrified by government for a long time and will probably never be innocent again. Hospitals frighten us and so does the military. Our economy is full of holes and our savings are leaking out. Black people, women and the aging suffer discrimination. Our men die young of heart attacks. Morals, if we can use such an old-fashioned word, don't exist: "What's mine is mine and yours is yours, until I take it away from you." Violence, drunkenness, drug addiction, thievery and murder can be found on every street corner, and out in the countryside. Both women and children are fair game, as are the old who can neither run nor stand and fight.

To top it all off, there is pain. Most of us suffer from one kind of pain or another and most of us hide it as a matter of course. When you attend your next meeting anywhere, know that at least 50 percent of the people in that room have back pain, shoulder and arm pain, headaches, or elbow, knee and foot pain. Some have two, three and even four painful areas, not to forget emotional pain, which eats holes in hearts both figuratively and literally. And we are full of fear. Whether we admit it to ourselves or not, we are all afraid of pain, both the kind we have and the kind we might get. So how can this be the best of all possible times? Amend that: It is the best of all possible times for us. That's because we are here, and it's the only time *we* have. That could be said of any generation since the beginning of life on earth, but for this generation there is a difference. There is a difference that wasn't here ten years ago. As far as we know it was never here before. *We know there is a way to get rid of most chronic pain and that that skill has not been locked away behind language or doors*. It is ours to learn and to use. Not only can we get rid of pain, we can *prevent* a good deal of it.

Something else. It's a good time to be alive because we have finally come to the realization that George isn't around anymore, if he ever was. We have been letting George do it, whatever *it* was, for too long, and look what happened. Everything is tumbling down and we can watch our own destruction nightly on TV.

It's a little like watching in a mirror while the doctor performs a panhysterectomy. There goes the best of your guts, not to mention the future, and you will be crippled with estrogen therapy, which, while you can't live without it, is a bullet with your name on it.

You knew and I knew there was no way government could go on borrowing and borrowing with no thought of tomorrow, which has finally become today. You knew and I knew the schools weren't educating the children. We had to hire the graduates who could neither read nor write nor research a subject as simple as why manufacturers are moving their plants out of the country and denying Americans desperately needed jobs.

I knew and you should have known that young bodies were disintegrating behind the hallowed walls of P.S. 9. As long ago as 1954 I went to President Eisenhower with the results of our study which proved American schoolchildren to be the weakest in the world. All America knew. All America was told by the President that he was going to *do* something about it. So George was called in. That was *six* Presidents ago, and I know and you might as well know that despite all the joggers, marathons and tennis tournaments, the physical state of those children as well as almost everyone else is much worse now than it was then. When the minions of the President turned the physical fitness of this country over to the physical educators, it could only go one way, and it did: down. We all know now that physical fitness is vital, but we don't know how to get it.

Not only were we unfit as children in school, we are unfit as adults facing troubled days. At no time since the twenties have we been physically educated by the schools, which are doing just as poorly with academics. Since we were provided with no background in things physical, we have no frames of reference. So we chase one fad after another in a vain search for fitness. Since those providing the fads (George again) know little about *their* bodies, they lead us jogging across America on ungiving surfaces of cement and macadam—surfaces that would spavin the strongest horse. You can imagine what they do to your frail pins.

Georgette has the women of America bouncing around on cement floors that support either tile or wall-to-wall carpet, never realizing that "dancing" on cement, no matter what its cover, is not one whit less destructive to feet, legs and backs than is jogging on cement. We spend millions on weight-training machines although we know absolutely nothing about stresses, strains, individual builds or built-in weakness. Neither do those who rent or sell them to us. We pedal around on spidery, unstable bikes meant for an age before there were millions of automobiles (many driven by frantic or homicidal freaks, junkies and lushes bent on self-destruction). We are fat so we diet. We are stressed so we eat. We are terrified of growing old.

We used to have frontiers. When our forebears didn't like the way things were going in the old country they came to the New World, America. When the East Coast became a little crowded, the venturesome opened up new lands in the West. Even when I was a little girl, people were still moving into the comparatively empty West, but now the stopper is in the bottle and everyone is trapped. When an animal feels trapped it develops another woe: stress.

The word stress got its meaning as we now use it from the Canadian doctor Hans Selye half a lifetime ago. He discovered that, given time, physical or emotional stresses, although varying in type, all cause disease in the human organism. Ulcers appear on the stomach walls, adrenals shrink, the victim *feels* bad. If we are healthy we become sick. If we are sick we become sicker. Worry is stress, fear is stress, anger is stress, and we have every reason to be worried, anxious, perplexed and angry. We have always been a young, hopeful, rather good-natured people until now. Now everything looks so bleak. There's no good news, ever. There is always a plethora of horror which we can hear about, read about and even watch on television. There we can see it all firsthand on the street, in the supermarket, even at home.

America doesn't have a corner on stress and distress; we do have a couple of things going for us. *Our* political stress is only a couple of hundred years old, and so far our cynicism is only skin deep. In other countries there is ground-in despair. We still have a modicum of control. We can look at the ruins around us, both at the edifices that have tumbled and those that are a-totter, and perhaps still do something about ourselves and our land. We cannot do anything much for America, however, until we have done a lot for our own physical selves.

There is an advantage to being alive today among the ruins. There is now a chance for everyone to get into the act. Our situation, while not yet critical, is dangerous. The man who has no bread knows his state is desperate. The man who can still buy bread on credit thinks he's OK until he can't pay the bill. We, unfortunately, are the second man.

But if we rebuild our physical selves, there is a lot we can do. We can rectify physical weakness, and we can erase most pain by ourselves. Strong and painless, we will be able to change our world for the better.

There was a time, and it wasn't long ago, when most people accepted pain as a natural part of living. Backaches, headaches, rusty joints, old war wounds, sports injuries, accidents caused by our jobs or our cars—all were to be expected, and borne with the aid of pills, hot soaks, slings and belts. As for fitness! Well, the doctor who represented the American Medical Association at the first meetings of the Advisory Committee to the President's Council on Youth Fitness com-

plained petulantly: "Fit! What do we need to be fit for?"

Of course medical training is not geared toward health and fitness, it is geared toward disease. And physical educators don't know what physical fitness is either, because their training is targeted to produce games for the masses and varsity sports for the few. The average person doesn't know what physical fitness is because he or she is, like the doctor, a product of the school system as a child and the media as an adult. Television, the press, magazines . . . what do they know? They're all staffed with average people who also came up through the school system. They get their information from advertisers and pass it along to you. It is advertisers who educate America, and we have come to accept their portraits of us as the most benumbed, bemused, absurd, banal, tedious, ignorant and just plain stupid people walking the earth. It's true that we're not as smart as the kids who dropped out of boring, inadequate schools, but we're not as bone stupid as the advertisers paint us. We can still learn, and troubled times may help.

It's impossible to stand in the rubble that's left of the American Dream and worry about constipation, bad breath, underarm odor and Maxi-pads. The last time we really faced hard times was back in the thirties, during the Great Depression. We didn't think it was "great" at all, but it did have some salubrious aspects. I was there and I remember.

One day we had a winter home in New York and a summer home on Shelter Island, a paradise off the end of Long Island. My father had just completed a development of ten beautiful summer cottages on a creek filled with crabs and scallops. Our house was in Dering Harbor and our forty-foot cruiser was anchored out front. There were two cars in the garage, two horses in the stables and a tennis court at the development, and we had the world by the tail. I didn't hear all the awful details because I was away at boarding school, but when I came home for Christmas vacation my parents were living in two tiny rooms in the Knights of Columbus Hotel and my sister and I slept on a foldaway in the parlor.

What was good about those terrible years? We were all in it together and everything became *very* simple. Food was simple, clothes were simple, parties were simple. And people became concerned about each other, and protective. The Depression hit us about ten years after we brought our "doughboys" home from World War I. The stockmarket crashed, the banks closed, people lost fortunes and jobs. Many veterans were in a fair way to starve. Then the Apple Shippers Association took a hand: the unemployed men were given apples on credit. They sold them on street corners.

One bitter winter night I left Columbia University, on 116th Street, on Manhattan's Upper West Side, where I took night courses while still going to high school. I passed one of those fellows standing by his tray, which was set up on a couple of empty crates. He was stamping his feet and flapping his arms as the icy wind off the Hudson blew his breath back over his shoulder. "Buy an apple, lady?" "I would if I had a nickel, but I don't. As it is I have to walk all the way to Seventieth Street."

"No foolin', you don't even have carfare?" Without a second's hesitation he put an apple and a nickel into my hand. That's the way it was. We *noticed* one another.

During easy times we have a way of forgetting about that just as we forget about fitness. Try asking, as the AMA doctor did, "What do you need to be fit for?" I have, and the answers vary, but they boil down to "Because it makes me feel good."

But, in the past five decades as our national fitness level has sunk lower and lower, we have developed a kind of en-nui. We don't want to make the effort that makes us feel good. We're too tired to do anything. It's so much easier to get a beer and a snack, turn on TV and sit down to watch George do it. The price of such abdication is high. As Arthur Godfrey used to say, "If you don't use it, you lose it." You've all seen the guy with both hands pressing on his lower back as he arches and groans softly before ambling down the hall or up the walk. For a lot of people, that first spasm has been the beginning of the end, and your sex life is not the only thing you lose through sedentary living. It is merely one of the last.

Being physically fit and free from pain is like being protected by a magic aura that keeps danger away. Life hurls us into many situations in which we must face up to problems that can cause both physical and emotional pain. The only times we can't handle the problems are when we are sick or in pain or trying to escape them through drugs or alcohol. Nobody has to tell you that we are a half-bombed society, but did you know that one of the major causes of alcoholism is pain? Certainly one of the reasons for drug addiction is pain. These are both vicious circles. The man with constant back pain can hardly wait for the five o'clock whistle that signals a stiff martini and the start of the numbing process that will make the night bearable. Very quickly he will prescribe for himself more than one or two martinis to get his pain down. To numb it he would have to (and often does) numb his mind.

And drug addiction is often *prescribed* drug addiction. The lady in pain is offered Valium. (Valium is suggested far more frequently for women than for men, perhaps because a woman's pain is often *thought* to be psychogenic, rather than somatic.) Whatever the reason, one Valium, like one martini, is not enough, and the lady is soon hooked. And Valium addiction is no fun. Read Barbara Gordon's *I'm Dancing As Fast As I Can.*

If the pain should one day go away all by itself, the sufferer is still left with the addiction, which by that time is worse than the original condition. The backache made life miserable; the pills or the booze makes it unlivable.

There are two reasons for this book. One is to share something called Myotherapy with you. It is a method *you* can employ to get rid of pain that may interfere with living. The second is to suggest ways in which you may raise your level of fitness . . . and keep it there. The two are interdependent. You must be pain free in order to exercise and you must do specific exercises to keep pain at bay. Getting rid of pain is far more simple than you might imagine. Getting into and staying in shape is far more fun and rewarding than you might think. And neither your age nor present condition should preclude it. As a matter of fact, if you are over forty it is easier to get back into condition than it is for the average teenager to achieve it in the first place. After all, the older person walked to school during the formative years before twelve. The teenager, unless varsity material or a cheerleader, never walked anywhere.

Discovery

There are some people who either can't catch up with the times or don't want to. If they want to but can't quite make it, they are always a little out of step. If they choose not to, they don't even bother to march. Then there are people like me, who, whether we like it or not (and it's not always the berries), are usually ahead of the times. We often see ten years down the road, and while it's exciting it can be very frustrating. Occasionally it is lethal, as it was for Ignaz Semmelweiss, who tried to get his surgeon colleagues to wash their hands between patients . . . they destroyed him.

In the forties, I discovered two things that changed my life and the lives of many others: 1. American children were the weakest in the world. 2. Physical education in the public schools was totally inadequate. President Eisenhower believed me, the physical educators did not, and the YMCAs took what I'd uncovered and ran with it.

After the study was proved true, there was a lot of interest in physical fitness, but prior to that no one had ever heard of it. In 1960 someone wanted to give me a gift of a book on the subject, but there were none on the shelves. Last year Americans spent fifty million dollars on fitness and diet books. In the fifties and sixties I had a weekly column on exercise in *Sports Illustrated* and a weekly pro-

gram on the "Today" show. It was ten years more before the spate of exercisers hit the airwaves and exercise articles started appearing in women's magazines.

In the fifties I launched my first class for people over seventy. That was almost thirty years ago, and at the time no one noticed. It wasn't until 1977 that the government started to take an interest in the fitness of the elderly, and it would have been better if they hadn't, because what has evolved from that interest is a disgrace. It's probably going to take another ten years before the proper format is presented, or until the "old guard" of physical educators (many are chronologically young) is replaced.

Back in the fifties we started fitness fashions, which caught on at once. Now, thirty years later, it is fashion, not fitness, that sells.

In the fifties I wrote a book called *Is Your Child Really Fit?* It told people how bad things were for their children and gave them a program that would work at home. In that same decade we compiled the *Sports Illustrated* articles into *Bonnie Prudden's Fitness Book* and launched a program for women as well as children. In 1960 I brought out *How to Be Slender and Fit After Thirty* and made history. It contained the first really vigorous program for women, the forgotten sex in sports. In that book we showed the first full-length, skintight exercise clothes seen outside of a circus and off the stage. We gave out the first word ever (in oh so proper America) on *sexercise*. There was a program for postcardiacs in a day when even *healthy* men were told not to shovel snow. Also a program for the handicapped confined to wheelchairs. There was a weight-training program for women —unheard of!—and exercises to be done anywhere: in the office, the kitchen or the living room. And there were exercises for the old. Not one of those innovations took hold for at least ten years, but all of them are here now, let's hope to stay.

Back in the sixties I introduced baby-exercise programs to America, and again *Sports Illustrated*, which for a few years was way ahead in the fitness field, published it month by month. The baby had been selected for the program before it left Mount Sinai Hospital and grew from a neonate to a very aware youngster under *Sports Illustrated*'s cameras. At the age of four he was already a trilingual athlete. Soon the book *How to Keep Your Child Fit from Birth to Six* came out, but it was years before we could make baby exercise popular. It is now, of course, as is swimming for babies. Revised and published together with three other books in paperback on children's fitness, *How to Keep Your Child Fit from Birth to Six* will be available for the children of the children for whom it was first written as this book makes its debut.

As for swimming babies, we started with one mother, one baby and one teacher in a YMCA in Detroit. With the help of the Detroit *Free Press* we launched the first Baby-Swim-and-Gym program, on a Friday. By the following Tuesday the program was full. Smart mothers thought it was wonderful. Fifteen years later, when I wrote *Your Baby Can Swim*, the "experts" were still fighting the idea tooth and nail, but it was too late. The young mothers had won.

About that same time I launched the first exercise class for pregnant women and men. That was not a misprint. The women were pregnant and looked it, the men just looked it. The doctors at Wesson Maternity Hospital, in Springfield, Massachusetts, felt women needed more than just breathing exercises if they were going in for "natural childbirth." I agreed and we started the class. Since the fathers-to-be kept peeking, we invited them in—not to watch, to take part. That was the first time I saw fathers involved with anything to do with babies. Now interest in prenatal programs is everywhere, but mothers-to-be, still without any physical education preparation for childbirth or anything else, are not getting what they need. *Some* exercise in the third trimester is too little and too late. It may take another twenty-five years to get what is needed.

In the sixties I released two exercise records which sold more than any exercise record in history and are still going strong. But in addition, I also put out four other records and their titles will show you that the future had been foreseen. *Fitness for Baby and You* was the closest to realization since prenatal exercise was already being used. *Executive Fitness* was well ahead of the times. Only in the past few years has there been an interest in corporate fitness, and most of what is available is wall-to-wall machinery, stress testing and running. *Fitness for Teens* was released fifteen years *before* Title IX made co-ed exercise a possibility. *Fit to Ski* preceded by eleven years the understanding that getting in shape to ski was a less traumatic way to go than skiing to get in shape. The message in the book *Fitness from Six to Twelve* fell on deaf ears, because the schools were uninterested in that age group. They weren't varsity yet, and besides, 50 percent were girls. The book *Teenage Fitness* would be right on target now, nineteen years after it came out; *How to Keep Your Family Fit and Healthy*, written in 1975, is just right now for parents who want to do something for and *with* their children.

Seeing ahead is fun, but pushing is very hard work.

So what have I done *lately*? In 1980 I released *Pain Erasure: The Bonnie Prudden Way*. It, too, works; this book includes what I have learned from the thousands and thousands who have used the technique also shown here, and also what I have learned about myself in the past three years.

I have been deeply interested in the study of pain for the past forty-seven years. Why? Because I was smashed up on a ski slope and started on the long, twisting trail of pain in search of surcease when I was twenty-two. For many years I was a guinea pig, as are most back-pain sufferers. When I was thirty-five I began to minister to patients who also had back pain, and took referrals from orthopedic surgeons, internists and general practitioners, for both preoperative and postoperative exercise. Much later, when I was fifty-six and lost my right hip joint due to posttraumatic arthritis, I again became the patient. Midway between that operation and the same operation for the other hip, ten years later, I discovered Myotherapy[SM], but this time—and for the first time—I believe my timing is right.

There is a new wind blowing through the medical world. Acupuncture has been accepted (reluctantly) by the medical profession, because it certainly does relieve pain. Today researchers are finding scientifically acceptable reasons why acupuncture works. That yin, yang and meridian business bothered the sawbones something fierce.

Rolfing, Pfrimmering and the Alexander Technique made inroads into what had been an empty field. Massage parlors (definitely de trop!) reappeared as "massage clinics." Masseuses and masseurs, once completely legitimate, but out of favor due to the "parlors," became "Certified Massage Therapists." We were back to square one, my mother's day, when you could get an excellent massage

Myotherapy[SM] is a service mark of Bonnie Prudden, Inc.

in any first-class hotel or "spa." Of course the word "spa" in those days really meant "spa," not clip joint.

Hypnosis, like massage, has been brought out, dusted off and given a new respectability. Back to square one again. Biofeedback, however, is something brand-new. In Germany there is a saying that "In America everything works electrically" ("*In Amerika alles ist electrisch betrieben*"), and biofeedback is the electric way to get your own attention. Then there is Transcendental Meditation, straight out of the East. It is on a par with biofeedback for getting attention, but after the initial expense for instruction, it isn't as costly and it takes only forty minutes a day. Behavior modification rolled out of the psychology labs. And nutrition, long an orphan in this poisoned land, began to come into its own. The word for this combination is "holistic." And believe me there's a lot more of it. Kinesiology, clinical ecology, iridology, reflexology and herbology, homeopathy, touching, juice fasting, yoga, shiatsu, gestalt, Jacobsen, herbalism, meditation, chelation, Bates-Vision, transpersonal psychology, polarity, Feldenkreis, megavitamins, hair analysis, acupuncture, acupressure, chiropractic, colonics, bioenergetics and autogenics are some. The tenets of holistic medicine are as follows:

You are responsible for your own health or illness.

Dis-ease is caused by stress.

Mind and body make up an indivisible unit.

Illness is a "healing crisis," an opportunity for psychological, spiritual growth.

Preventing disease is better than fighting it.

It is better to treat underlying "disease" than alleviate symptoms.

The goal is wellness, not just the absence of obvious disease.

The patient is not a lone organism.

A physician is a guide or partner, not an omniscient worker.

One of the interesting things about this new development is that many of the holistic centers which provide these "new" methods are run by medical doctors who have come to feel that merely medicating the patient is not the answer. Either that or they have a very sensitive finger on the patient's pulse as more and more patients take a dim view of medication.

In any case, into this climate of rejection and change came the wonderful discovery of Myotherapy, and it *is* wonderful, as you will soon be able to see for yourself. Not just see it for yourself, but *do* it yourself. It didn't begin with me, of course; *all* discoveries come down from someone else's discoveries, which were made because someone discovered something else, and so on. Discoveries are often the result of simple observation, and observation is often forced on the observer, as it was with Myotherapy.

While we were going through the Depression in America, a German by the name of Max Lange discovered, as had many others, that there were tender areas in muscles and that the tissue at these sites seemed harder than that of the surrounding areas. He had used a sclerometer, a gadget for determining the relative resistance of measured tissue to outside pressure. He found that the tender areas were up to 50 percent harder than the surrounding tissue. He also discovered that when he used intensive exercise on the extremities, while these muscles increased in volume and strength *they did not get harder*. That's one myth that's been around a long time, that strong muscles should be hard. A *healthy* muscle when at rest is soft as butter.

In 1948 Dr. Janet Travell, the White House physician during the Kennedy administration, began her pioneering work in the same subject, which by this time had a name. Those tender areas were called myofascial trigger points (TPs). Dr. Travell had begun her work on these points with injections, so the technique was called trigger-point injection therapy for myofascial trigger-point syndromes. It was from Dr. Travell's work that the discovery of Myotherapy came.

Put simply, a trigger point is a highly irritable spot in a muscle and is identified by exquisite tenderness. We believe there are two kinds of trigger points, matrix points and satellites. Although both can cause deep, aching chronic pain, matrix points refer pain to distant sites. The satellites have their own way of contributing to discomfort: they seem to have the power to excite the matrix points back into action after treatment has neutralized them. Trigger points can be both active (causing pain) and latent (silent for the time being, but with the potential for action at any time).

For those of you who would like a more scientific description of a trigger point, here's how an abstract of a Janet Travell article is worded in the *Archives of Physical Medical Rehabilitation*.

Myofascial trigger points (TPs) in a muscle are usually activated by acute or chronic overload of the muscle. They are identified by objective and subjective findings. Objective signs include a palpable firm, tense band of muscle, production of a local twitch response, restricted stretch range-of-motion, weakness without atrophy and no neurological deficit. Subjectively, the patient reports stiffness and easy fatigability, spontaneous pain in a distribution predictable for that TP, an exquisite, deep tenderness specifically at the TP. Sustained pressure on the TP induces referred pain in the predicted pattern. Some muscles are likely to produce additional objective and subjective autonomic concomitants. Laboratory and radiographic findings are negative.

As with so many things I have done, my discovery of Myotherapy was an accident. My skiing accident had left me strung up in traction for three months thinking about the prognosis and never realizing that traction was doing even more damage. I would always limp, would never ski again, could no longer climb mountains and should not have children. I was weak as a kitten and my legs were so atrophied that my husband could circle my calf with his thumb and forefinger. I looked like something grown under a rock and *almost* believed the doctor's grim predictions. Two days after I was freed I went to Florida for six weeks of sun and surf. I should say here that I went with my mother-in-law, who was a most unusual lady. Not once did she say, "Careful, you'll hurt yourself" or "I wouldn't do that if I were you." *Stress was minimal.* Keep that in mind. Returning from Florida limpless, I had already made up my mind as to the prognosis. It was wrong.

In July my husband and I hied ourselves to Estes Park, in Colorado, for a vacation, where we made several first ascents of routes on 14,000-foot peaks. That made two parts of the prognosis that were wrong. I didn't actually go for three, but in the fall there was no question about it, I was pregnant. Baby number one was born by C-section in May, and the following winter we went to Sun Valley to do what I should have done *before* I took Suicide Six straight: learn to ski. So much for the things I was told I couldn't do. So much for the doctors!

Four years later my marriage started disintegrating, and although I wasn't wise enough to understand it, I was about to learn what the stress of unhappiness can do. I began my long affair with back pain. I did what many of you have done: made the rounds to various doctors, tried pills, infrared, X rays, braces, heat, ultrasound, diathermy, traction, rest. Nothing helped until I found out about trigger-point injections. Many injections later I was better, and for the next twenty-seven years I would be all right, then get messed up emotionally or overstressed physically, start a new back attack and have

more injections. Every time my stress level rose, my back would respond like a trained seal. Somehow I never saw the connection between the stressful crises and my pain. Had I seen the connection I might have taken steps to remove my vulnerable self from my very untenable situation.

At that time in my life I was spending every Saturday working with a doctor who had joined the then new specialty called physiatry, or physical medicine. He was a consultant at the hospital and there were patients with every back problem I'd ever heard of and several I had not. They had had laminectomies, fusions and fat-pad excisions. Some just had pain. It didn't seem to matter whether they had been operated on or not, the pain was equally severe, and I was glad I'd never allowed an operation on my back. Actually the doctor I was working with didn't allow it. What did *I* know? If he had said go ahead, I would have. But now I *do* know, and soon you will too.

There were a lot of compensation cases; we said they had "compensitis," and were rather scornful of their *unwillingness* to get better while someone else was paying them to stay sick. Since then I have learned that the percentage of patients getting well even though on compensation seems to be in direct proportion to the length of time they are away from work. I think that is because while on compensation and in pain they learn a different kind of life. That may be similar to the current problem that afflicts people out of work for a long time. It is called the discouraged-worker syndrome. Those who can't find work for weeks and often months finally give up and just stop hunting. The longer they are out the greater the chance of joining that unenviable group. A new way of life and a new way of looking at things is learned. Fortunately, now with Myotherapy, which does an excellent job on the newly injured as well as with chronic pain, we may be able to prevent "compensitis."

In 1976 I was chasing down trigger

points in a lady's neck which were causing her a lot of pain and pulling her head over toward her shoulder. I had been working with Dr. Desmond Tivy for some time and we had an excellent system. I would find all the troublesome spots, circle them in ink and send the patient to him for injection. He would inject procaine and saline into the circled trigger points and then ship the patient back to me for the necessary stretch exercises. It was a good system and quicker than anything else around.

While I was probing the lady's neck I evidently hit a matrix point in full flare. I may have pushed harder or held longer than usual, or perhaps I was absolutely on target, but whatever I did the patient screeched like a scalded cat and her head bounced straight up off her shoulder. A few seconds later she said she was fine and "Thank you very much, that's a great relief. I can hardly believe it." I was in shock. What had I done?

The next patient had a "tennis elbow" that we'd been working on twice a week for a fortnight. She was much better but still had some pain when she rotated her arm inward. The same thing happened to her when I hit the trigger point just below her elbow. In those days I didn't even know we had a technique, let alone how hard to press or how to use the patient to direct me.

The third patient really tied it. She was an older lady with "bursitis" of the shoulder. Cortisone hadn't helped, nor had the wearing of a sling, and just getting out of her jacket and shirt was difficult. She would slide the good arm out first and then, letting the hurt arm hang, drag the garments down and off. Getting back into them was even worse. She would lean over to let the arm hang free and then slide the sleeves back up. Being independent, she permitted no assistance. It was through her that I learned that the body *will* do whatever it *can* do and you don't have to think about it. When there is either substitution or the need for assistance, *there's a reason.*

I had gone through the usual warm-up procedures for a shoulder, which Dr. Travell had taught me, a hot, moist towel covered by plastic, an electric pad, two more towels (dry) and ten minutes of cheerful conversation. The next step would have been passive stretch and as much range of motion against resistance as I could manage without too much discomfort. Instead I said, "Just a second, I want to see if I can find some sensitive spots in your shoulder." I had no trouble finding plenty and she allowed that they did "smart some." *Then* I tried the stretch. What joy! Almost full range and no tight lips. We went through the entire series of exercises without *any* pain and she was ecstatic. So was I. It was when she went for her shirt that I learned my lesson. No leaning over, no dragging a sleeve. She just picked up her shirt and put it on as you or I would have. "Did you see that?" Yes, I'd seen that. "You know, that's the first time I've been able to do that in three months."

Yes, I knew. The movement had been totally unconscious, just as there had been no unconscious effort to protect the shoulder. *There was no longer any need for protection.* Today, all certified Bonnie Prudden Myotherapists^{CM} are trained to watch for any change from protective movement to free movement. The degree of success, other than freedom from pain, is determined by the degree of *unconscious* free movement. Often habit persists in hampering such movement, but the right exercise takes care of it. A limp is trained out with simple rhythmic steps set to music, *step, step, stop,* for example. We do this both forward and backward. Muscles respond to music far better than to voiced commands.

There is another use for unconscious movement. Train yourself to *observe.* Does the driver have to twist his upper body in order to see to back up? You might ask him when he hurt his neck. There are three possible replies. "How

Certified Bonnie Prudden Myotherapist^{CM} is a certification mark of Bonnie Prudden, Inc.

did you know I hurt my neck?'' is one. ''I had a whiplash . . . fall . . . operation'' or some other traumatic experience is another. And lastly but most important, ''There's nothing wrong with my neck.'' Limitation caused by pain is easy to detect. Limitation caused by trigger points in action but not yet to the point of pain make habits. Start watching your family, your friends and *yourself*. Is your range of motion circumscribed anywhere? Are your shoulders rounding? Does one foot turn in even a little? Do all your fingers work equally well? Are both wrists and ankles equally supple? Can *you* turn your head freely? Myotherapy when used to correct such limitation is called *prevention*.

Sooner or later in my lectures someone will ask why medical doctors didn't discover Myotherapy if they've known about trigger points for over fifty years. Part of the answer is training. Doctors are trained to use medication, and when medication must be delivered to a localized area the most effective form of delivery is by needle. Lacking that training, I was not encumbered by habit when faced with something different. Another part of the answer is serendipity. Serendipity is the gift of making fortunate discoveries by accident. A great many people have it, but it only works if they possess the other side of that coin, observation and tenacity. The opposite is seeing what you expect to see, which is one of the negative sides of training. The doctors I learned from also knew about pressure, as do doctors using acupuncture. Injection seemed easier and quicker and probably was. It took longer to do a pressure job, and in order to get the desired results the area had to be covered thoroughly, and not just in one or two key places. And therein lies the major difference between trigger-point injection therapy, acupuncture, acupressure and Myotherapy. We found *hundreds* of trigger points in our searches along muscles, and since we were neither invading the body with instruments nor infiltrating it with chemicals, we were at liberty to be thorough.

While being thorough in a trigger-point search on a very tall, well-muscled ophthalmologist, we discovered that the body has an interesting protective device with unique qualities. The protection is called *armoring*, or *splinting*. The body limits its own action without any external confinement. The doctor had a hip that had been pinned after fracture, and his armoring covered just about every muscle between his foot and his neck, *but we couldn't find a single trigger point*. He had pain and limitation of movement but no trigger points. Unheard of! I asked him if he could come back the next day. He did and he had literally hundreds of trigger points. By what magic had he hidden them and what point finally released them? Impossible for me to say. Then there was the barrel-chested man with painful shoulders. Trying to make a dent in those spasmed muscles was like attempting to make an impression on a saddle with your little finger. Suddenly the Myotherapist hit a key point. We knew it was a key point because the entire shoulder girdle relaxed. He could even breathe easier.

Armoring may protect the body from additional pain, but it is usually carried too far and too deep in chronic pain. It builds up in layers. One day a ''protecting'' layer is removed by Myotherapy only to reveal underlying layers the following day. The easiest to erase, of course, is the last laid down. The last trigger points to give up are usually the ones that were laid down years before in some long-forgotten accident.

Armoring prevents full range of motion and full function of muscles. It also locks in metabolic wastes. Emotional stress, which causes its own armoring, acts as an accessory to that caused by physical damage and pain. When we started using me as a guinea pig for Myotherapy, which still in 1976 didn't even have a name, we found very telltale patterns of pain and distribution of trigger points. They followed the kind of damage that would have been sustained in each of my accidents, operations and occupations. And it was then that we began to pay attention to the *life* histories of the patients sent to us. It is not enough to know the patient's age, general health *now*, his current complaint, date of the pain onset, the name of his insurance company and its address. To find out how to get rid of the pain it is necessary to know what actually caused it and when. He may *think* he hurt his back carrying his current wife over the threshold. Actually he set the stage for this back attack as he was tackled while carrying the ball over the goal line twenty years before. The emotional stresses of separation, divorce and now a new marriage turned the trick. The precipitating incident was merely that. If he mentioned football in his history our search would take a different direction. We would check out his legs as well as his back. By the same token, had he said he was a jeweler by profession, a hurry-up job (which is what he needs right then) would start in his neck.

Knowing what has gone on before in a person's life, including your own, but now from another slant, often makes the difference when sleuthing after pain.

What is it we want to know and what is it we want the other person to know? We want to know about birth and any stories that can be dredged up about early childhood. We want to know about accidents, operations and occupations starting with the first job, as paper boy or magazine-subscription salesperson. We want to know about sports in school and out, and about hobbies. We want to know, or at least have our friend examine for himself or herself, emotional stresses such as losing a love, a job or possessions. It makes sense to know what the person's diet is and whether or not he or she is on drugs or alcohol, and why. We need to know what the minimum fitness level is and where it needs raising. To that

end we will need a simple muscle test (page 131). Speaking of tests in general, we are often asked if we give the exercise stress test. No we do not. First, what is it? In the exercise stress test the "client" at a Y or health club, or a "patient" in a doctor's office, is asked to pedal a bicycle or walk a treadmill while an electrocardiograph monitors his heart. The machines are said to provide clues as to how the heart is functioning while exercising, clues that are not seen when the heart is resting. Each year since 1975 a different medical journal has reported on the unreliability of the test. In 1979 a study in the prestigious *New England Journal of Medicine* criticized the test for sounding alarms for healthy men and women and giving false assurances for sick ones.

A team led by Dr. Thomas J. Ryan, of University Hospital, in Boston, analyzed 1,465 men and 580 women with symptoms of heart trouble to see how well the stress test detected disease. They discovered that in patients who definitely had heart disease, a positive test tells the doctor little that he does not already know. More worrisome, however, was the finding that among angina patients that successfully passed the test, *one third of the women and two thirds of the men had coronary-artery disease that escaped detection*. Conversely, the tests produced false alarms for 12 percent of the healthy men and *54 percent of the healthy women*. Holy Toledo!

Those are figures on a piece of paper, but translate it into living tissue. A middle-aged lady with three children wants to lose weight and "get into shape." Her husband convinces her to take the exercise stress test they give over at the Y, the club or the company gym. They are also given in hospitals, colleges and doctor's offices. The cost is minimal, a mere two hundred dollars to know where your baseline is when you start your program. She takes the test and it changes her life all right, but not as she planned. The test says she has a heart condition and shouldn't even *think* of joining a class or running with her husband. Out of shape to begin with, she settles down to slow deterioration—with a perfectly healthy heart.

Then there's the fellow who gets a clean bill of health. "Your heart's as strong as an ox," he is told. He *knew* it was. Those occasional pains are surely due to indigestion. One day his "digestion" has an attack on the track.

Aside from the history and the minimum fitness test on page 131, you need to know your weight and measurements *and* a rundown on emotional stress insofar as you can pursue the hunt. Once this basic information is at hand, the next step is to determine just what kind of pain you are facing.

Acute vs. Chronic Pain

Two kinds of pain concern us here: *acute pain*, which is a valuable warning system, and *chronic* pain, which *seems* to serve no useful purpose. It feeds on itself to cause more excruciating pain over an ever larger area. In addition to accepting the warning provided by acute pain, we should also be aware that such discomfort not only pinpoints a damaged area, it also predicts future trouble from accumulating trigger points.

Chronic pain is involved with the millions and millions of people who suffer from backache, headache, "trick knees," aching feet, leg cramps, menstrual cramps, painful neck and shoulder syndromes, facial pain, TMJD (temporomandibular joint dysfunction, a pain in the jaw), heartburn, spastic colon, nervous stomach, arthritic pain, pain accompanying strokes, cerebral palsy, Parkinson's disease, teething, colic, asthma, eye, ear, nose and throat disease. To name a few.

Chronic pain has at least one very important aspect: *there does not seem to be a cause*. It comes on insidiously as a rule, and so quiet is its approach that we rarely consider it as real trouble. It might start as a slight stiffness after a long drive, a stint at the typewriter or a night in a strange bed. At first the stiffness may be blamed on a draft from an open window, or the result of any action that brought the pain to our attention.

We tend to ignore low-grade pain and to go about our business as usual at first. As time goes on, however, the pain does not dissipate as with acute pain once healing has taken place. Instead it continues to increase in severity and to attract similar response from adjacent structures. After a while, chronic pain reaches a point where it is no longer merely a nuisance, but a very real threat. Work is missed, needed exercise foregone, a drug pattern is set up and possibly an increase in alcohol consumption. Pain, plus either drugs or alcohol, interferes with sleep, and even when sleep is achieved it does not result in *rest*. Weariness merges into exhaustion, and stress mounts.

Chronic pain is too often misunderstood, misdiagnosed and mistreated. The truth of that statement is borne out by absenteeism, lowered productivity and the millions of hard-earned dollars spent on muscle relaxants, tranquilizers, analgesics, belts, braces, traction, hospitalization and surgery.

Modern medicine does a fine job of putting people back together again after injury, and there has been great progress in joint replacements. Advances in medication and organ transplants promise to be the contributions of our age. But Modern Medicine falls far short in handling chronic pain, pain for which there doesn't seem to be any real cause. Since chronic pain seldom produces anything "abnormal" in tests, it is often considered psychogenic. This is an error that causes enormous and needless distress. The headache may feel as though it is *in* your head and a suspicious doctor may confirm your feeling although pejoratively, when in reality the cause is *on* your head, trigger points in the muscle under the scalp.

The diagnosis ("trouble *in* her head"—it's usually *her* head) was wrong, the understanding was nil and the treatment will be medication which may work for a while, then there will be a switch to another medication. One headache specialist boasted on TV of having seventeen hundred new patients each year and twenty-six thousand patients return to him on a regular basis. If Myotherapy had a record like that, I would consider it a total failure.

Medication will eventually bring on other problems, but at least those are not as serious as some of the results suffered after back surgery for discogenic disease. Discogenic disease has to do with the disks that act as cushions between the vertebrae that make up the spine. One of the first thoughts to go through the mind of a back-pain sufferer is, "It's a disk." It is now known that many of us have ruptured, disintegrated, deteriorated, or whatever disks, yet never suffer a backache. Once in a very great while a sick disk actually impinges on a nerve, but most really good orthopedists don't want to chase a pain by causing a wound which contributes more pain. The disk is rarely the cause of the pain anyway, but, rather, trigger points in the powerful back and seat muscles. Most reputable surgeons prefer to treat back pain conservatively with rest, analgesics and, of late, exercise.

Then there is chronic knee trouble, which is often characterized by pain, swelling, cracking, "going out" and occasionally "locking." It has numerous names like arthritis, chondromalacia, slipped patella, Osgood-Schlatter, me-

niscus tears. If the injury were acute, a fall down the stairs, a football pileup, a sloppy *tour jeté,* or perhaps a bang against the dashboard, conventional treatment would be clear-cut. Ice, elevation, rest and probably a shot of cortisone into the suspect area, the knee joint. With chronic pain, a different tack will be taken. First the elastic bandage accompanied by heat, cold, diathermy, ultrasound, elevation, cortisone and rest. If the knee does not respond (and it rarely does) there is a "new" procedure around that has quickly become very popular. It is called "arthroscopy." It began as a sort of third eye. A tube containing a light and mirrors was inserted into and around the knee joint, looking for abnormalities. Pretty soon the tube was fitted with tools for the repair of such problems as were observed. In acute injuries it is apt to unearth trouble; in chronic injuries its success is less spectacular. One of the reasons is that the arthroscope cannot "see" a trigger point, and even if it could it is "looking" in the wrong place anyway. The cause isn't in the joint, but in the muscles called the *vastus medialis* and the *vastus lateralis.* These run up the leg from knee to pelvis under the inner and outer seams of your pants. There will also be trigger points in the *gastrocnemius* and the *soleus,* the calf muscles. Very few doctors consider muscle spasm when it comes to knee joints, even those in the new specialty, sports medicine.

Pain is never pleasant, but both acute and chronic pain have messages for those trained to receive. Acute pain's message is hard to miss: "You are busted, burned or bleeding. Get help." Chronic pain's message used to be like the ancient Egyptian demotic and hieroglyphic symbols before we found the Rosetta stone. Now we know it *has* a message, and that message is very simple: "There is too much stress in your life, more than you can handle without physical deterioration." By the time your pain has reached the chronic stage, so has your milieu, and the problems have been in effect for a long time. Chronic pain says loud and clear: "Make your life better or you won't have one."

Acute pain requires one of two things if it is to put in an appearance: threat of damage or damage itself. *Chronic pain* requires three: trigger points already in the affected muscles, physical or emotional stress, and lastly a precipitating incident. Most people already have "silent," or latent, trigger points. These have the potential for causing pain but rarely "fire" without emotional upset. There are many kinds of emotional stress; even falling in love is stressful. Nobody would miss falling in love, but under certain circumstances it can bring on a migraine. But positive stress, like winning and loving, is not what we have to worry about today. Today there's too much negative stress intruding into our lives. One of the most pervasive is the fear of unemployment. We can even put up with inflation and high interest rates if we know our jobs are safe, but who would have believed Japan could bury Detroit under a mountain of Toyotas? What about radios and TV sets? Could you have foretold a name like Sony? Most people can and are willing to tighten their belts *if* they have belts to tighten, but imagine what is happening to the backs and bowels of those who pick up pink slips with their last earnings. Try to understand what is going through the minds of car salesmen today. And how about the black lady with two unemployed teenage sons who have taken to the street? That's stress.

There are other ways of being stressed even without such extremes. Try teaching in a junior or senior high school. What about carrying two jobs *and* trying to get through school at the same time? Or marrying and living with a creep. Then there is getting a divorce and losing the kids. Or being allowed to keep the kids, but without financial help. What about having an old parent come to live with

you? Or worse, *being* an old parent and being forced by the new economy to go and live with the young ones? There are the everyday problems like being an athlete or a concert pianist and having to produce—win or else. These are all examples of stresses we face. Is there any wonder that pain in America is on the upswing and pharmaceutical houses are making money as never before?

We also have physical stresses that compound the problem. There is the need to work longer hours or take on two jobs, or sign up for work we are not trained to do. There is even the almost ridiculous situation of those who feel it is necessary to jog, join the racket club or go to an "aerobics" class because Jones and his wife are doing those things.

So, in order to produce chronic pain, we need trigger points and stress, which most of us have. The third ingredient is the one that fools most people, including doctors. It is the *precipitating incident*. The precipitating incident *seems* to be the agent of destruction, but is merely the finger on the trigger. The patient *knows* his back pain is due to lifting incorrectly. However, a lifetime of lifting "correctly" will not stave off the next episode of pain when the climate heats up again. The skater can train to a fare-thee-well and rest for a complete season, but given the trigger points *he has*, the stress of wanting to win, and the right moment of imbalance, and the muscle will go into a tearing spasm again. A great actress catches a cold and in a coughing spell throws the *intercostal* muscles (between the ribs) into a spasm because she activated trigger points in residence since a fall from a horse thirty years before. She can avoid colds, take enough cough medicine to blur her lines, but the problem of trigger points and stress will continue. Next time, the precipitating incident may be lifting her poodle. Then she will avoid lifting her poodle, so the next and the next incidents may be closing a window or sneezing.

Every day, you read in the papers of athletes sidelined for a week, a month or sometimes forever. All athletes have trigger points garnered in games or in practice. The stress of needing to perform well and, they hope, win is ever present. But what about Dad's backache? He hasn't played anything more athletic than gin rummy since he left the semipros in Dallas. No, but he *did* play once, and years don't matter. As for stress, he just learned that the junior partner was given both the job and the raise he was promised.

Ah, you think, but housewives don't get into athletic competition. Never did. Why should there be such a high rate of pain-filled, pill-filled women in that category? Take over a house for a week sometime, a house with three "littles" under five, a dog, a parakeet, a mortgage, inefficient plumbing, the cleaning, the shopping, the bills, the jitneying, the shots, the braces, the flu, the chicken pox, diapers and diaper rash, squabbling, TV and a belly out to *there* with little number four. If, when I ask an older woman with back pain what her profession was and she answers, "I raised four boys," I don't have to question further. She will have trigger points *everywhere*.

Myotherapy

The discovery we made in 1976 was a way for the average person to erase pain for himself, herself and others. It was given the name Myotherapy by Dr. Desmond Tivy, who was in on its development from the beginning and has championed its cause every step of the way. In the first book, *Pain Erasure: The Bonnie Prudden Way*, he wrote the Foreword, which every book of its kind needs. But he also wrote an Afterword. In the Afterword, Dr. Tivy tried to anticipate the questions readers, especially those with medical backgrounds, might ask. Since he did a far better job than I could have done, as I have a very different kind of mind and experience, I quote him from time to time in order to give you immediate answers to the questions you no doubt will ask.

To start with, *myo* means "muscle" and *therapy* means "service to." Myotherapy works with muscles. Nerves and vessels are included, of course, but for the most part they are secondary in our thinking. Once we realized what could be done to relieve pain, we felt we owed it to people to get the news out. Dr. Tivy wasn't so sure. At first he wondered about the advisability of publishing a medical discovery directly to the lay public. Medical discoveries are normally published first in the medical literature "step by tedious step." That is so they can be exposed to "harsh peer criticism."

I must say, however, the only "harsh" criticism came from two headache specialists on "Kup's Show." That is a TV show out of Chicago, and on it I was called everything that the two men could think of. There was no real criticism of Myotherapy, just of Bonnie Prudden, which boiled down to plain bad manners.

There were some snide remarks re my contention that most headaches were due to trigger points in muscles causing spasm. That wasn't too surprising, since they advocated medication as a treatment mainstay augmented by getting up at the same time even on weekends, biofeedback, and relaxation. Not very long ago there was a newspaper article heralding some interesting news. Some doctors had declared that "To get rid of headaches caused by muscle tension, simply locate the headache's trigger point—the muscle where the pain is coming from—then gently massage it." Aside from the fact that they didn't know how to locate the trigger point or what to do when they found it, they *had* admitted that, yes, trigger points did cause headaches. And whose name was attached to that amazing statement? The doctor who had jumped all over me on "Kup's Show."

While Myotherapy has a medical discipline as its forerunner and model, it really isn't a "medical discovery" reserved for the medical profession, as is medication or invasive work like injections. It can be done by almost anyone, and once your doctor says, "No, you don't have any anatomical pathology such as a fracture, a tumor, tuberculosis of a bone or an aneurism," you can be pretty sure Myotherapy will help. We have a class of six-year-olds who do very well with it, especially on "growing pains," and we teach it in our nursery school to three- and four-year-olds. Dr. Tivy said about discoveries, "That which can be readily refuted is probably false; that which many can find little fault with is probably true; and many shades of gray exist between the two."

You should know that neither Dr. Tivy, who has been hoping for controversy, nor I, who have not, have had communication saying Myotherapy does not work. We have had thousands of letters from the public attesting that it does. While on tour with the book, which in essence means going across the country doing TV and radio spots, giving lectures and signing books for people who had innumerable questions about their pain, I encountered many doctors other than the two "headaches" on "Kup's Show." Their only complaint was that I might miss something pathological since I lacked that training. Missing something pathological isn't tops on my worry list, as none of our clinics accept patients without a medical referral from doctors who *do* recognize pathology. Since we have made that clear to the medical and dental societies we have addressed, there has been no further question on that aspect of Myotherapy.

The major "complaint" against Myotherapy is that it has not been "scientifically researched." True. We had not taken several hundred patients (or several thousand) and given them Myotherapy while withholding it from an equal number. This second group would then be treated by conventional methods: muscle relaxants, analgesics, traction, heat, whirlpool baths, rest and surgery. As of this writing such studies are under way.

Dr. Tivy says that one of the reasons I wanted to release Myotherapy now is that I am no longer young, and kindly adds, "Except in heart and in demeanor." And while the slow dissemination of the work might be better served where the medical community is concerned, "I haven't got time for the waiting game." Neither do millions of sufferers who have already tried everything else available and are still living and dying in pain. I don't have the time or the will, either, to stand by while valuable careers in sports and the performing arts go glimmering when some muscle work would save and probably augment them.

Dr. Tivy also said, but in far more elegant phrasing, that if I dared to stick my head up there would be many who would take potshots at me. I'm used to that. I've been fighting entrenched ideas for a long time, and I'm not afraid of controversy. I said American kids are weak. They are. I said there is nothing the matter with American girls and therefore no reason to have them doing modified physical fitness tests. There isn't, and the girls now taking weight training are making the physical educators who broadcast that fallacy (and those who, sheeplike, went along with it) look foolish. I said running on cement would hurt legs. Fifteen million has-been runners have borne that out. I said "aerobic dance" done as it is would cause "shin splints" and calf-muscle cramps; it did. I said curtailing deep knee bends was wrong and that warm-ups had to be done *before* running and stretch afterward and that most older people can be put into *good* shape in a matter of weeks when challenged and *properly taught*. No, I'm not afraid of controversy.

Today we have medical doctors offering to do the research in exchange for the opportunity to learn about Myotherapy and experience the work. We have nurses coming to school to add myotherapy to their other skills even though Myotherapy has never been reported in a medical journal. How does the medical community learn about it? The same media that offer the advertiser's *mis*-information tell all about Myotherapy, too. Dr. Travell discovered years and years ago how to stop hiccups with a spoon. It appeared in the medical literature and no one ever saw it. I never met a doctor who had read about it. A few months ago an article about it appeared in one of the tabloids and everybody read about it. Even more recently, Myotherapy got a big boost from an article in the New York *Times* telling how it helped bring pianist Leon Fleisher back to performing after more than a decade on the shelf with muscle damage. Now everybody knows about that too.

Doctors learn about Myotherapy from their wives and their patients, neither of whom are bogged down with piles of medical literature or waiting rooms filled with patients. Patients ask doctors for referrals, and many thousands have said, "Well, it might be worth a try."

Dr. Tivy said he never believed that those patients whose pain his profession could not explain or cure were victims of an overzealous imagination, or neurotic, or psychologically sick, or whatever. I feel he is absolutely right and that those who are the most scorned are usually the least deserving of that scorn. All too often when patients are sent along for Myotherapy they have previously been treated with "behavior modification" because they were "undoubtedly reaping secondary benefits from their illness." They may even have been referred to a psychiatrist for pain, which is much like being sent to a dentist for bunions or a podiatrist for tooth extraction. There *is* a connection of a sort, but there are more direct ways to go. When such people finally find us and, after checking for trigger points, I say, "No wonder you hurt, you have enough trigger points for two people," they often burst into tears. Nobody believed them before. It is one thing to hurt and receive attention and sympathy, and quite another to hurt equally while being treated as beneath contempt.

You may wonder about the high success rate claimed for Myotherapy. Roughly 5 percent of the people we see show no change whatsoever. Those are invariably the people who have had the problem for a long time and been downed by it, or who have pathology which has not yet been discovered or which has not reached that point where it can be. In the first instance we will try for several sessions, and in the second, send the patient back to the doctor for more tests. Myotherapy is not yet for them. The stress fracture has to heal, and the tumor or aneurism has to be treated medically or surgically. Only then will it be possible to relieve the pain of spasm. For the other 95 percent, we have found that we can alleviate all of the pain in most, most of the pain in others and at least control the pain in the rest; that is if they will continue with their exercises at home for the rest of their lives.

Exercise in America is a misunderstood entity. It did not do too badly prior to the thirties, while the influence of Sweden, Germany and Czechoslovakia was still in effect, but when a group of American physical educators decided to outlaw it in favor of "play," the doors opened for every half-baked theorist in the country, and they were like locusts in a cornfield. Destruction was everywhere. "Children," they said, "want to *play*, not sweat over unimaginative exercises." "Exercise," they said, "makes girls muscular and masculine." "Exercise," they said, "isn't *progressive*. We don't need muscles anymore, we can push buttons." They never knew that muscles are needed for living comfortably and that healthy muscles assure freedom from most pain.

It should be noted here that nobody ever asked the children. I was one of them, and we loved our Indian clubs, wands and marching. We thought tumbling in formations was great, and everybody wanted to be the top man on the pyramid. Girls were considered normal human beings then, not fragile reproductive organs encased in weak, undependable frames. It was the perennially menopausal types who did us in (both male and female, but—would you believe it—mostly male). *Now*, over fifty years later, we have graduated four generations of schoolchildren who were denied the exercise *and the attitudes* they need for health and freedom from pain. Now, fifty years later, we are going back to jump ropes and running, and wands, mats and action, *but not in the schools*—outside, where grown-ups are trying to make up as best they can for the lost joys that should have been theirs as the right of children.

About the theory of Myotherapy, Dr. Tivy says theories are good predictors of future data, they give us a "handle" to hold on to while we think about the subject. He suggested to me that I not get into them, because that is not my forte, and besides, my theory might well be proved wrong, as have been most other theories on pain, and in that event they might throw the baby out with the bathwater.

Aside from Dr. Tivy's very legitimate concern, I also have to remember that, while most theories come first and the proof later, we came up with a method for getting rid of pain first, and I feel quite comfortable that someone else will no doubt find out *why* it works, as the government is now trying to find out why chiropractors get their results. Meanwhile people are getting well.

This is a time of skyrocketing medical costs. Hospital bills are astronomical, many physicians charge about $2.50 a minute and chiropractors roughly $1.00 a minute. That sounds like a better deal until you realize you go to a doctor occasionally, but to the chiropractor every Tuesday, often for years. Medication is costly at best and becomes both dangerous and addictive at almost worst. At worst it can kill you. Nobody today can afford to be sick or in pain.

There is another reason to avoid sickness and pain. We've already touched on it, but it looks as though we'll all have to deal with it for some time to come. So let's talk about unemployment. Unemployment is a problem now, but it is going to get a lot worse. Between the Depression and the eighties we have almost come full circle. Back then, if you were out of work, well, tough. And there were no jobs for teenagers. None. Any job around was filled by a head of household. There were no guarantees of any kind, and there was a lot of "genteel poverty" as well as the out-and-out kind. In between then and now, despite three wars, most people got along fine. That's over.

Not very long ago, most unemployed could count on unemployment compensation. At the height of the 1973–75 recession, more than 75 percent of the jobless were on it. In 1981 only 37 percent received any help. Fewer are finding themselves eligible for benefits, and those who are get less. Those may be straws in the wind, but they weigh like bales for those affected. Shoplifting in this country used to be done for kicks. Now it's for real. Management passes its losses on to the customer and it costs the average family over $350 a year in higher prices, and the thieving population is no longer confined to kids seeking kicks. The old are getting *hungry*. Hungry and scared. They, too, are stealing.

While trigger points are garnered by everyone, the stress of fear, anger and despair coupled with precipitating incidents as people try to do work for which they are unprepared will lead to more pain than this country has ever seen. *You* can't afford to be numbered among that tragic legion, nor can you carry friends and family on your back. The time to *do* something is while you can prevent it and the side effects that accompany sickness, injury and pain.

Dr. Tivy on the subject of safety and

the known side effects of Myotherapy gave the following list:

1. PAIN.   The treatment by pressure hurts for a few seconds, commensurate with the pain of an intramuscular injection of a mildly irritant substance, but often less than the pain involved in injecting saline or local anesthetic into exactly the same spot [trigger point]. It certainly seems less than the pain of injecting around an inflamed tendon, as in "bursitis" of the shoulder.

I can add a little to that. I have had hundreds of trigger-point injections, and every one of them was exceedingly painful. I've probably had thousands of trigger points extinguished by Myotherapy. I am the prize guinea pig and have been for years. Not one of those came close to even the least painful injection, but the best part is that *you* control the job. You can always say, "Hold it right there."

2. BRUISING.   Bruises at the site of pressure do sometimes occur. They are very small in extent and occur more often in women who are known to bruise easily. They are less common and less extensive than would be likely were the same spot to be injected. Those on anticoagulants will bruise more readily of course. Our experience with such patients is limited, but it has not so far been a problem.

I'd like to add something to that. If you are on large doses of aspirin, you are on an anticoagulant, whether it is called that or not. Recently I worked on a lady who had been treated with radiation for cancer of the lip. She had been on massive doses of aspirin to control the pain in her mouth. She bruised if I said, "Good morning."

3. INCREASED FUNCTION LEADING TO CARELESS BEHAVIOR.   A few have celebrated their newfound mobility and freedom by going dancing or engaging in some other form of activity inappropriate to their degree of control, thus ending up falling and doing themselves harm.

True, the incredible relief felt by the patient who has suffered for years and suddenly is pain free does lead to *some* lighthearted, not to say foolhardy escapades. But in every instance in which this has occurred another session undid the damage and in every instance the patient said, "It was worth it!"

4. PAIN SHIFT.   A unilateral pain which switches sides after treatment; or it may shift from one area to another. Our experience is that, the fact that it can do this at all confirms the probability that the disorder is functional, not structural. Further treatment to the new areas usually results in further pain relief.

To this I would like to add that quite often the pain in one area is of such intensity that though other areas ache too, the sensation of the lesser pain is superseded by the greater to the point where it is not noticed at all. When the high-intensity pain has been cleared out, then the other painful area calls attention to itself. A good example of this is the pain in the noninjured leg. The leg, which has been overworked for weeks, often months as a support for the nonfunctioning leg, actually has pain which goes unnoticed until the injured leg feels painless. The surprise and dismay shown by the sufferer, and the distressed remark "But now my other leg hurts," say it well.

5. PAIN EXACERBATION WITH OR WITHOUT SHIFT.   Usually this means either structural disease, such as herniated disk which has been overlooked, or severe superimposed inflammatory reaction and/or psychological overlay. In any of these cases medical treatment is required. With careful selection of cases this is rare in our experience.

6. TEMPORARY   RELIEF   . . .   NO LASTING BENEFIT.   Here the diagnosis may be wrong or there is more than one diagnosis; or the patient is improperly motivated (for a multitude of possible reasons) to continue exercises and other home treat-

ment to prevent recurrences; occasionally the reasons are undetermined.

To that I would add that if the diagnosis has been right and success is achieved at first but the pain recurs, it is very possible that a trigger point or points have been missed. As we will show in the *Permanent Fix* section of this book, when you have searched the area close to the pain, made headway and then lost ground, you must move on to adjacent areas, those next in line for that specific pain.

7. DOLLAR COST. (This is assuming that you want a more skilled person or you want firsthand instruction and must therefore seek out a certified Bonnie Prudden Myotherapist.) Though the Bonnie Prudden Institute for Physical Fitness and Myotherapy's charges are equal to or slightly less than the going rate for physical therapy, the number of sessions required is usually far fewer. And if by taking a gamble, expensive testing is also obviated, then the cost is often less than the testing process itself. But, at present, the absence of third-party insurance for Myotherapy does deter a significant number of people from the initial cost.

To that I would add that there are eighty-eight Myotherapists in the world today. As each year more and more graduate from the Bonnie Prudden School for Physical Fitness and Myotherapy[SM] there will soon be many more certified Bonnie Prudden Myotherapists available. One notable exception to the rise in unemployment is in the service-producing sector, which includes health care. They have added 737,000 jobs in the past year. Myotherapy comes under health care.

8. IF THE INDICATION TO USE MYOTHERAPY IS WRONG, IT WON'T WORK.   This applies to almost everything else of course.

Dr. Tivy had some thoughts on other disciplines too, and he said about acu-

The Bonnie Prudden School for Physical Fitness and Myotherapy[SM] is a service mark owned by the Bonnie Prudden School for Physical Fitness and Myotherapy, Inc.

puncture: "Acupuncture went through quite a vogue a few years back (though I never had any of my patients use it), and then the public interest died down. Why? It would appear it often relieved pain, after innumerable treatments, and after enormous expense, but seldom lastingly. I begin to see why relief was temporary, for if acupuncture relieves the same kind of pain that Myotherapy does (and maybe the frequent coincidence of acupressure points and trigger points is more than coincidental), then unless you treat the cause of the pain, it will return. And if the cause be, for instance, posture muscle function, function related to posture, unless you *teach* the muscles better subsequent habits, the cycle will start all over again."

To that I would add that the exercise portion of Myotherapy is of extreme importance, as is the use of those exercises on a continuing basis. According to Dr. Janet Travell: "Myofascial pain (from trigger point activity) may be perpetuated for long periods of time after the initiating event by self-sustaining neuromuscular mechanisms, aggravating metabolic factors, mechanical stresses and emotional stresses. The injured skeletal muscles differ from other tissues because skin, bone and joint capsules heal, whereas *the muscles learn to protect themselves* [italics mine]. The better the musculature, as in the athlete, the more likely other muscles are to guard and splint the injured muscle indefinitely, so that it is not used serendipitously in the course of daily activity. Stretch to maximum normal range interrupts the self-perpetuating mechanisms that maintain trigger point activity."

If daily living does not provide considerable activity, including full range of motion for the injured muscle as well as the rest of the body, pain is apt to become the expected condition. The American way of life certainly does *not* provide opportunities for such activity; the only way to achieve it for the vast majority is with a well-designed exercise program conscientiously pursued.

Dr. Tivy on internal organs: "Myotherapy does not pretend to influence internal organs, as I believe acupuncturists claim to do. But I can now understand why they thought they could. I have seen a number of cases of abdominal pain, for instance, that patients were persuaded were due to gallbladder disease, and the patient could not understand why the X rays were always negative. After Myotherapy and relief for a year or more (whereas previously pains occurred almost every week, which is unlikely periodicity for gallbladder disease anyway), it seems to me the pain was musculoskeletal in the first place, secondary to postural deficits. But I can quite understand that the patient and her therapist might imagine that it was her gallbladder that was cured."

A second example of musculoskeletal masquerade was even more confusing. The patient who, after years of suffering, had her gallbladder removed. Imagine her chagrin when the pain continued at regular intervals (usually when stress was at a high level) with the same intensity as before the offending organ had been removed. In desperation one night just before the ambulance arrived to take her back to the hospital for pain control and then tests and observation, she had Myotherapy done on her *back* and the pain was eased at once. After several applications to back and abdominal muscles, the spasms ceased, *never* to recur. The question to consider here is . . . what would have been done in the hospital if Myotherapy had not been available?

Dr. Tivy on acupressure: "I think I now understand why Kurland's acupressure only sometimes works in cases of migraine. He advocates the same sort of pressure used in Myotherapy on only four of the trigger points used by certified Bonnie Prudden Myotherapists, and subsequent exercises are not stressed. If only a *part* of the full treatment is used,

no wonder it fails in some cases! This too is a check for the unwary reader of this book. Anyone who tries Myotherapy and doesn't do it right can expect failure, as can anyone who takes only one penicillin tablet to rid himself of a sore throat."

On physical therapy, transcutaneous electrical stimulation and biofeedback: "I think I now understand, for the same reasons as given regarding acupressure, why physical therapy works and fails when it does, though its results tend to be more long-lasting than acupressure. And why TENS (transcutaneous electrical nerve stimulation) and biofeedback (both very time-consuming and expensive) succeed and fail when they do, for analagous reasons. And certainly why proponents of multiple injections into trigger points only sometimes succeed: *You just can't treat a few trigger points* [italics added] and do nothing about the rest. It just doesn't work. To my mind Bonnie Prudden's greatest and key contribution here has been the discovery of in just how many places unexpected trigger points may lurk."

And what does Dr. Tivy have to say about chiropractic? "I know little of their work and methods, but anecdotal evidence of good results is just too overwhelming to ignore. The overtones of the word *manipulation* do conjure up the image of possible dangers that a certified Bonnie Prudden Myotherapist could never encounter. But I must say that if the medical profession could produce as relatively few disasters as one hears from the chiropractors, I would be more ready to criticize the methods of the latter. Even if there were twice the rate of incompetence among chiropractors as among doctors (for which I have no supposition or evidence), their toys seem a lot less dangerous to play with than ours.

"It would seem entirely that certified Bonnie Prudden Myotherapists and chiropractors succeed on the same types of pain via different approaches, possibly via the same mechanisms. But several differences arise. First, chiropractic is a passive therapy, which the therapist does on you while you lie back. Little attempt is made to prepare the way against recurrent pain, so you return week after week for a dose of the same medicine. Myotherapy, at least as practiced by Bonnie Prudden, though passive at the start, demands continued patient effort to reeducate the patient into non-pain-producing habits. The necessity for multiple visits would be deemed a failure of the method, or the therapist, or the patient's resolve. As a rule I find that it takes as many visits to a certified Bonnie Prudden Myotherapist, to ensure full pain relief, as the first figure of one's age. This reflects the concept that pain erasure seems to be an unlearning process (followed by relearning) and that children have less to forget than their elders, and learn faster afterwards. Subsequent repeat visits are necessary when time, new bad postural habits, or new injuries supervene. But some patients, apparently unweanable from passivity, will still prefer the chiropractic approach. And I must admit that the flock does seem to behave better if a visit to the pastor is required at regular intervals."

There is one group of patients who return for Myotherapy on a regular basis without apology. These are the stroke patients, who need more and longer care, and also the patients with frightful injuries, usually due to automobile accidents that have affected both body and brain. Unfortunately at this time we usually get them after the rehab center has either given up on them or refused to take them because they are considered hopeless. Such patients not only need to be systematically freed of trigger points, they also need to know that someone has hope for them and that someone actually cares what happens. There is a vast difference between being left alone to yank on a pulley, turn a wheel or walk your fingers up a wall and having someone's undivided attention while exercising for an hour to the music of the Top Ten.

Dr. Tivy on the limitations of Myotherapy:

> Another difference is that certified Bonnie Prudden Myotherapists (insofar as I can influence them) are under no illusions that they are treating the spine and its nerves, and do not hypothesize unsubstantiatable theories about their work. I have always thought that if chiropractors would keep quiet about their theories, the doctors might listen to them more, but I wish I and my colleagues were blameless in this respect. I understand *why* they theorize; it has its uses, but is counterproductive at present.

As I have said before, Dr. Tivy has been most insistent that certified Bonnie Prudden Myotherapists keep *their* theories to themselves. So we do. Dr. Tivy says:

> The final difference between chiropractors and certified Bonnie Prudden Myotherapists is that the former take X rays, the latter do not. This upsets the doctors more than anything else, as we feel we have the best training around in diagnosis, and this is really indisputable. A properly trained certified Bonnie Prudden Myotherapist will not treat a case not checked by a physician (or as in the case of TMJD [temporomandibular joint dysfunction], a dentist) and will only give an opinion as to the advisability of continued versus further medical treatment after the first session.

I would carry that one step further. *If* you find a person claiming to be a certified Bonnie Prudden Myotherapist who takes you for treatment *without* a medical referral, you are visiting a fraud and should be warned. Certified Bonnie Prudden Myotherapists go to the Bonnie Prudden School for two years and graduate as certified Bonnie Prudden Myotherapists and certified Exercise Therapists. Every two years they must attend renewal sessions in order to be recertified.

Dr. Tivy on arthritis:

> A word should be said about arthritis. There are ninety-odd forms of it listed in the medical literature and doubtless more to follow. Most people know about degenerative osteoarthritis, which may develop with age

and after injury, and which shows up on X rays. And they usually know about the inflammatory types of arthritis, such as rheumatoid arthritis and lupus erythematosus and gout, which can occur in younger patients. Of the less common types they remain in fortunate ignorance.

But the type not mentioned among the ninety-odd, the commonest type of all is the-arthritis-that-isn't, the type the doctor says you have when he really means pain. My patients sometimes ask whether it is true that Bonnie Prudden really "cures" arthritis. Certainly not, but she does often relieve the diagnosis of arthritis-that-wasn't, or at least wasn't the cause of the symptom. For if your sixty-year-old painful neck is X-rayed, osteoarthritis will commonly be found, but that is not to say that the arthritis is the cause of your pain. It may be, but more commonly it is setting the stage for improper muscle function, which can usually be relieved by Myotherapy. And since the pain is relieved concomitantly, and the X rays still show arthritis subsequently, one can only conclude that it was the muscle dysfunction that caused the pain . . . which will return unless the muscles are "taught" to behave more comfortably in the future.

To the above I would add that the word "cure" is not in the lexicon of the certified Bonnie Prudden Myotherapist. Myotherapy has two major functions: to get rid of pain and to reeducate the muscles into healthy, pain-free habits. There are of course some additional pluses that go along with Myotherapy: you learn to care for yourself *and to think about yourself.* Selfish, according to the dictionary, means *too much concerned with the self*, but Ayn Rand has written an entire book on *The Virtue of Selfishness.* I'm with Ayn Rand. There probably is such a thing as being *too* concerned with the self, but most of the time I find people are too *little* concerned with the self and rather too much concerned with other people. The way your body feels and looks should be of prime concern to *you.* It's the only thing *you* own and it is your only means of attaining whatever

makes you glad, joyous and fulfilled. It is the author of your freedom. It is your safety and your home. Only you can keep it pain free, strong and ready for tomorrow. And tomorrow is now.

Dr. Tivy on disease:

In similar fashion, Myotherapy can achieve pain relief in a number of organic, structural diseases that are episodic in nature with quiescent periods between flare-ups. It would seem that not all the crippling that occurs in rheumatoid arthritis, or even multiple sclerosis, is due to the disease itself (much as not all the pain associated with osteoarthritis is due to the arthritis itself). While only physicians can (or at least attempt to) deal with the acute flare-ups, Myotherapy can sometimes relieve the pain, probably due to disuse and stiffness that occurs in the quiet intervals. Physical therapists know this too.

If Myotherapy can be safely developed for preliminary use *before* consulting a physician or if physicians can ever feel safe providing it before engaging in a series of expensive, definitive diagnostic tests, then Myotherapy could make a significant contribution toward solving the problem of the escalating cost of medical care. I find Myotherapy sometimes useful as a diagnostic test; I find it teachable to other therapists and even, in limited fashion, to patients; I find it remarkably effective and largely predictable; and I find it safe. I hope the world will agree, and can use it.

When Dr. Tivy wrote those comments, in July 1980, *Pain Erasure: The Bonnie Prudden Way* was just going to press. No one knew if just-plain-people could really use that book except me. I knew they could because even before the book was written there were articles in magazines and newspapers about Myotherapy and people were following those very limited directions and making them work. The patients who can learn to use Myotherapy in only "limited fashion" are often people who have been all but destroyed by the disease and sometimes the treatments prescribed for the disease. *You* can learn and *you* can use it. Just be sure that you or your friend or relative has no pathology such as an unhealed fracture or a tumor or an aneurism, or something requiring medical attention. Of course if you've gone the whole route and haven't improved, you already know your problem and have already consulted at least one physician.

Trigger Points and Pain

Trigger points get into muscles when they are "insulted," which means damaged, and there are many opportunities for such damage from before birth to life's end. The placement of the trigger point conforms to age, activity and chance. We have grouped these opportunities under five major headings:

> BIRTH
> ACCIDENTS
> SPORTS
> OCCUPATIONS
> DISEASE

While that list seems to progress according to age, the only heading that is really age-related is number one, birth. Accidents can happen at any time, and sports, once considered the province of the young, now attract people of almost all ages. Occupations, which used to be the responsibility of adults, are now being embraced by the young. There is no other way for most of them to get the money needed for the expensive wants of today's youth. Disease, like accidents, can strike at any time, but increases as the years wear down the organism.

BIRTH

Trigger points can be laid down in the womb as well as during the birth process. Babies are born neither equal nor equally. There are forceps births and vacuum extractions, both of which cause muscle damage to tiny heads. Then there is Pit-ocin, a "hurry-up-kid" medication. It is often given for just that, to speed or even induce birth. Or it can be given to counteract the Demerol provided routinely to "spare the mother's strength" during the first stages of labor.

Birth is not really the first opportunity to pick up a trigger point. If the baby takes the wrong posture after its uterine swimming pool gets overcrowded with itself, it is possible to lay down trigger points in several areas. If the head is tipped to the side and the position maintained for a period of time, spasm may be initiated in the neck, upper-back and chest muscles. If the feet are turned inward, they may be locked into that position, later to be treated with casts, braces and corrective shoes. If the back is bent forward unduly or curved laterally, you may not see the results until puberty. At that time the posture anomaly that surfaces may be diagnosed as "idiopathic scoliosis" or "kyphosis."

The birth process is something else again, since the American way of birth is just plain out-and-out *abnormal*. Many other countries treat birth as a normal part of life and allow their women to have their babies without interference. We do not. We don't even let them believe they *can*. In spite of Read, Bradley and Lamaze (normal-birth advocates whose proponents do try to counteract our beliefs), we continue to attack both mothers and babes. *Routinely* they are provided with fetal monitoring, medication, slit vaginas and forceps. America seems to be one of the most dangerous places in which to have a baby, while Sweden is the safest.

You can protect yourself *and your baby* by learning as much as possible about birth in these United States and what *could* be done to you, and by shopping for the doctor ahead of time, and by having in your hands a list of "routines" you will *not* permit. When "D day" comes, be sure you go to the hospital accompanied by a *man* as knowledgeable as you are about birthing procedures. A woman might be protection enough *if* your doctor respects women, but you'd better find that out ahead of time.

Demerol, a pain-killer, affects the fetus and slows labor, sometimes to a standstill, necessitating the use of forceps. *Pitocin* is a hormone that speeds labor and affects the baby, too. It can be administered over and over in the IV and you'd never know it. That is one of the reasons for looking with a jaundiced eye on that bottle that is wheeled into the room almost before you get your shoes off. However, there is a greater danger connected with that IV. The nurse has been told to tell you that you will be dehydrated, which will certainly be true if you are not allowed any water by mouth. But *why* aren't you to be allowed a drink of water or many drinks of water? The answer is as simple as it is ominous. "You may require a cesarean section, and for that you need an empty stomach." You haven't been in the room long enough to unpack and they are already measuring you for a cesarean. That is American birth thinking, and you have to protect yourself against that *well* ahead of time. Find out what your proposed doctor's rate of cesareans is and also the rate done at his hospital. The hospital's rate will reflect your doctor's habits, so you have a double check, and don't think you don't need it. Some hospitals have a cesarean rate of 5 percent and some go as high or higher than 35 percent. The higher the rate, the greater the knifing habit.

Someone may tell you that a C-section is the painless way to go. Don't you believe it. Not only is there a lot of pain connected with it, but you don't get connected with your baby when you should, *which is at once*. Also, cesarean babies have difficulty getting their systems started. The powerful contractions that propel a baby down the birth canal also inform its whole organism that it is time to plug in, to get with it. Cesarean babies don't get a clear message, perhaps because the transition is so fast. One second they are being zonked with anesthesia, and the next having their protective sleeping bag unzipped. One minute it's quiet, and the next, uproar followed closely by bedlam. Sometimes they are so crocked with drugs they can't breathe on their own. These babies often suffer with breathing problems and digestion problems. Don't have a cesarean if you can possibly avoid it; one way to avoid it is to stay away from hospitals where medication is given *routinely*.

There are several ways to damage a baby's head, and one of the more common is by breaking the bag of waters to induce labor. This takes away the cushion that is supposed to protect the head as long as possible. Your baby knows when it's ready to bid for life. Neither you nor the doctor knows. There was a time when birth was induced routinely for the convenience of somebody, but mothers are getting smarter now and they are asking questions, and fewer are replying, "If you say so," to anybody at all. And it's going to get worse—or, rather, better.

If the baby's head is damaged due either to Pitocin and forced labor or forceps, it may have a pointy head or be bruised and even bloody. If it has been vacuum-extracted, it may have a lump on its crown. In either case you may be holding a future migraine sufferer in your arms. Keep this information in your mind. (Or better, in your baby's records along with the birth certificate. It could be very useful someday.) There may be a more urgent need for you to be both observant and knowledgeable. The headache may not be deferred until a later time. It may start at once or within days.

Babies who cry a lot are called "colicky babies," and the first effort to correct this situation is usually with diet. If the baby is being breast-fed, the commissary will be suspected of giving lightweight milk. However there may be a much simpler reason for the screams: a headache. If a baby has pain, it screams, and when it does, it swallows air. When enough air is swallowed, it develops a stomachache and the screams increase, making the typical jerky almost panicky movements of babies with true colic. Very often it has so exhausted itself that when the breast is offered the baby it is too tired to make the most of the opportunity. This will affect the milk production and the baby's weight. A supplementary bottle will be suggested, but since the headache continues the crying continues. Full formula is next, but that won't help either, because of the headache. However, *you* may be able to help. Wait until the baby is awake but not crying, and press lightly on the forehead, temple or almost anywhere on the face or back of the head. See page 142. If the baby puckers with discomfort, you may have found a trigger point. If the second press elicits another look of discomfort, you can be almost sure you have found at least part of the cause, and if you held the light pressure (See Zone 1, Segments 3 and 4) for about three seconds . . . you will have erased those two trigger points. There are more, but you are on your way. Also you know a good reason, besides a *possibly* deficient diet, for your baby's all too obvious distress.

Check your new baby's neck, shoulders and hips. All three can be injured during birth. A wry neck can result from pulling the baby out. Shoulders too can be strained. Stringing the baby up by the ankles while walloping its insignificant bottom has the potential for dislocating hips. Don't wait until you hear someone say it's a boy or girl before you *ask* to see and hold that baby. Make that part of your contract with the doctor as your right *and* your baby's right. We have come so far from *normal* birth in this country that the most *normal* sequences are overlooked. After all, who *had* that baby anyhow? Nobody but you.

If you do find trouble, call it to someone's attention at once. A baby's head is supposed to be on straight and the shoulders even. Some heads will be out of shape through no fault other than birth, but remember it. Always write what you observe in the baby's records . . . always. If it *has* had its head injured by forceps, pixied by Pitocin or lumped by vacuum extraction, you just lost the fight for *normal* childbirth, never mind *natural* childbirth. "Natural" is the buzzword for the eighties and means nothing when attached to anything.

There will be something you can do about your baby's injuries and your own if you had an episiotomy. The need will arise later, probably much later, but at least you will be alerted. Check "Seeking Massage" on page 229 in the *Sports in America* section. You may even be able to *prevent* future distress.

The lithotomy position (lying flat with legs lifted and strapped apart into stirrups) even if you escape episiotomy, which is done routinely unless you specify otherwise, will put trigger points in your lower back and legs. It is an abnormal position and the major cause for anyone needing an episiotomy. Both mother and baby are forced to work against gravity and tightly stretched tissue. If your hands were manacled, check your shoulders, chest and arm muscles for pain or stiffness. If your baby's birth was long ago and today you have pain in those areas but cannot recall an accident that might have laid down trigger points, remember the delivery room. Remember twisting against restraints that should never have been there. Such restraints might well have been the cause of your present "bursitis."

As soon as you get your baby home, do "Seeking Massage" and have it done on you. Start the baby's exercise program and your own. You both need some rehabilitation. You will find your program in the *Sports* section, and read the book *How to Keep Your Child Fit from Birth to Six*, Dial Press, 1983 (paperback).

ACCIDENTS

No accident, no matter how *seemingly* trivial, is inconsequential. The accidents sustained during the birth process can remain hidden for many years, only to surface when physical or emotional stress reaches a critical point. Falling down stairs or off swings, slides and seesaws are all accidents with the potential for bringing on chronic pain. After the laceration has healed or the cast been removed, always use the Seeking Massage to find out if any fifth-column moles have been left behind: sensitive areas denoting trigger points. Look also for lopsided growth. If the diagnosis is "idiopathic scoliosis," or spinal curvature, it may mean the doctor doesn't know what caused it, but if *you* remember a fall sustained by that youngster years before, you *could* have the clue as to what caused the trouble and what to do about it as well. If you are aware of what falls *can* do, you may also be able to *prevent* posture anomalies.

Whiplash injuries can occur from something as mundane as hitting the curb with your bike wheel. They occur almost universally in auto accidents, even the accidents that are so mild as to go unrecorded. They can affect everything from the crown of the head (headaches), down to the face (TMJD, or jaw pain, tinnitus, facial neuralgia, tic douloureux, Bell's palsy) and on to the neck (pain and stiffness, torticollis, hoarseness, difficulty in swallowing, aching teeth and ears, double vision, dizziness) and still further to affect the arms, chest and upper back.

A fall caught by one or both arms can put trigger points in the chest, upper back, shoulder girdle, arms, hands and,

very important, the armpit (*axilla*). Trigger points can direct spasm upward to affect the neck and head muscles.

A "prat fall," or "banana-peel fall," in which the person lands on the seat, can set up pain in the lower back, upper back, neck and head. If the pain skips from seat to head, few would suspect the real cause. Such a fall often refers pain from the back to the front: the groin. Impotence and frigidity are rarely considered to have a physical cause. The psychiatrist running down clues leading to maternal inadequacies would be surprised (and possibly chagrined) to learn that Mr. Doe's mashed coccyx was at fault.

A fall on or blow to the knees could, at some later date, cause hip pain, aching legs and swelling. The reverse is also true. Injury to the *quadriceps* muscles, in the thigh, may cause knee pain mistakenly diagnosed as a meniscus tear or osteoarthritis.

Falls account for 14,000 deaths annually, and roughly 360,000 such accidents make it to emergency rooms and hospitals. Imagine how many lesser falls go unreported even though the victims are far from all right. The real damage may not put in an appearance for years.

The products we buy for our health's sake often have Jekyll-Hyde potentials. Deaths from bicycle accidents are second only to deaths occurring in auto accidents. But as in falls, deaths are secondary at least in numbers and suffering to the injured. Bikes are involved in thousands of concussions (then and future headaches) and fractures which will always have to be watched for trigger points collecting at fracture sites *and* at the attachments of any muscles involved. In addition, if there is traction used, other than for setting the limb, there will be further damage. And then there are cuts. Cuts are wounds, and wounds heal, marking their passing with scars. Scars house trigger points. Bike accidents are long on amputations, usually caused by irreparable damage to blood vessels or infection. Amputation sites sustain hundreds of trigger points, many causing phantom-limb pain and resistance to prosthetics.

A header taken off a bike and onto cement causes damage to teeth, which is expensive to begin with, but if a rider hits hard enough to break teeth he has done more than just that. He has laid down trigger points in face, jaw, head, neck and shoulders.

Automobile accidents are so astronomical in number and catastrophic in effect that statistics are obsolete before the ink is dry, but there are other types of accidents that should be noted. Accidents involving garage doors, cleaning agents, table corners, rugs, box springs, frame beds, climbing sets, diving boards, windows in bath enclosures, wax floors, glass doors, to name a few. There are also dogs, horses, guns and stairs.

Every one of the above accidents will lay down trigger points, and every point has the potential for causing pain, disability and misery. Many accidents could not have been avoided. Some could have been with a little care. Almost all of the trigger points can be found and neutralized even *before* pain warns that damage sustained long ago is about to erupt again.

the lower legs, heels and low back *and* the thighs. The competing swimmer damages shoulders, neck, chest and *axilla*, or armpit. The basketball player usually hurts knees and ankles and occasionally shoulders. What the ice-hockey player and football player do to their bodies is a crying shame, not so much at the moment of injury, but later, about twenty to twenty-five years later. In adult recreational sports, we see the tennis players with arm, shoulder and knee damage. Where downhill skiers used to sprain ankles more than fracture, the new equipment seems to protect the ankles. But since the force must go somewhere, it fractures the leg or tears out a knee. While the varsity football player *may* get a shoulder separation, the woman taking up "aerobic dance" *will* get calf-muscle spasms, "shin splints" and probably low-back pain. Every sport must be considered risky as far as trigger points are concerned. Some are riskier than others, but that's no reason to avoid sports. It only means that you should take measures to avoid collecting trigger points where possible, be aware of any picked up in the pursuit of health and pleasure, and make efforts to neutralize them and keep them neutralized.

SPORTS

Sports are the elite level of physical activity, but few Americans are either trained for them or fit for them. Later, in the *Sports* section, you will see how this happened in a once-fit country; for now, just accept that although sport is an ideal way to stay in condition, it is a major contributor to trigger points and chronic pain. We begin to see sports injuries down in the Little League set, with a condition called "Little League elbow." Later on, this painful problem will be termed "tennis elbow," whether the sufferer wields a racket or a screwdriver. In high school the soccer player starts laying in a supply of trigger points in the thigh muscles, the jogger and the track man in

OCCUPATIONS

Occupations too are fraught with danger, even the most sedentary, simply because they *are* sedentary. It is easy to see and understand the perils connected with using a jackhammer or working in a mine or as a longshoreman. *Over*-use resulting in strain is obvious. However, sitting at a typewriter or computer terminal eight hours a day five days a week is just as dangerous, as is practicing the piano. The body is held in a restricted position while the same muscles are used over and over in exactly the same way. This results in a condition known as micro-trauma. The dentist and the violinist court the pattern of pain as they twist to the left with arms raised, performing minute movements under complete and stressful concentration. I was once asked by a cardiologist if I could fix his lower back. Fifteen minutes later he was fine, and I said, "Your back was more like that of a violinist than a cardiologist." He replied happily, content that at least something held over from a different time, "Oh, but I *was* a violinist before I became a doctor." Nothing we *ever* do a lot of is lost. We never forget how to swim, ride a bike and drive a car, and muscles don't forget either. No trigger point we ever garner gives up its *potential* for causing pain. With your pain or the pain of your friend, leave no possible trigger point unturned. When you come to your history, remember *all* your occupations, not just the last.

DISEASE

Disease is usually thought to come to us as we advance into old age, and a lot of it does as tissues deteriorate from multiple causes. But disease can start in utero, and predisposal toward various diseases is given us at conception. The aftermath of some disease is catastrophic, as with sight and hearing impairment following measles. But there are silent problems after disease too. Trigger points laid down by high fever or seizures can cause exactly the same kind of pain as that due to sports, accidents or occupations. The noxious products of disease will lay down points *and* fire up already existing ones, as will alcohol and drugs. It is not yet clear whether the spasticity following a stroke is caused by trigger points laid down by the condition or by already existing trigger points responding adversely to a new condition. In the event that the latter proves to be the case, one preventive measure that all middle-aged people could take would be to sweep the body clean of known trigger points on a regular basis.

Diseases such as lupus, rheumatoid arthritis and multiple sclerosis can set up new trigger points and even activate old ones. This causes spasm and pain, and since the pain accompanies the diagnosed disease, the sufferer thinks of the pain as an unavoidable accompaniment of the disease itself. Since many believe that the only way to control pain is to take medication, they fall into a deadly trap. Anti-pain medication is just that. It is against pain, and to a greater or lesser degree controls it. It does not, however, get rid of the cause of the pain, so without it the pain continues. Thus the medication must be continued, usually in ever-increasing dosage until some side effect worse than the disease develops. This is called a trade-off. You get rid of one kind of pain only to develop something else, for which another kind of medication will be prescribed. That medication will be taken until yet another side effect develops, etc. This goes on until the heart, constantly assailed by toxins, gives out.

There is another facet to such cyclic diseases. They are sometimes in "flare" and sometimes in remission. When they are in flare, the disease is active. The lupus patient hurts, the rash is all too apparent. The patient with rheumatoid arthritis has swollen, extremely painful joints, and the multiple-sclerosis patient may lose control of the extremities and even sight. Then comes the long, slow climb to a semblance of health. However, just because the disease takes a holiday does not mean that the trigger points will go along. Far from it. Once activated and kept activated by toxins, the trigger points continue to function, as does the need for medication. *But* if the trigger points were erased, much of the pain would cease, as would the need for medication . . . and so too would the deterioration *caused* by the medication. The *painless* individual could then pursue a physical-fitness regime that would *prepare* to meet future onslaughts of the disease with a much higher level of health as an aid.

The Technique

What does a trigger point feel like? Lay your forearm on the table in front of you and with the *knuckle* of the middle finger of the other hand, press straight down on the surface of the arm one-half inch from the elbow crack. Press in *slowly* toward the table. As you press you will find a very sensitive spot which will become more painful the harder you press. Hold that pressure for seven seconds. Release slowly and evenly, as though your knuckle were operated hydraulically.

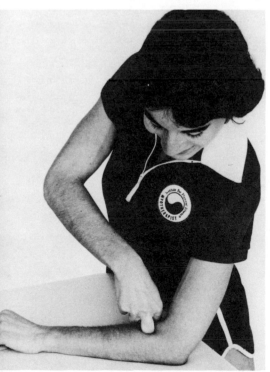

You have just found and "erased" (at least for the time being) one trigger point. As you will learn in the next section, *Quick Fix*, that trigger point is one of the major villains in "tennis elbow."

You may be tempted to say, "Well, I'd hurt anywhere if I pressed that hard." Not so. Move your knuckle halfway down your arm and repeat the same pressure. Unless you have a chronically painful wrist or hand, you will experience pressure, but no pain at all.

In addition to learning the hiding place of an important trigger point, you have just become acquainted with the first of five major tools used in Myotherapy techniques: the *knuckle* used in *straight-on pressure*.

Next, your forefinger. The *forefinger* is the second tool in Myotherapy. Place it against your temple as though your hand were a gun and you were about to shoot yourself. Repeat the *straight-on pressure* into your temple. There *may* be a trigger point there, and if so, hold it for five seconds. Face, neck and head areas require less holding time. Do not release the pressure even if there is no painful response, but learn the second technique, the *compass*. Think of the area under your finger as being a compass, with your finger covering the center of the dial. Keeping the pressure steady, press the skin straight north, toward the top of the head. If you have a trigger point, hold it

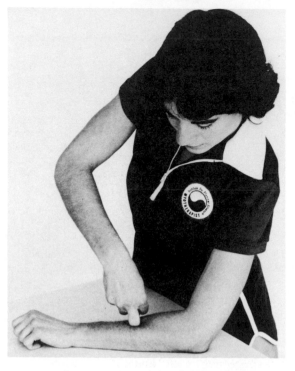

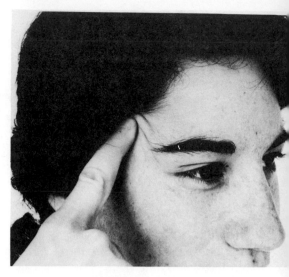

If you have either headaches or TMJD (temporomandibular joint dysfunction, a pain in the jaw), you may have found four.

You now know two Myotherapy techniques and have already used two tools. Pressure is what Myotherapy depends on to erase pain, and the compass technique is required for most trigger-point hunts.

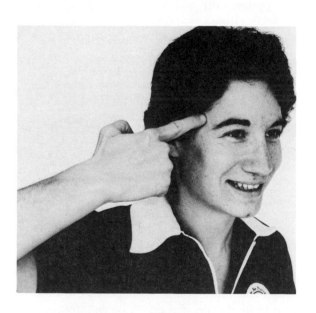

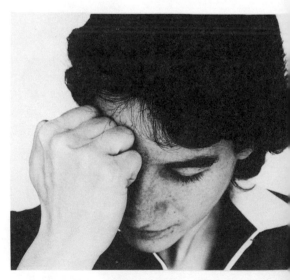

for five seconds and then press due south, toward your shoulder. When you have checked that compass point move east, toward your eye, and then west, toward your ear. Somewhere on that compass dial you will have found a trigger point.

The *roller technique* combines a new tool, your *fist*, with a new technique. It is used almost exclusively on the head and is the most precise method of working on the curved conformation of the skull, where there are apt to be many trigger points. Place the first knuckle of your right hand on the side of your forehead at the hairline. Roll the fist inward knuckle by knuckle, pressing on each of the four evenly placed spots. The last contact will be made by the knuckle of your little finger at the hairline mid-forehead, above your nose. If any one of the rolling knuckles hits a trigger point, hold the pressure for five seconds and then execute a compass: press north, south, east and west. If any are unearthed, hold those as well. At the end of the "roll," drop the fist half an inch and repeat. It should require three rolls to cover the right side of the forehead; then do the other side, using the left fist. *Always do the other side*, even if only one side, one eye, one leg or one part of the back hurts.

Now you have three techniques at your command: straight-on pressure, the compass and the roller; and three tools: knuckle, finger and fist. Your next tool is your *thumb*.

The muscle called the *splenius capitis* introduces you to one of the key trigger points in most headaches; among certified Bonnie Prudden Myotherapists, it is known as a "zinger." You will find it at circle 66, Figure 1, page 48.

Place your thumb on the back of your neck over the spine at the hairline. Slide outward two and a half to three inches on the hairline and you will find a hollow just beneath the curve of your skull. Press upward against the bone to trap the trigger point and hold for the required five seconds. Keep the pressure on and execute the compass holding for five at each sensitive point.

For the person with weak or damaged thumbs, there is an alternate tool, *two-finger pressure*. Place the index finger on the spot and then cover it with the middle finger. You will find this alternate helpful also in small spaces such as the *intercostals*, between the ribs.

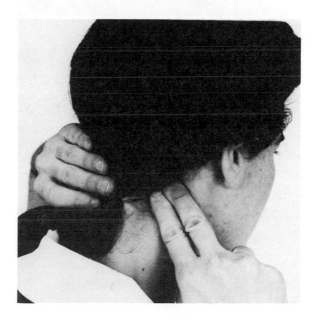

The next technique is the *wraparound*; with the finger, it is used to circle the eye on the *orbicularis oculi*. Place your middle finger on the top edge of your eyebrow next to your nose. Put the pressure on and *then* push the skin covering the muscle down and over the edge of the eye socket. Hook back against the socket edge to trap any trigger points in the muscle against the bone. That one *will* hurt. Hold for five seconds.

The wraparound is also done on larger surfaces, as for example over the ribs if you want to erase a "stitch" while running.

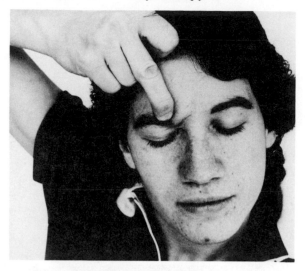

Place *three* fingers at the edge of the lowest rib and, pushing the skin and muscle beneath it over the rib into the chest cavity, pull up under the rib to trap the offending point against the bone. Hold for seven. This will be a good tool for use around the pelvic rim.

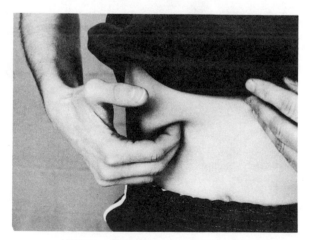

There is one tool left, the *elbow*, and one technique, the cutback. For both you need a partner. You already know what trigger-point pressure *feels like*, which means you are ahead of the Ob-Gyn man, who never had either a baby or an episiotomy. Now when somebody yips you will know full well why and you will be neither sharp nor impatient.

While many trigger points can be done on oneself, the work goes far better when a friend is involved. This is especially true for the back, which, without additional tools, is impossible to get at. When I was describing how to get rid of backache on a call-in radio show, a lady got on the air saying she was a widow living alone and how was *she* supposed to get rid of hers. There's a way, and it gets rid of more than a backache. I told her to get out of the house and find another widow and they could swap help. Widowhood usually comes along late in life. Older people have had longer to rack up trigger points from illness and accidents and much more than a little medication. *They need each other*. It could be a kind of "You do me, I'll do you" arrangement. That can be carried a step further. Get your whole club involved. It's not much fun to play bridge with your back in spasm or when you can hardly shuffle the cards. And 95 percent of pain is unnecessary.

People get frightened by low-back pain because they think (have been taught to think) it comes from the spine. Most of it is caused by trigger points in the huge muscles in the seat called the *gluteals*. Have your partner lie prone on a table. If you use a bed, put a pillow under the hips so they won't arch downward. If they do, that bed is too soft and can *cause* backache.

No matter what your subject's attire, pretend that you are seeing blue jeans with two back pockets. *The trigger points are in the upper halves of those back pockets.* Now comes your last technique, *the cutback under*, and with it the last new tool, your *elbow*. Reach *over* your friend's body and place your elbow on what would be the outside edge of the pocket, near the top. Holding the hand of the working arm for extra power, press down toward the table and then cut back under the edge of the muscle toward the median line. You don't have to feel the muscle, and if there is a lot of padding you won't, but your friend will! In most

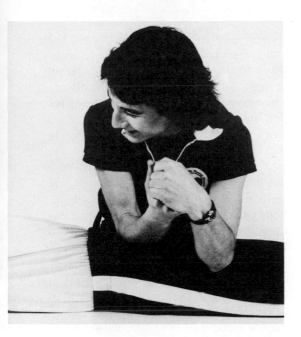

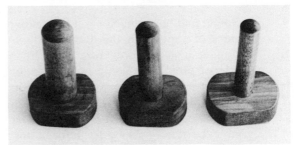

instances the subject will react vocally, because all of us have put at least some trigger points into the seat muscles. Sport will do it, as will having a baby. A fall lays down trigger points, but so does running, walking or even standing on a hard surface over a period of time. Hold the pressure for seven seconds and then execute a compass. If you didn't hit anything with the first pressure, you certainly will with the compass. Hold each sensitive spot for seven seconds. Release as you went in, *slowly*.

Now you know all the techniques and have tried out all the permanent tools, the ones attached to you and which you will never be without. The only additional one is not attached; we have named it, rather inelegantly, a "bodo." This is a small, wooden dowel with a handle. It is used in small places such as the hands, feet and between the ribs. There are also two additional sizes which are helpful for people who must live or travel alone. For the drivers of cars and trucks who suffer from recurring neck stiffness they should be a permanent fixture in the glove compartment. See the *Permanent Fix* section for ways the bodo can be used for the back.

"How hard shall I press?" will be answered by the subject. It is your job to listen and watch and feel. Before I start working on anyone, I explain what a trigger point is and demonstrate on the elbow, where there is bound to be a tender spot. I explain that while all trigger points hurt, some are worse than others. I tell them I want to know on a scale of 1 to 10 just how bad the pain is and that I don't want them to *let* me go past 10. I make it perfectly clear that past 10 is too much and that he or she can say, "Hold it!" and I will. That takes the fear away at once. Most people feel relaxed when *they* can call the shots. I also explain that in time the area will be less sensitive and that we have that time, so there is no reason to go for broke, ever. It is also true that it will never again hurt quite as much as the first time, and usually much less.

Make it abundantly clear that you do not want or need a macho hero. Bearing pain is not what Myotherapy is all about. What you do need is a map. You want to know *where* it hurts, *how much* it hurts and whether or not your pressure refers pain to somewhere else, and if so, where. Later, in the section *Permanent Fix*, you actually will make maps, and those maps will help you to get rid of the pain, prevent pain and allow your friend to continue with whatever work or sport desired.

Myotherapy is something special. It is a very real and mutual partnership between subject and therapist. It is very different from trigger-point injection, in which the subject lies passively (if you can call tight as a drum and quivering passive), waiting for that needle to find its target and home in. Nor is it like taking a piece of paper from the doctor and exchanging it at the drugstore for a little bottle of pills, then going home to wait and see what they will or will not do. You are not alone. In Myotherapy there is someone right there with you sharing your experience, asking for information while offering skill and understanding. Soon you begin to ask your own body questions and you will get answers. After a while you will be able to say, "You're close but if you will move a little more to the left, the right, up or down . . . I think it's there." And sure enough it *is* there.

You are just about ready to start, but let's recap: When a trigger point goes into action, it causes the muscle to increase tonus until it may induce a painful spasm, or cramp. This can be felt as sharp, disabling pain, a deep muscle ache or even unbearable agony. Spasm causes pain, and pain causes more spasm, until a spasm-pain-spasm cycle has been set up. When you experience a headache, most of the time trigger points *on* your skull or *in* your neck, face and shoulders have been activated. Those trigger points may have been laid down in the muscles last week, when you hit your head on the counter; last year, when you fell on the ice; or forty years ago, when you were born in two and a half hours. *When* it happened doesn't matter. It's there and needs attention.

When the muscle housing the offending trigger point goes into spasm, pain is felt and a message travels along nerve pathways to the autonomic nervous system saying, "We've got trouble in the attic." The nervous system has just the thing for that, more spasm, which of course causes more pain. After a while the muscles in the immediate vicinity or even on the other side of the head will be drawn into this unlawful caper, and the headache will settle in for hours or even days. One patient who came to the clinic had had unremitting headache for *twenty years*. And I once met a little boy who was seven before he learned that not everybody hurt all the time, the way he did.

Active trigger points can do more than cause pain. Muscles in spasm can entrap nerves (sciatica), limit circulation (cold feet, slow healing and leg ulcers), pull muscles into a shortened state (spasticity in stroke victims), cause weakness ("the athlete's legs go first") and interfere with coordination. Even when they are so mild that they go unnoticed, they are dangerous. Given the right combination of physical and emotional stresses, they can magnify into a massive, tearing spasm that has the capability of ruining a career or even costing a life.

Relief from pain is achieved by interrupting the spasm-pain-spasm cycle. Conventional medicine does that with medication, etc. Myotherapy does it with pressure. You now have your tools and the basic techniques. Next you need to know where.

Quick Fix

For a better understanding of the mysterious and wonderful organism which you are, examine the nature of organisms. Organisms are structures composed of many parts, bound together and working for a common purpose—in your case, working and, we hope, enjoying life in a very unpredictable world. While each segment of the whole enjoys a certain autonomy, there is no escaping interdependence. Although your legs most certainly carry you, your torso holds you erect to facilitate locomotion. Where pain is concerned, you may *feel* as though it is isolated and label it a "headache," a "toothache," a "bellyache," "bursitis" or a "bunion," but none of those conditions really exists alone. *All* involve other areas near or even far from the sites for which they are named.

In all corporate structures the entire company will be influenced to some degree by moves made by the president; say, a salary raise or cut. However, lesser decisions made by department supervisors are apt to affect employees more directly. It is within their power to hire or fire. Still more basic to the health of each worker is the mood, attitude and rate of absenteeism of the co-worker at the next desk. That is because day in and day out there is no escape from proximity. On the other hand there is no escape from at least the possibility that a disgruntled stock boy might set fire to the loading zone in the basement and burn the whole place down with you in it.

While everything affects everything else even when the connection is remote, co-workers and family members have the best chance for irritating one another. If this principle is applied to the human body, then a pain starting in the back of the head can soon bring in both the forehead and the eyes. Neck spasm often moves upward into the jaw, to be named temporomandibular joint dysfunction, or it can project downward to take the form of stiff and painful shoulders or chest pain that mimics angina. The shoulders have the power to involve the elbows in pain that will be called "tennis elbow," or the elbow can set things in motion to bring on "bursitis" in the shoulder. Either one or both can affect the wrists and fingers and be called "carpal tunnel syndrome" or "arthritis."

The muscles strapped over and around the chest as well as the upper back can influence the lungs, *inside* the rib cage. Pain in the upper back can set up a jangling in the head or refer pain down to the lower back. That pain in turn can bring on either abdominal pain, groin pain or both. The *gluteals* (seat muscles) have an inordinate amount of influence on the legs, and the reverse can be true. Since the feet are the base for posture, they, like the arsonist stock boy, can send fire straight up through the structure to the top floor, giving the president a headache which may be called a "migraine" and treated as a "migraine" and kept going for a lifetime.

A simple rule of thumb when dealing with chronic pain is to view it as you would an antisocial co-worker at the next desk. The structure closest to your pain is *apt* to be the most active contributor to the misery. However, if firing the co-worker doesn't clear up the dissension in the department, and erasing trigger points in adjacent muscles doesn't get rid of pain, even temporarily, one must find the ringleaders. There are always followers who can heighten pain and even spread it, but as in life, leaders are fewer and more important. They start things. So that the search for the initiating trigger points will not be a hit-or-miss affair, we will provide maps which will save time in what we call "quick fix" and assure thoroughness in what we call "permanent fix." And somewhere between the two you will discover what you need to do on a continuing daily basis to stay pain free.

The quick fix, like first aid, is something to do immediately and on the spot in order to be rid of pain. It is a stopgap measure to be used until you have both the time and the place in which to do a complete job of hunting for the trigger points causing pain.

In the war on pain, a quick fix is like knowing your way through a minefield. Since you know where each mine is buried, you can defuse the ones that are immediately threatening. But the job is not finished until you have cleared the whole field.

There are many occasions when a quick fix is indispensable. For example, you are at the concert hall at seven thirty to play with a chamber-music trio and that old pain that periodically attacks your left shoulder has begun. You can't hold the violin properly, let alone concentrate on the subtleties of the music. A quick fix properly applied to your arm, chest and *axilla* (armpit) will render you

pain free for the evening and perhaps longer. Of course it will return after you have practiced too long, driven too far or slept all night on your left side. But at least, right at this moment, you can perform.

The trucker with a load to deliver, though in pain, is a prime candidate for a quick fix. It may save his life, perhaps several lives. The insurance salesman who drags into the motel, his face gray with fatigue and a grinding pain in his back and leg, is another. A quick fix may keep him from falling asleep at the wheel and so improve his self-confidence that he makes the important sale. There is nothing quite like pain to undermine a personality. The teacher who has murder in her heart after a painful day with a raging bunch of uneducated, undisciplined, unhealthy fourth-graders, is also a prime candidate, and she should not be allowed to leave the teachers' lounge without a quick fix. Had one been available in the morning, she might have discovered she had *children* in her classroom.

There is still another group: those beautiful people, the athletes and dancers who give us so much delight. They have been *educated* to expect to work through pain and to bear pain while executing maneuvers that most people approach only in dreams. *They* are candidates for quick fix, permanent fix and, above all, prevention. Instead, they get ice, whirlpool, liniment, cortisone, rest and tape. We shouldn't be too surprised when we hear that one or another of them is on drugs or that some theater "great" has died of an overdose. "The show must go on" is a rule of life for those people, just as losing by default is anathema for athletes. Both groups will do just about anything to "play," and for that reason will accept almost any help that is offered even when the same help has done nothing whatsoever for other members of the company or the team. One can only wonder if some of our high-ranking government people might not profit from a quick fix for pain. It is possible that, pain free, they might be a little slower in making decisions that put the rest of us in line for the same.

The quick fix is just that. It's *quick*. It almost always works for people who, though in pain, are able to get to work and stay through the day. Last year we put a call through to a large organization and were unable for a full week to reach our contact. She was "out sick." When we finally did get through we learned that, yes, she was back at her desk but that, no, she wasn't better. Her neck was just as painful as ever and she guessed she'd just have to wait it out. "Nonsense," we said. "We'll send a certified Bonnie Prudden Myotherapist down right away." "Better send two," she joked, "everybody around here's got *something*." So we sent two. On an afternoon, they cleared up four headaches, two backaches, the stiff neck and the chef's thumb. In addition, one of the executives was almost frantic. She had left her asthma spray at home and was starting an attack and had an important meeting in fifteen minutes. Fifteen minutes was exactly the time needed for the certified Bonnie Prudden Myotherapist to abort the attack.

No, those people were not likely to be pain free permanently, but at least each one knew that there was a way to get rid of discomfort. They were no longer doomed to work all day in pain, leave the office in pain, travel home in pain, only to take a couple of Extra-Strength Tylenol (and who knows what *they* will do?) and fall into bed still in pain. What kind of life is that? No life at all. But it's the way thousands live every day, year in and year out.

We start with quick fix because it is a quick course in the vocabulary of pain, in making maps (and reading them) and also in understanding the kind of fifth-column activity indulged in by trigger points. Practice the quick fix on yourself and complaining friends and relatives

after the doctor has ruled out any anatomic pathology. If you have already gone the route with the muscle relaxants, pain-killers, X rays, injections and physical therapy and still hurt, you are a great subject for a quick fix.

There will come a time when you will be able to work on people who have had pain for a long time, really desperate people, and you will want to be successful. However, for the sake of your self-confidence, which by the way is catching, develop your skill on easy things such as backaches and headaches.

In our first book on pain, we tried to cover all the areas where trouble might lurk, and we demonstrated Myotherapy done under ideal conditions. Ideal conditions are those in which the subject, clad only in underwear, shorts or leotard, is stretched full length on a padded massage table that is exactly the right height for the Myotherapist. That's a lot like going to a physical-education college to become an instructor. The future teacher learns to work in beautiful surroundings with attentive students dressed appropriately. All the accoutrement is there: balls, mats, parallel bars, barbells, the track, the pool, showers and time. Then the student graduates into the real world. He finds his gym is the playground and his equipment limited to one ball and the school wall. He has eighty-five boys in each thirty-five-minute class twice a week, and the only uniforms are running shoes. He has those because running shoes are the style.

It would be delightful to have all the advantages shown in my book *Pain Erasure the Bonnie Prudden Way*, and you should have the book in your library, because it helps to know how to use the ideal as well as the impromptu condition. The more you know about various aspects of a subject, the better you will be able to assess the whole. In this book, especially in this *Quick Fix* section, you will be shown how to work with the absolute minimum while faced with the maximum in adjustment problems. There will be no massage tables but, rather, the things that would be available in the office, the waiting room, the car or even on Main Street. You will be using a couple of filing cabinets, two chairs, a box, a railing, a park bench or a low wall. You will learn how to use the *edge* of a table or desk, and you will even know how to help a friend while sitting in a plane. We do it all the time. It will also be possible to work in front of others in such a way as to intrigue them and inform them that there *is* a way to help.

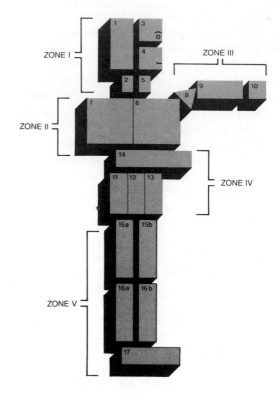

THE QUICK-FIX MANUAL

Everyone needs an owner's manual for the car and the house. Now we have one for the body, but if it shares the fate of most owners' manuals, a place at the bottom of a drawer, you will not profit very much. If the owners of such manuals read about the care, repair and maintenance of their possessions, there would be fewer ripoffs, less disaster, not to mention totaled mechanisms. Where the human body is concerned, this is trebly true. Most diseases are inflicted by less than healthy life-styles, but most pain could be eased or erased if there were a thorough understanding of how pain progresses as well as how to prevent it in the first place.

In your manual the body is divided into seventeen *segments*, which fit neatly into five *zones*. Each segment represents an area needing attention, and each zone contains the segments most likely to refer pain to each other. That is not to say that trigger points in distant zones will not invade. They will. But at least you will have a starting place for the immediate problem of teammate, co-worker or family member.

Zone I contains the head and neck and is divided into five segments numbered according to the progression we have

found most rewarding and easiest to follow.

Segment 1 is the back of the head.

Segment 2 represents the structure most likely to be involved with the back of the head; it is the back of the neck. Whatever part of the body we are working with, we must remember not only its abutting neighbor, but the one opposite.

Segment 3 is the front of the head and includes the forehead, temples and eyes.

Segment 4 is the nose, cheeks and jaw.

Segment 5 is the front of the neck.

Zone I is referred to as "the headache zone"; and the head has many options when it comes to pain. There are tension headaches, migraines, clusters, sinus and a dozen others. As far as Myotherapy is concerned, a headache is a headache, and the technique is the same no matter the name. In addition to headaches, Zone I can house tic douloureux, Bell's palsy, tinnitus (buzzing in the ears), eye, ear and tooth pain and jaw pain, the one called temporomandibular joint dysfunction (TMJD). Stuffy nose is often caused by trigger points, as is *some* double vision. In Zone I there are even trigger points that cause loss of taste and smell. The neck muscles in Zone I often cause dizziness and referred pain to the teeth, ears and head. They are known to cause a stiff and painful neck, torticollis and a forward head. Trigger points in that area can pull the lower jaw into a subluxation, making it impossible to either close or open the mouth to its full range. They are often responsible for hoarseness, difficulty in swallowing, wrinkles and a squint.

Zone II houses two segments: the chest and the upper back.

Segment 6, the upper back.

Segment 7, the chest.

Trigger points causing all manner of distress can lodge in the chest. There is, for example, simple spasm that *mimics* angina, and then there *is* angina, the real thing. Trigger points have the power not merely to refer pain and spread it, they can also *augment* pain. Asthma is a chest disorder, as is emphysema, and so is the pain called heartburn, which is often attributed to hiatus hernia. Muscle spasms in the *intercostal muscles* can cause agonizing pain after a siege of coughing. If there are latent trigger points in the *intercostals* just waiting for an excuse to fire, a sneeze would be enough.

The upper back, which is the back of the chest, in Zone II, forms part of the shoulder girdle and participates in much of the pain suffered in its opposite wall and even in Zone IV, below the chest. Gallbladder pain is known to refer to the back, and *sometimes* taking trigger points from the upper back will ease abdominal spasms that *appear* to be from the gallbladder. There is of course the classic upper-back pain that accompanies so many occupations and also shoulder injuries such as partial or full dislocations and separations. The upper back is a nesting ground for many trigger points garnered in falls, lifting, whiplash injuries and accidents that didn't quite happen, because the arm and upper-back muscles

held the car on the road (while taking on trigger points that would become a plague later on). There are also posture anomalies such as round back and kyphosis, which is the extreme of that condition, and a forward head, which is the natural adjunct.

Zone III contains three segments.

Segment 8, the *axilla* or armpit.

Segment 9, the arm.

Segment 10, the hand.

If any of the above runs into trouble, it is almost certain that at least one of the others will be in on it. At the distal end, the hand, there is the ache often attributed to arthritis or carpal tunnel syndrome. There are also trigger points in the vicinity of old scars, thumb dislocations called "skier's thumb," numbness or tingling often suffered by musicians (if the two come together we call it "numbling"). There are of course all the ballgame fingers.

Moving up into Segment 9 we have wrist sprains and swelling, aching arms, "tennis elbow" and what is called "bursitis" (although it rarely is). The word "bursitis" means inflammation of the bursa. *Bursa* comes from the Greek and means wineskin. In medicalese it is a sac or saclike cavity filled with viscid fluid. The bursa is situated at a place in the tissues where friction might develop. *Itis* means inflammation, and the word alone indicates one of the treatments often given for "bursitis," a shot or two of cortisone into the shoulder joint. Most of the time the trouble is not an inflamed bursa at all, but, rather, trigger points at work in the muscles of the arm, chest, upper back, neck and armpit. This potential involvement of so many powerful muscles is the reason why shoulders are often hard (but not impossible) to fix. The armpit, or *axilla*, is one of the most important areas for trigger points in the whole body. It, like the *splenius capitis*, at the back of the head, circle 66 and the circle on the surface of the shoulder blade (scapula) and labeled 13 in Figure 5, page

71, are at junctions where several muscles abut or cross. For that reason all three, *splenius, axilla* and *scapula*, have considerable potential when it comes to trigger points and pain.

Zone IV has four segments.

Segment 11, the lower back. Of all areas this one contributes most to *disabling* pain.

Segment 12, the side of the pelvis, the *gluteus medius*, which stabilizes the standing posture.

Segment 13, the *groin*, the front of the back.

Segment 14, the *abdominals*. The abdominals, too, are the front, but they are also the bottom of the chest and the top of the groin. Inside are many organs that are quite capable of giving abdominal trouble, and vice versa. The pain called "menstrual cramps" is actually caused by abdominal, groin, and back spasm and is a good example, as is the spastic colon. The pain attributed to hemorrhoids is often a combination of gluteal spasm, groin-muscle spasm and spasms in the floor of the pelvis stretching from back to front.

Zone V contains five segments covering both legs and feet.

Segment 15a represents the backs of the upper legs, highly important when it comes to back pain.

Segment 15b, the fronts of the upper legs and a contributor to groin and abdominal pain.

Segment 16a, the backs of the lower legs, a wasp's nest for athletes.

Segment 16b, the fronts of the lower legs, favorite for shin splints.

Segment 17, the feet.

Any muscle in the legs can refer pain downward into the feet, and the reverse is also true. Pain in abused or structurally inadequate feet can be transferred to the legs. Between the ankles and the hip joints lie the knees, which seem to suffer the most pain from spasms in the muscles, and not nearly so often from trouble

in bones and ligaments, as is suggested by the names given knee pain: meniscus-ligament tears (rarely), chondromalacia (softening of the bone, also rarely), floating patella, slipping patella, arthritis and so on. *Most of the time* the pain is due to muscle spasm in the huge *quadriceps* muscles of the thigh, pulling upward, and the calf muscles, pulling downward. Leg pain is usually blamed on "tears," "tendinitis," "shin splints," "growing pains," "spurs," "calf-muscle cramps," "lack of potassium," etc. *Most of the time*, you can count on trigger points to be the main villains.

The human body is much like the person who owns it: human. As such, nothing is ever black or white and there are no absolutes. So it is with our zones and the segments within the zones. There are no permanently set frontiers; they all overlap. Zone I can overlap into both Zone II and Zone III. That means that the headache, while affecting all the segments within Zone I, could also send pain down the arms or into the back or chest. Or trouble can (and often does) originate in Zone II, the upper back, moving upward to cause a headache. Zone IV is almost always involved when a person is said to have sciatic pain or pain running down one or both legs, but then the runner's powerful thigh muscles can affect first the lower and then the upper back, causing a debilitating condition that excludes him or her from further running and may, in addition, interfere with productivity and even attendance on the job.

While we know that nothing is certain, we have set up zones and segments in the order we have found to be most helpful. If your subject says, "I have a headache," that at least tells you that Zone I is your starting place. Thousands of headaches have shown us that the back of the head, Segment 1, is the place to start, at least the first time.

We start at the back of the head because *most* headaches seem to originate there and are often augmented by trigger points in the huge *trapezius* muscle, rising from the shoulders and upper back. One has only to sit at dinner or a writing task or simply remove a sliver from a finger to discover in what position the head is held a good part of the time and how its weight drags on the neck and shoulder muscles.

While the headache may get its *start* at the back of the head, there is nothing to prevent it from moving straight over the top via the *galea aponeurotica* to settle down in the forehead, back of the eyes or on either side. In this last instance it would be called a "migraine," which comes from the Greek *hemikrania*, which means half a head. With this exotic designation and from truly bizarre prodromal symptoms that seem to accompany half-head pain: nausea, vomiting, auras, and flashing lights, to name a few, it will be treated with drugs served up in a darkened room. Trigger points in this area are often laid down early in life, in fact as early as birth. This is more than merely possible if the birth is a hard one or made unnaturally fast with Pitocin. Forceps, needed or not, can also set up the new little head for a lifetime of pain.

Headaches *feel* as though they are inside the head, but *almost* all the time the cause and the ache are *on* the head. They are due to trigger points in one or more of the many muscles that cover the skull and facial bones and form the supporting pillar that is the neck. We know already that trigger points get into muscles when they are "insulted," or damaged, in some way. It is the trigger points that cause the spasm, which in turn causes pain. Falls contribute more than their fair share to head injuries. Whiplash injuries, prevalent in automobile accidents, cause headaches often referred up from the damaged neck muscles. Even more likely to damage the muscles of head, neck and shoulders is *micro-trauma*. There is no

sudden blow, but a gradual buildup stemming from occupations that limit range of motion and call for thousands of small, precise, repetitive movements. The muscles are hurt a little every minute of every hour of every day, for years. Typing is a good example, especially when the head is turned in one direction in order to copy material. The same goes for computer work. The head, neck, arms, hands and back are held at unnatural angles while doing concentrated work. *What* one does is not as important as *how the body adjusts to it* and for how many hours a day. To this we should add, *what one does to counteract the restriction.* Accidents are accidents, and there is nothing to be done afterward to prevent them. We must accept the fact that trigger points are now in residence, but be content in the knowledge that we *can* find them, neutralize them and keep them under control with exercise. Where occupations are concerned, we will give you the information you need in order to avoid piling up trigger points, plus the exercises that *prevent* spasm and pain. We will do that in a section later on.

Myotherapy is something very new; *Pain Erasure: The Bonnie Prudden Way* was the first book written about it. There we gave the body a new kind of map. While the muscles, like mountains and rivers, cities and towns, kept their names and certainly their relationships to one another, we gave you a new way to look at them. We demonstrated new relationships among them *where pain was concerned.* Hundreds of thousands of people have read that book and used the new maps. Many of those same people will read and use this book. They will be on familiar ground now. The names of the muscles will not change, of course, but neither will the numbers we gave to them. Number 66 on the map in *Pain Erasure* will always be the *splenius capitis* muscle, and number 13 in that book will always be a vicious trigger point on the scapula. No matter which book you are using (and you should have both), the same numbers will apply.

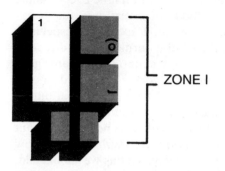

ZONE I

ZONE I, SEGMENT 1: THE BACK OF THE HEAD

Zone I is divided into five segments; Segment 1 is our first concern. Look at Figure 1 and you will see that the huge *trapezius* muscle, which covers the upper back, reaches up to the head and is anchored on Line D. Note too that the powerful *sternocleidomastoid* muscles (SCM) also tie in at Line D. If your car has a head-on collision, your head will snap forward to pull mightily on Line D (the back of the neck), the *occipitalis* (at Grid C) and, of course, all down the back. Nor need you wreck your car in order to sustain these strains. The same potential for damage in those areas would be present in a simple fall forward onto one or both arms.

Note the circles numbered 66, on Line D. You became acquainted with them when you learned to use your thumbs on the *splenius capitis* (page 37). Circle 66 is one of the most sensitive spots, not only because it is in use so much of the time and in danger of overload, nor because a forward fall almost guarantees damage to that area. It is a "zinger" because circle 66 is a junction where at least three muscles come together and each can contribute to muscle spasm. In addition to the *splenius capitis* you have the

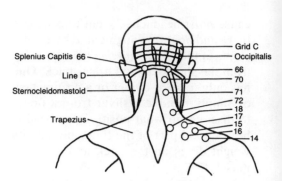

FIG. 1: BACK OF THE HEAD, NECK, AND SHOULDER

semispinalis and the upper reaches of the *trapezius*. The *splenius capitis* is the captain of this team, as you will soon see and understand.

Trigger points seem to cluster at the attachments where muscles begin and end, and the *splenius* attaches to the *cervical vertebrae*, in the neck, a spot noted for the designation "cervical arthritis." At the other end it attaches to the three upper *thoracic vertebrae*, in the upper back. That is the spot that often aches after a long day on the job requiring eye/hand coordination. You can just touch this lower attachment if you reach over your shoulder and as far down your back as possible. It is the spot most people rub intuitively when the upper back aches.

As tools for working on *splenius* and company, you can use your fingers, thumbs or knuckles—whatever suits you. Every hand is different and you will develop your own style in time. Use of the bodo will be demonstrated for those who live or travel alone, but while the bodo will work, a friend works better.

If you are in a place where there is a desk or table of some kind, it would be easier for you if the subject could lie prone. Place a small rolled-up towel or hands under the forehead to protect the nose. Stand to one side and, reaching *over* the subject, place your thumb or fingers on 66. It is just below the hairline and two and a half inches out from the spine.

Press slowly and gently but *firmly* upward against the curve of the skull and hold the pressure for about five seconds. Think as you press that it may be the shock of the discomfort or possibly oxygen deprivation to that one spot that interrupts the trigger-point action long enough to break the spasm-pain-spasm cycle. Patting gently or rubbing the spot isn't going to do the job.

When you release after a five-second hold, do so *slowly*, as if controlled by hydraulic pressure. Keep in mind that the skull is quite durable and you are nowhere near the more fragile spine, nor will you ever be. You are not ''manipulating,'' you are *pressing*, and you could do that with considerable power almost anywhere on the body and not even raise a bruise. You don't bump the blood vessels, you *squeeze* them for five seconds.

When you have held the pressure against the skull for the required five seconds, use the compass technique (page 35). Keeping the pressure steady, press outward toward the *mastoid process* (behind the ear), inward toward the spine and finally downward toward the shoulder. Be sure to hold any trigger points noted for the full five seconds. If there is no *pain reaction* where you press, there is no trigger point *right there*. That is not to say there are not several lurking in the vicinity. Success with Myotherapy depends on getting *all* the little horrors, at least temporarily. If you are thorough enough, the muscles seem to lose the habit of going into spasm as the patterned reaction to stress.

The purpose of this *Quick Fix* section is to first show you how to get rid of pain quickly and on the spot, so the subject is free to accomplish painlessly any task or pleasure of the moment. The painlessness may last for hours, days, weeks or even for always. But if it doesn't, you must realize there was more work to do. See the *Permanent Fix* section to learn the next steps to take.

Getting rid of pain at the office, in a

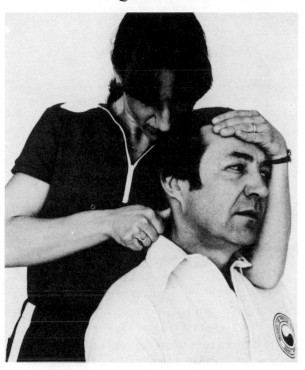

classroom or the teachers' lounge is not really difficult. Merely substitute a chair for the table. Have your subject sit comfortably in the chair with feet flat on the floor and empty hands relaxed in the lap. Stand behind and rest your left elbow on his or her shoulder. Place your left hand on his forehead and gently pull the head back to rest against your chest. Place the left side of your face against the subject's head and apply pressure to circle 66 on the right side with your thumb. When you have completed the initial pressure plus the compass, place the heel of your hand over the area and massage with moderate pressure in a small circle. Slide the skin over the muscles, not your hand over the skin. Do the other side at once even if the headache is on the side you have just worked. Finish with a minute or so of massage to that side also.

If it's your own head that aches and you are alone, use the bodo. Grasp the handle in your hand on the side you will be working. Turn your head away and down a little to put the muscles on a slight stretch. Press as you would using your

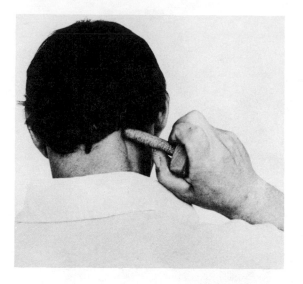

thumb on someone else. There are people who can't bear to cause themselves even the slightest pain. Self-administration works best when the pain of the headache or whatever is really worse than the bodo pressure, but even if the pressure applied is lighter than it ought to be, some good will be accomplished. When the trigger points are so painful that they can barely be touched, we start work on the periphery of the given area, *or* we apply such light pressure that while there may be some improvement, it is far from a finished job. The next time we try, however, the trigger points will be less sensitive. So, if you are very sensitive to pain, be kind to yourself. Take a little longer to get the work done and realize that if the pain persists, it probably wasn't the technique that failed, but the application. Go find a friend to help.

The reason for enclosing the subject's head within the circle of your arm, hand, face and thumb is, first, to stabilize the head so that you can work, but also to provide a sense of security and caring. You *are* going to hurt to a degree, and the more you can spread the contact between your body and that of the subject, the more pain you will dissipate. One of the reasons injections hurt so much is that there is no sensation other than that caused by the needle.

Something should be said right here about personality, attitude and reasons for doing Myotherapy. If you don't like people in general, especially little people and animals, both representing helplessness, don't try Myotherapy. You won't be successful no matter what your reason for wanting to help one particular person.

I can remember lying stripped to the buff (uncomfortable to begin with because it makes one feel so vulnerable) and waiting for one of those ghastly trigger-point injections of procaine and saline to go into my seat muscle. Now, understand this. The pain of the trigger point being invaded comes *before* the action of the local anesthetic, so it isn't like having a local to numb the area *before* a procedure. In addition, there are doctors who use plain saline (salt water) and some who "dry-needle" the trigger points. If you've had *one* such injection it's enough to set up a sweat for all the ones that come after.

There I was, a mass of quivering nerves doing what I so often do when terrified, talking up a storm. The doctor turned to me, sword in hand, and said curtly, "Oh, you're just scared, keep quiet." At that second he cut any good he was trying to do in half. I went quiet and as rigid as stone. He was right, I was scared to death. I'd been through dozens of those excruciating sessions before and I knew all too well what to expect. Where he was also right was in his knowledge of what was needed for my pain and how to administer it, if not painlessly at least effectively. Where he was wrong was in his unfeeling attack on *me*. It happens quite often with doctors who start out as surgeons. In surgery they work on patients who have been rendered into senseless, *silent* meat by anesthesia. Later, they tend to treat the bodies of the conscious patients as though all feeling had been zonked out. They have no time for the terror that ensues as their callousness comes through. When you come on such a person, move on. There is no excuse for inhumanity, which is usually visited on the helpless, especially the poor, the old and women.

When I finally met Dr. Janet Travell I was in such a state of disintegration that there wasn't much that could be done, but she tried. At her hands I won't even say I *suffered* dozens of injections. I had them all right, and they were painful. But her kindness and care and, yes, humor made them bearable. All the while she worked, she taught, and so intriguing were her ideas and thorough her technique that I learned what I needed to know to develop Myotherapy. If you are kind *inside*, not just for effect, and if you are caring, and if you are both concerned and gentle, you will be successful *most* of the time.

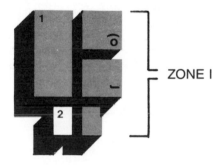

ZONE I

ZONE I, SEGMENT 2: THE BACK OF THE NECK

The second segment to be explored is 2, the back of the neck. It is the area adjacent to the back of the head, and while it can entertain trouble in its own name, "a pain in the neck," it also refers pain and, acting as a bridge, brings spasm up from the shoulders and passes it on to the head itself. When looking for spasms causing headaches, remember that the neck is a minefield.

Check with Figure 1, on page 48, and you will see three small circles marked 70, 71 and 72. Those do not represent separate muscles, but, rather, three sta-

tions on the same line. They are close enough to each other so that when the whistle is tooted at town 70 it can be heard at town 71 and quite possibly at town 72 as well. The potential for shared pain becomes even more apparent if you draw additional circles on Figure 1 directly across from the three already there. The "tracks" aren't very far apart and any warnings tooted on one line will most certainly alert those on the other. That is one good reason for doing both sides of everything.

If your subject is lying prone on a table, the best working position will be from the end of the platform facing the subject's head. Stabilize the head by placing your free hand alongside of the head just over the ear. As you examine each of the three spots for tenderness (they are about three quarters of an inch apart on the average adult neck), press downward but slanted slightly in toward the medial line. Aim for the Adam's apple. When you have completed your first five-second hold, keep the pressure steady and begin your compass by pressing toward the ear, then up toward the hairline and finally down toward the shoulder. It is easy to move the skin around on the necks of kittens, puppies, and children, but as we grow older it thickens and often develops a condition we call "fibrositis." Fibrositis seems to be connected with emotional stress. It shows up on the thighs, hips, arms and upper backs of women, but the neck attracts it in both sexes. Pinching that tissue elicits exquisite tenderness (try it, you probably have it). To get rid of it calls for pinching first, followed by massage, and then exercise. If you are overweight, diet and step up the exercise program farther on in this book.

When you have completed 70, 71 and 72 on both sides of Segment 2 (the back of the neck) you are almost done, but not quite. Each muscle has at least two attachments; the distal attachment for the *splenius capitis* is 18, down in the back.

It is on the same line and guaranteed to provide you with a very excitable trigger point where the muscle ties in to the three upper thoracic vertebrae.

To find the spot with the subject lying prone is a cinch. It is usually about one inch out from the spine and four inches down from the shoulder. If it hurts in the first place you press with your knuckle or elbow, use your compass technique, moving north, south, east and west. Hold the pressure for *seven* seconds, two more than for head and neck structures.

To do the back of the neck in a chair, simply hold the head as for the *splenius capitis*, circle 66. Press with the knuckle or thumb or, if *you* are the patient and you're alone, with the bodo, on each of the four circles 70, 71, 72 and the lower end of the *splenius* (18). Hold each of the points for *five* seconds, use the compass on each and release *slowly*.

To get at circle 18, have the subject lean forward to rest the forearms on the knees, allowing the head to droop. Stand

to one side and, using the elbow nearest the head as a hunting tool, hold the subject against you with the other hand placed under the armpit. From this position it should be possible to get at circle 18 on both sides of the upper back.

Using the bodo for circle 18 is next to impossible manually. If you have a job or hobby that calls for constant use and overuse of the upper back, you will need continuous help in the form of Myotherapy at the end of each trying day. Screw a bodo to a doorframe at a height that brings it in line with circle 18 as you back up against it. If your house or apartment does not have wooden frames, there is a plastic tape used for indoor/outdoor carpet which will hold onto a metal surface such as a refrigerator.

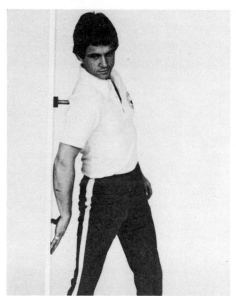

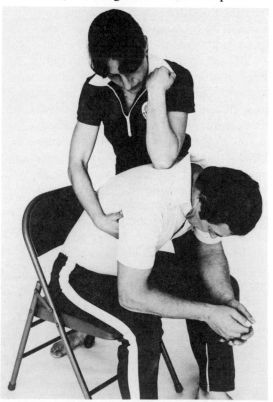

Or you can make yourself a kind of shepherd's crook with half-inch aluminum conduit, bent to curve over your shoulder or around your waist or pelvis. You will have to cement little rubber stoppers to the ends or they will slip out. Both can be bought at the hardware store. Some stores will even bend them for you. If your hardware store doesn't have the tools for bending, plumbers do. Seems like a lot of bother? I agree, unless you have neither kith nor kin living close

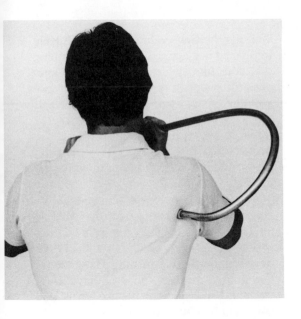

driving anything at all. That includes tractors, cranes, cars, cabs, trucks, buses, trains or planes. Of all of those vehicles, however, cars have the most drivers (almost everyone over sixteen), so we show you how to fix the aching shoulders of the drivers of cars.

The cushioned seat back of a car will do the job of supporting and stretching admirably. Have the subject kneel and lean over the back, which will support the chest. Allow the arms and head to dangle into the back area. From the back seat area lean over the subject's body with your free hand stabilizing by holding the arm. Capture circle 18 under your elbow and proceed as though the subject were either prone on a table or resting in a chair. Don't forget to do both sides even though the discomfort is on one side only. If the driver has the habit of resting his or her elbow on the windowsill, that may be a contributor to the pain. See if the habit can be broken.

enough to help you when a muscle back there goes into spasm. Then, of course, there are those of you who have both kith and kin within arm's reach or at least a holler down the hall, but you wouldn't dream of asking at three in the morning, when the spasm hits.

The crook can also be used in the seat muscles (*gluteals*) for low-back pain. Place the end where you think the trigger point is. Some of you *know* where it is. Either pull forward with the shaft or lean the curve against a wall and back up (see page 184, where the bodo is used in this way).

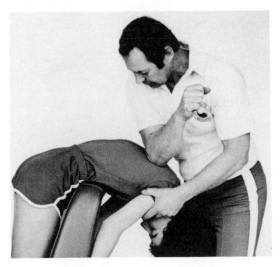

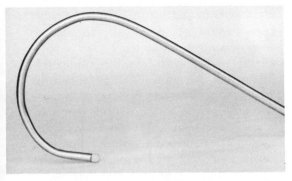

Circles 66, 70, 71, 72 and 18 are involved in eye/hand coordination, especially in action that is repetitive and engaged in for long periods. That would apply to any kind of craft and also to

Passive Stretch for the Neck

You have now found at least *some* of the trigger points causing the pain in your subject's neck, head or shoulders, and now the muscles in Segments 1 and 2 need to be stretched. Incidentally, Myotherapy itself *warms* the muscles by increasing the circulation, so you need not worry about *stretch* before *warm-up*. Pressure that neutralizes the trigger points also releases the muscular spasms and takes the squeeze off the blood vessels. The stretching is part of teaching the muscles new habits.

Have the subject sit in a chair (or the front seat of a car) with shoulders facing straight forward, feet flat on the floor. Place your hands on his shoulders to keep them in position and ask him to turn his head as far to the right as possible. Then place your hands on either side of his face, providing blinders limiting his lateral vision. Ask him to note and remember whatever it is he can see at the farthest reach of his vision to the right. Then do the same to the left. *Both of you should remember what it was he could see on each side.* If, when you're finished

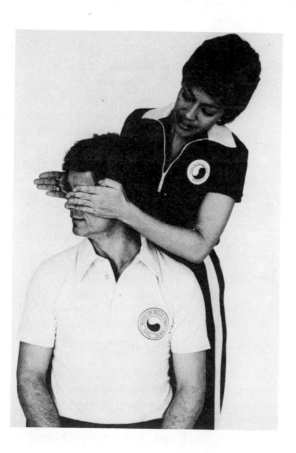

working, he can see farther, you will have improved neck range of motion. Nothing succeeds like success. Even a *little* success provides a positive outlook and willingness to work harder for more. If the subject (and you) discover that the range of vision has improved, there will be a change in attitude. This is especially true if there has been little cause for rejoicing in the past.

The subject then rests his hands in his lap as you place yours on either side of his face. Turn his head from side to side, setting up a slow, gentle rhythm. If the head responds well, turning easily within the limited range, you will have little trouble. If the movements are jerky, you may require the use of music. Just turn on the radio and find some music slow enough for your needs, and let it help get the rhythm through. We all have rhythm, and music is often able to help us bypass whatever is interfering with coordination. This works even with the spasticity caused by cerebral palsy, multiple sclerosis, strokes and other conditions.

Resistance exercises contribute to *flexibility* as well as strength; the ones you are about to do work on a well-known but often ignored principle. When you bring a cup of coffee to your lips you know that the *biceps* in the front of your upper arm will contract. What is less well understood by the average person and often overlooked by those who should know better (doctors, physical therapists and trainers) is, while the *biceps* is patterned to respond to your command "Bring cup to mouth," its antagonist in the back of the arm, the *triceps*, is responding to another command, one that is not consciously given. That command says, "Give up contraction." All the muscles are patterned to respond to their antagonists by letting go, and they must let go *before* the contraction takes place. The degree to which the paired muscles cooperate determines how smooth your movement with the cup of coffee will be.

People who suffer from conditions that interfere with this pattern of action and reaction have jerky movements. Then the distance between table and mouth is fraught with peril, often ending in spilled coffee.

For our purpose, when one set of muscles is in spasm we facilitate spasm release by calling on this pattern of relaxation prior to contraction. We deliberately force the antagonists to work against resistance. By turning the head to the left, the antagonists on the right (even though in spasm) will respond to a degree and at least try to let go.

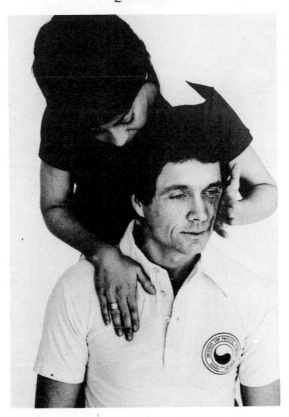

Lateral Neck-Stretch Exercise

Grasp the subject's right shoulder with your right hand for stabilization. Place your left hand on the subject's left cheek and ask him to turn his head to the left, pushing through the *slight* resistance you will offer with your hand. Be sure to make the resistance light at first or you will discourage effort. You want the subject to be able to turn his head from side to side, and you can always increase the resistance little by little, once the action is understood. When the turn has gone as far as possible, hook your fourth and fifth fingers under his chin to hold the head at its farthest reach. Put a *little* pressure on the chin to turn the head a *little* beyond the end of the turn. Keep the pressure firm. Release the right hand from the right shoulder and place it against the subject's right cheek, taking over the pressure from the left *at the farthest reach of the turn*. Don't let it get sloppy and begin just anywhere. The key lies in starting at the *outside reach* on each turn. Place the now free left hand on the subject's left shoulder for stabi-

lization and have the subject turn as far as possible to the right. Take over at the end of the turn with the fourth and fifth fingers of the right hand under the chin and encourage a *little* more reach.

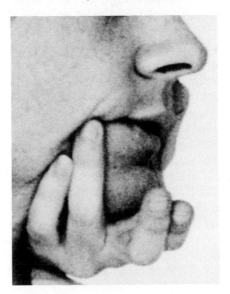

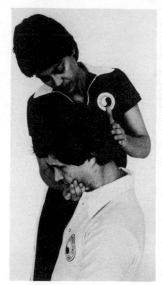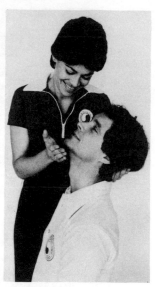

Forward-and-Back Neck Stretch

Stand to one side and place one hand under the subject's chin and the other on the back of his head. Ask him to look down into his lap as you give resistance under the chin. When the extreme stretch has been reached, use the hand in back to start resistance *before* you ask the subject to raise his head to look at the ceiling. As in the lateral neck stretch, there are two crucial points, one when the subject reaches the extreme stretch forward, the other at the extreme stretch backward. The success of the exercise depends on keeping the pressure steady so that the return can always begin at the absolute end of the stretch. This signals the antagonists to "let go" at points farther along the spasm line. Alternate, four stretches forward and four back.

When you have finished the stretch, check the range of motion again while using the hands for blinders. Your friend should be able to see farther in at least one direction, probably both.

When you have finished the stretches, ask the subject if the pain has moved. Perhaps it has changed its shape from a roundish spread to a thinner line or is less intense. Perhaps it has moved to the other side. *Do not ask if the pain is gone*. I usually say, "Where is the pain now?" However, to the subject's amazement (and probably yours) it may well be gone. One of the commonest reactions following any work with Myotherapy is surprise. I get letters all the time, from people who have read *Pain Erasure*, saying, "You won't believe this but I got rid of my husband's (boss's) (cab driver's) (teacher's) (minister's) headache." But I *do* believe it. Nobody was more surprised than I was the first time and the second time and probably the fortieth time I was able to get rid of somebody's pain. Now, seven years and thousands of pains later, I'm not surprised at all unless it happens after working on something I've never worked on before, such as spastic colon, which first showed up two summers ago, and heartburn said to be a hiatus hernia, in the fall. By next year you won't be surprised either. And if something comes your way that wasn't mentioned in this book, please, by all means let us know so we can tell others.

When the work is finished, the subject's usual reaction is to sit still while looking at the ceiling or the floor as if trying to *feel* if the pain is still there or at least *somewhere*. If it really isn't, then you have had a successful day as a sleuth/slayer of trigger points. One of those trigger points may have been Papa Bear. Your friend may be painless for the evening, for a few days or even longer. I took away a headache for one of the B. Dalton bookstore salesladies when I was on tour with *Pain Erasure*. Three months later I met the same lady in another bookstore, in another town in another state. She was delighted to tell me that the pain had never come back, and we had worked for less than three minutes. You could get lucky! Now at least you know how to stop that kind of headache in that person and you will be able to do so in minutes anytime, anywhere.

If the pain went but returned in short order, then you know that while it is a headache amenable to Myotherapy, there are some very uncooperative trigger points nearby, and the law of facilitation has come into play. The law states: when an impulse has passed through a certain set of neurons to the exclusion of others, it will tend to take the same course on future occasions; and each time it traverses this path the resistance in the path will be smaller. In essence this means that the longer the pain has been in effect the easier its return to that state will be. That is one good reason for considering all chronic pain an enemy, even when it is almost insignificant. It won't stay that way.

The muscles develop habits, and starting up a spasm-pain-spasm cycle becomes easier and easier. This is especially true if your stress level is on the rise. What has probably happened is that some of the muscles in Segment 1 have been cleared and quieted but there are trigger points elsewhere in the same zone that are referring pain. Go on and find them.

And what if the pain moved? It may well have shifted to the other side or settled behind the eyes, or is now squatting like a toad on top of the head. What then? You simply move on to Segment 3, the front of the head.

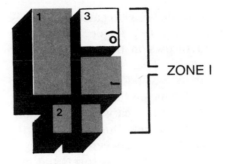

ZONE I, SEGMENT 3: THE FRONT OF THE HEAD

The front of the head can harbor many trigger points, and in *Permanent Fix* we go after them all. In *Quick Fix* we don't have time. The concert is about to begin or the important meeting has already begun. If the headache is at its pounding worst in the back of the head, you will have to start there. But if time is of the essence and the pain is in the front or on either side, you may find your answer quickly in the *orbiculares oculi*. They are the muscles around the eyes, numbers 60 and 61, on Figure 2.

Trigger points have an affinity for the attachments of muscles and also the edges, rather than the bellies. The *orbi-*

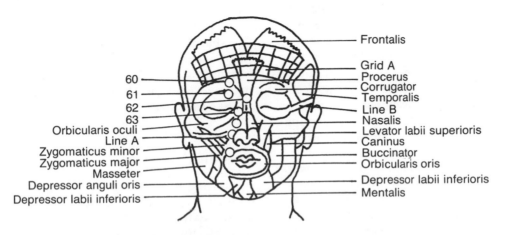

FIG. 2: FRONT OF HEAD AND FACE

60
61
62
63
Orbicularis oculi
Line A
Zygomaticus minor
Zygomaticus major
Masseter
Depressor anguli oris
Depressor labii inferioris

Frontalis
Grid A
Procerus
Corrugator
Temporalis
Line B
Nasalis
Levator labii superioris
Caninus
Buccinator
Orbicularis oris
Depressor labii inferioris
Mentalis

cularis oculi allows us to catch both edges under one questing finger at the same time and throws in the *corrugator* for good measure. That means we will have a good chance of finding several trigger points. It also means that the chances are excellent that the area will be very sensitive. To compound this, there is little protecting tissue between the trigger points and the bone that forms the eye sockets. You are going to use that bone for trapping the trigger points between it and your finger as you did while learning the technique on page 37. Remember, the *orbicularis oculi* is very sensitive. So you be sensitive too, to the subject's reactions.

Like the *splenius capitis* and company, in the back of the head, the *orbiculares oculi* are overworked all the time, and this is especially true for people who have poor eyesight or who have very mobile faces and exhibit much expression using the muscles around the eyes. Attacking the trigger points in the muscles circling the eye sockets would be a little easier if the subject were supine, but the chair will do nicely in a pinch, and in a pinch is when the quick fix exhibits its greatest value. If you do have a table handy so the subject can lie supine, stand at one end *above* the subject's head and reach down over the forehead.

If the subject is in a chair, stand behind the chair and, holding the shoulder to stabilize, press the head back against your chest. With the other hand reach over the top of the head with either the second or third finger and press down firmly on the top of the eyebrow. You have now caught the upper edge of the *orbicularis oculi*, 60. Put the pressure on and start to push the eyebrow (and whatever is underneath it) down over the edge of the socket. In addition to 60 you will have caught 61, the lower edge of the *orbicularis* and the *corrugator*. When you know you are over the edge, hook your finger around it and press up against it, using the wraparound technique you

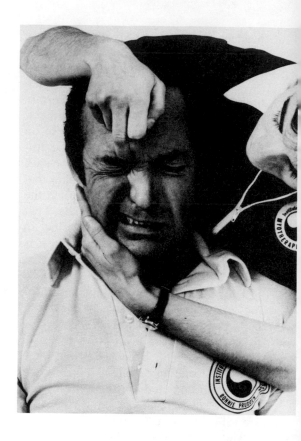

learned on page 37. The trigger points are now between the bone and the finger. The subject will let you know at once both vocally and with a grimace. Hold for the required five seconds and then release slowly. Move your finger outward toward the edge of the eye one finger-breadth at a time, hunting and holding at each spot where a trigger point is unearthed. The second position is usually worse than the first, but the others less so. Press at the same intervals back toward the nose along the lower edge of the socket. Do both eyes and then have the subject do the eye-muscle stretch.

Eye-Muscle Stretch

With the eyes closed, raise the eyebrows and hold the stretch for three seconds. Next, scrunch the face as though eating lemons. Relax and repeat three times. Then, with the eyes still closed,

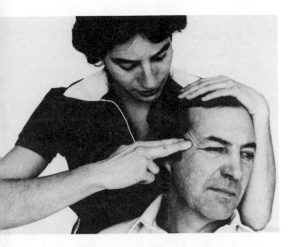

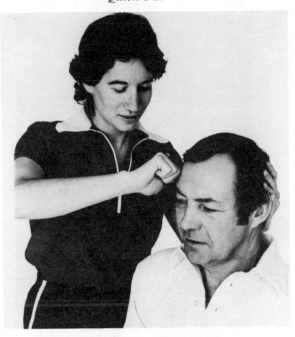

roll them to the right, left, up and down. Do that set three times.

Next, check out the temple area, on Line B. You were introduced to it back in the *Technique* section. With the subject's head held against your chest and rotated to the left, use your left hand to hold it in place as you work with the second and third fingers of the right hand. Press straight in close to the eye socket on Line B and then use the compass. When you have completed that, move on toward the top of the ear at half-inch intervals. Do the same thing on the other side by reversing your hands. And do reverse your hands. As you learn Myotherapy *use both hands alternately* whenever possible. Like any other repetitive movement, pressing constantly with the same elbow and hand can put trigger points into the muscles and give *you* pain.

Temple Stretch

Use the fingers flat against the side of the head to move the skin over the muscles in small circles along Line B. There is room for three: one at the eye, one near the ear and one in the middle, between the two.

On page 36 you learned about the roller technique, which is used on the forehead and, if needed, over the entire head. No-

tice Grid A. All those squares represent places where trigger points could lodge. Make a fist and, rolling your knuckles like a slow-moving set of gears, try to hit one small square at a time on the line just above the eyebrows. If a knuckle causes pain, stop and hold the pressure the required five seconds, make a compass and move on. There are lines of squares representing three passes of your roller across the *frontalis* muscle, in the forehead. Do both sides.

Forehead Stretch

Use the heel of the hand on the forehead, massaging in small circles, three to a side. Keep the pressure firm so you massage the muscle, not just the skin.

Here is another opportunity to ask the subject, "Where has the pain moved to?" If it was still there after working in Segments 1 and 2, but is gone after doing 3, you may want to *start* in Segment 3 should your subject have another headache before you can get to *Permanent Fix*. There is a good chance that the main troublemaker is in *that* area and you could save time.

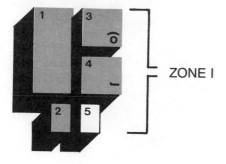

ZONE I, SEGMENT 4: THE FACE

When people say they have a "sinus headache," it usually means they feel pressure in the facial sinus (in back of or around the eyes). It may or may not be connected with a cold or an allergy, but trigger points in the face can be the initiators, even of that stuffed-up feeling. Start with the subject's head against your chest and turned to one side. Use your thumb and place it between the eyes on circle 62, the *procerus*. Press straight in and then execute the compass. The upward pressure is usually the worst. Massage with one finger, making small circles.

The sides of the nose come next. Look at Figure 2 and notice the three small circles that run down the line next to the nose. Start with the one at the top and press *in* toward the nose. Hold for five seconds *even if there is little or no response*. Then press away from the nose into the *malar* (cheekbone). That usually causes some commotion, especially if you are given to smiles and laughter. It is a small price to pay for such a sunny disposition! Hold for five and then slide the finger down to a point midway between the corner of the eye and the corner of the nostril. Repeat the press into and away from the nose. Lastly, the circle at the nostril edge. Press in toward the center of the nose and then outward and *up under* the malar. There is almost always a trigger point there, however latent.

Hold the pressure for the required five seconds and then execute a compass.

The jaw muscles are extremely complicated, and the problem mentioned most often is called TMJD, or temporomandibular joint dysfunction. The trouble makes itself felt in the jaw, but the jaw is like the knee and the shoulder and the elbow: the trouble is rarely *in* the hurting joint, so injecting into the joint itself rarely helps. Often the trouble is spasm caused by trigger points, and they can be anywhere in Zone I. They have also been found in Zones II and III. We have not had much luck with quick fix to the jaw. We do have success, however, with permanent fix, so, rather than disappoint yourself and your subject by thinking that *one* trigger point might be the cause, turn to *Permanent Fix* and do it right.

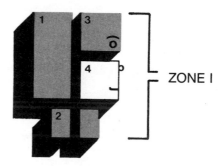

ZONE I, SEGMENT 5: THE NECK

Segment 5 in Zone I houses a pair of muscles that have tremendous influence on your well-being and are in danger from the moment you start down the birth canal, if not before. The *sternocleidomastoid* (SCM) starts in the side of the neck at the *mastoid process*, that curve of bone just under the ear. Squeeze the lobe of your ear between your second and third fingers and then press in against your neck with the second finger. That is the *mastoid process* you feel under it. From there it runs down to the *sternum*, or breastbone (circle 73), and the *clavicle*, the collarbone (circle 74), in the front. You may balk at that long name, but it's very easy if you know what it means. We could remember the name Sistermaryjoseph when we were only five, and it has the same number of syllables. All I could get from the word Sistermaryjoseph was that she was a nun named after St. Joseph. Most nuns have Mary in their name anyway. Sister also meant that she was not a man, who would have been called Father. But look what you can get from *sternocleidomastoid*. Place of residence, the neck. Has three attachments: the *sternum*, the *clavicle* and the *mastoid process*. Furthermore, it is a muscle. Here are some of the facts you will *not* get from its name. Starting, as it does, at the *mastoid process*, it is very close indeed to the *splenius capitis*, the *semispinalis* and the *trapezius*, at circle 66. That means that spasm in that area can affect the neck. It also means that spasm in the *sternocleidomastoid* can affect the head. Check with Figure 3 and you will note that it is a thick, strong muscle and splits into two heads at its distal end. These two heads attach to the borderline between Zones I and II. That means that

the neck can affect the chest and the chest can affect the neck. As a matter of fact, both the *clavicle* and the *sternum* are a part of the chest, which should tell you that the *sternocleidomastoid* may wear two hats and affect structures in both directions. The *sternocleidomastoid* has the power to give you pain, make you dizzy, and cause you to fall down, and even allow other people to take away your car keys.

While most of your work with the *sternocleidomastoid* will take in the whole muscle, including the main body and both sides of the division, it might be helpful to know how various parts of one muscle can affect vastly differing structures. If any part of the *sternocleidomastoid* harbors trigger points, pain can ensue, but so can other troubles.

Circle 74, the head of the *sternocleidomastoid* that attaches to the *clavicle*, or collarbone, refers pain across the forehead and deep into the ear *on the same side*. It also refers pain to the *postauricular* region, right behind the ear. Can you see the connection between the collarbone broken during a football game and headaches starting in the *front* of the head ten years later during divorce pro-

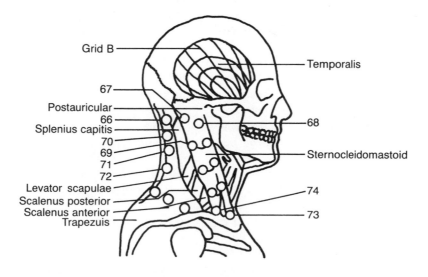

FIG. 3: THE NECK

cedures? How about trigger points behind the ear referring pain that *feels* like angina in the chest? And how about the woman who broke nothing at all when she fell and merely bruised her collarbone? Why should she be driven to distraction with *tinnitus*? And quite aside from those buzzing noises, she has a constant pain deep inside her ear and has been told that if the noise doesn't let up she will need a "masker" to drown it out and quite possibly an operation for the pain. And can you see why the operation on the ear wouldn't help?

Nor is that the limit of the muscle's influence. The same head of the *sternocleidomastoid*, circle 74, has a still more disabling dysfunction to offer, postural dizziness (spatial disorientation and impaired weight appreciation). While such a problem would interfere at any age, it is most devastating for the elderly. To begin with, it feels strange, and the first thought will be "Oh, no, not a brain tumor!" That's if there is time to think anything at all before falling and possibly breaking a hip. Dizziness and impaired balance in the old gives a false impression of senility and incompetence, not to mention suspicion of drug addiction or alcoholism. At best this means giving up the car and at worst, a nursing home. Of course there is always another medication to add to the stuff you may already have been saddled with, and the combination, while slow-acting, is still medical poisoning.

The elderly population has become both guinea pig and pharmaceutical garbage pail. If one medication doesn't "cure," another and yet another will be tried. Very few doctors, trained in dosing, would suspect that the little old gentleman who sits so patiently waiting to be seen because he has been having "spells" got the trigger points that are causing them driving racing cars when he was thirty. Antivertigo pills will be added to his medication for high blood pressure, angina, back pain, headaches, emphy-

sema, arthritis and, not surprisingly, depression. Almost all medicine has the potential for causing depression, and his already has a multiplication of seven. Multiplication is the right word to describe his plight because those medications not only work on *him*, they work on each other. With Myotherapy applied to his neck as well as all the segments in Zones I and II, you might get rid of the dizziness and the headaches, and the neck and upper-back pain. In addition you might be able to make his angina attacks less severe and certainly ease his breathing. He would look and feel fifteen years younger. If he could throw out at least some of the junk he has become addicted to, the depression would lift.

There is a special medication we should mention here: the medication that doesn't work. It doesn't *do* anything for the patient, but he is assured that without it he would be even *worse*. This medication serves three purposes: It assures the patient that someone knows what he has (which is not always the case) and is doing something about it. Since he doesn't get well, he has to keep coming back for repeat visits. And lastly, the misery can be blamed on him, because he doesn't get well even though the right medication is being given. It serves him right for getting old.

Circle 73, the sternal division, is a major source of pain in the throat, the face, the bony cavity containing the eyeball, the top and back parts of the head, and the sternum. This last you already know can refer pain *into* the chest as well. Since the front of the chest influences the upper back and also the organs within, there is every reason to treat the *sternocleidomastoid* with great consideration and a thorough investigation.

Whether your subject lies supine or sits up in a chair, the trigger-point work will be the same. However, everyone stands before the bathroom mirror several times a day. We will use the *sternocleidomastoid* to teach you more about working on yourself. You need to know how it feels when a trigger point is trapped and squeezed and also what stretching does to bring comfort *after* the trigger point has been neutralized. Then there is the raising of your *level of expectation.* When you discover you can get rid of your own pain, you will expect to be completely pain-free, and most of the time you can.

Starting with the level of expectation, dysfunction often comes on insidiously. It may start as a little stiffness which responds to a hot shower, a massage or just shrugging the shoulders a few times. There may be—and this is harder to note—a retreat from full range of motion. If there is an accident and the subject suffers a whiplash that immobilizes the head for a few days or even weeks, the limited range is highly visible. The neck may even be treated to a collar, which applies additional limitation to the already damaged muscles. This often compounds the problem.

But the range of the neck muscles can be lost *imperceptibly* over the years, and it is only when someone asks you why you have to turn your entire upper body when you want to back the car up that you know something is very wrong. By then you have been patterned to believe that age has overtaken you. Age, at any age, is rarely the cause, and the cure begins by not accepting age as an excuse, but from now on *preventing* small losses which could one day add up to a very big loss. *Expect* to be fine, insist on it and then keep yourself that way. *You can.*

Standing in front of the mirror, turn your head as far to the left as possible. The *sternocleidomastoid* will be easily discernible running down from the ear to the center of the chest. Once you have found the muscle, place your thumb on the side toward the back and your fingers to the front. Relax the tension by allowing your head to droop toward your waiting hand. Grasp the muscle firmly, separating it from the underlying tissues. That

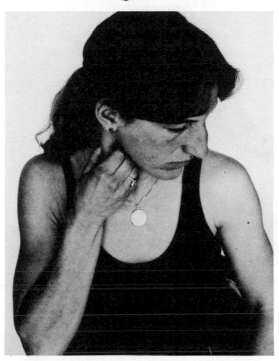

sounds more complicated than it is. When you have the muscle separated out it will feel about the size of a chicken's neck and fit neatly between thumb and fingers. Check with Figure 3 and you will note that you have grasped the *sternocleidomastoid* about one third of the way up. The trigger-point circles are paired, as are your thumb and fingers. Squeeze to put pressure on the trigger points that may be trapped. If they are there, the squeeze will hurt. Hold for the required five seconds and then slide the fingers up about one-half inch. Squeeze again and hold if painful. Now slide down to one-half inch below the original squeeze and repeat. Most necks require three squeezes.

Your next move should be up at circles 67 and 68. Start with circle 67, the trigger point on the back edge of the *sternocleidomastoid.* With two fingers, press forward to locate any hidden points. Follow that with pressure to circle 68, which is on the front edge of the muscle. *Some* squeeze may be possible up that high, especially in a thin neck, but usually those two circles, though paired, must be done singly.

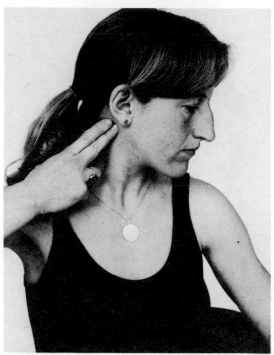

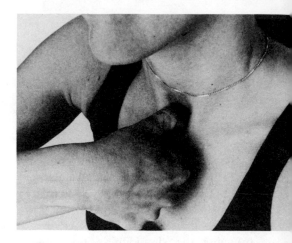

the bone and then over the edge, *wrapping around* into the hollow where the ends of the *clavicles* come together.

To trap any trigger points at the clavicular end of the *sternocleidomastoid*, slide the first and second fingers out about one inch from circle 73 *on* the

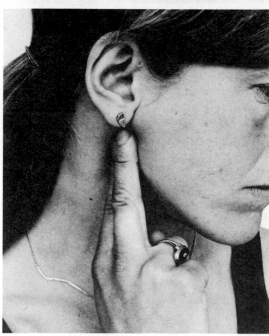

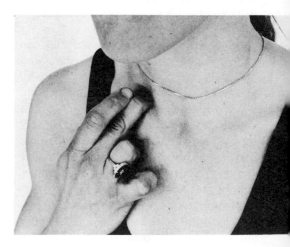

clavicle. Your fingers will be right over circle 74, the clavicular head of the muscle. Repeat the wraparound. Then slide your fingers along the clavicle, pressing at one-inch intervals out to the point of the shoulder.

There are still two points left: circle 73, which is the *sternocleidomastoid*, which attaches to the *sternum*, and circle 74, attachment to the *clavicle*. To entrap any trigger points at the sternal end, place your thumb at the top of the *sternum*, right at the start of the neck. Press onto

The Sternocleidomastoid Stretch

To stretch the *sternocleidomastoid*, stabilize yourself by sitting in a chair and grasping the handle of a door in your right hand. Using your left hand on your right cheek, turn your head as far to the left as you can manage, and then, tipping the head slightly upward, draw the head still farther and hold the stretch for a few seconds. Let up and then reapply in a slow, gentle rhythm about eight times. Switch hands and do the other side exactly the same way.

You have now seen the word *sternocleidomastoid* fifteen times in the past few pages and must know it by now. Certainly you remember Sistermaryjoseph!

Chronic pain comes on slowly as a rule and there may be mild spasm in effect for years before the three necessary components come together: trigger points, emotional or physical stress, and the precipitating incident. You won't get rid of it like a flash, either, except temporarily perhaps, with a quick fix. It will be necessary to keep the muscles stretched

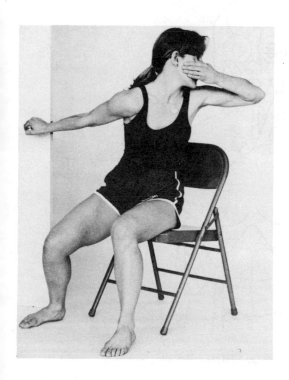

so they function properly without substitution.

Reeducating muscles is like reeducating children. You show them what to do and then you keep after them day and night until there isn't another way to do it. They, both muscles and children, will grumble all the while, and you may feel it isn't worth the effort, but it is. Well-educated, self-disciplined young people (self-discipline is an outgrowth of gentle, unwavering discipline) are nice to have around, and they are productive. So are well-educated, disciplined muscles. Having a job, keeping a job, or being employed at all often depends on whether or not your body can get *to* the job, keep you *on* the job . . . and do the job better than the next one. Staying alive or dying can also depend on your body if you are threatened with an accident. Having a healthy baby or a sad-little-sick-little-thing also depends on your body, as does something overlooked bringing up that baby.

Trigger points you already have, and tension is daily. The opportunities for precipitating incidents are everywhere, and you've met up with that terrible trio at least once or you wouldn't be reading this book. What's your protection? Exercise. You need all kinds of exercise, but for your neck you meet fire with fire. Every time you must hold still for any length of time, warm it up with some shoulder shrugs and stretch it with side-to-side turns.

Don't wait for the warning signal of pain. Tie in your shrugs and stretches with something you do all the time: changing the paper in the typewriter, going down the hall to the bathroom, stepping over to the sideboard for a cup of coffee, putting down the receiver, changing the station, opening the refrigerator, stopping for gas. Long ago I said that muscles were like women. They'll take a lot of guff, but they won't stand for being ignored and they have a lot of ways of getting even.

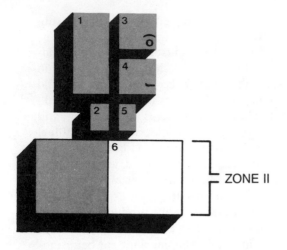

ZONE II

ZONE II, SEGMENT 6: THE CHEST

Segment 5, the front of the neck, brought us to the end of Zone I, the zone containing *most* of the trigger points apt to cause headaches and neck and facial pain. Zone II encloses the chest, 6, and the upper back, 7. Always keep in mind that each zone is like a box. Where there is a top to the box there must be a bottom, the front has a back and one side has the other side. Any one of the six can affect one, two or even *all* the others.

The front of the box that is Zone II is made up of the sternum, ribs and *pectorales major* and *minor*, the muscles of the chest. Since attachments usually house trigger points, you will be interested to learn about those of the "pects." It's important that you realize just how many structures offer pain to the chest and how many can be affected by the pects in return. Just knowing about these will clear up a lot of mysteries and turn you away from a goodly number of medications that come under the heading of "medicines that don't work" or those that will be better at the bottom of the sea. The great Dr. Oliver Wendell Holmes had something to say about that. He said it would be worse for the fishes.

The *pectoralis major* also attaches to the sternum and the clavicle at circles 73,

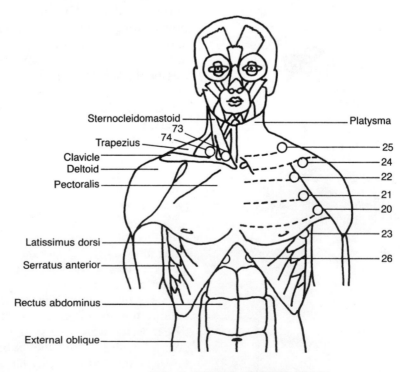

FIG. 4: TORSO, FRONT VIEW

in Zone I. This means you should entertain a little uneasiness about the neck muscles when you are trying to locate the cause of a pain in the chest, just as Zone II would not be considered above suspicion when it comes to a headache or jaw pain or even throat spasms.

The pects are also attached to the six upper ribs and the *aponeurosis* of the *external oblique* muscle. An *aponeurosis* is a flattened or ribbonlike expansion serving mainly to connect a muscle with a part it moves. It can also be a party to muscle spasm and referred pain. In addition—and this information is crucial—the pects attach to the *humerus*, the single bone in the upper arm. In other words, as the much-used arms go, so go the pects. Spasm in one can refer to the other.

Chest pain can be very uncomfortable and *frightening*, as anyone who has ever had either a real or mimicked attack of angina or even "heartburn" can tell you. But trigger points that reside in the chest seem to be much kinder to the home place than they are to such neighbors as arms, armpits, the neck, the upper back and the abdomen. There are three notable exceptions: asthma, angina and emphysema. Most people who suffer the crushing pain of angina go immediately where they should go: to a hospital. There something can be done. Others, the asthmatics and folks with emphysema, whose pain is usually not so dramatic or insistent, may just bear the pain or dose themselves, hoping the latter will help, at least temporarily.

Occupations put trigger points into the chest muscles and often light up those already in place as a result of falls or repetitious movements such as pipefitting, weaving, or operating a machine as heavy as a pneumatic drill or as light as a typewriter. Since *any* occupation at *any* time in life does this, one should not be content with examining the life-style of today. One must go back to the beginning. See "Your History . . . For Yourself," on page 119.

The trouble with trigger points in the chest is that they are so seldom recognized as the cause of the trouble. An elderly widow came to us with excruciating chest pains which had started about six months after her husband had died of a massive heart attack. He had suffered for years with the same kind of pain, and she was convinced that her days were numbered. Her personal physician and two cardiologists had assured her that no, her heart wasn't sick. It was just fine. She thought they were lying. She still had her pain, she was still scared to death, and she kept calling the doctor. Knowing her heart was not involved, the doctor sent her for Myotherapy.

The trigger points were everywhere in both arms and armpits, her chest, her upper back and shoulders, even in her hands. When we finished erasing (or at least damping) the trigger points we said, "Now, don't go doing anything other than your exercises for ten days. No gardening, no bread-making, no long-distance driving. Let yourself heal a little and give the muscles time to lose their bad habits. Just the exercises, understand?" Yes, she understood. Off she went and I didn't hear from her for eight days. Then she was back with exactly the same complaint: chest pain. "What in blazes did you do?" I asked her with considerable dismay, and I guess my tone was accusatory, because her back went up at once and she was quite indignant as she said, "Nothing! Absolutely nothing! I didn't even go out of the house. All I did was sit in front of the TV and crochet. I made a whole layette for my grandchild." That's *all* she did! She had gotten the trigger points from a lifetime of knitting up her entire family and *all* she did was the worse thing she could possibly have done: more of the same. The end of the story is we cleared the trigger points again and she has given up handwork for walking and cross-country skiing. She could have bought a lot of sweaters for the money she spent on doctors and tests and the psychiatrist who told her she was just emulating her husband and could do with some behavior modification.

Sometimes one *has* to switch hobbies or even work. If it hadn't gone on for so long, the problem could have been controlled even though she continued to aggravate the overworked muscles. But if you *have* to give up something, there's one sure cure for the void that is left: take up something else.

While working on the face, head and neck, you used a five-second hold. Now, in the chest and also in the rest of the body, with the exception of the feet and hands, you will use a seven-second hold. Still working on yourself, place the third and fourth fingers on the top of your sternum and, with your thumb and first finger, probe the chest muscle on both sides, looking for tender spots. As you work your way down, hold any tender spots you can reach and use the compass.

Once you have cleared the inner edges of the muscles, where they attach to the *sternum*, you will need to check the outer edges, where they approach the arms. This area *can* be done alone, but it is a lot easier if you have, or can get, help. If you must do it alone use your bodo.

Stand in back of the subject and place your fingers on circle 22 on Figure 4. Stay close to the chair back to give body contact. Press slowly and gently and watch for signals that tell you you have gone far enough. Once the pressure is on and the first seven-second hold is completed, use the compass in all four directions.

Using circle 22 on Figure 4, page 66, as your guide, move toward the *sternum* at half-inch intervals. When you have completed that line, start inward from circle 21 and finally inward from circle 20.

If the subject is female, have her move her breast out of the way. They do move, you know, and that old wives' tale about blows to the breast causing cancer has been disproved. Besides, you are press-

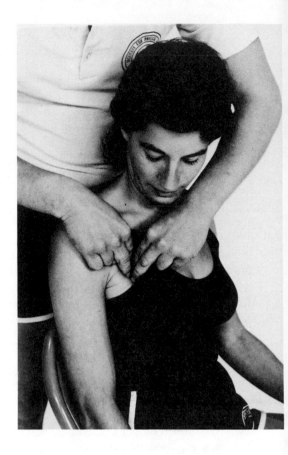

ing, not hitting, and there's a vast difference. Trigger points in the chest can be extremely sensitive, so be sensitive yourself.

Agonizing chest pain can result from bouts of coughing, and if enough trigger points are present or if they are in the right place, even a sneeze will start the action. The muscles hiding the trigger points are the *intercostals* (between the ribs). They can garner a flock of trigger points for such active people as athletes and dancers and those doing heavy work. Merely cracking a rib will leave behind a residue of trigger points after the bone has healed which may not be heard from until long after the incident is forgotten. A fall against a table that does nothing more than bruise is very apt to mark its passing with at least one small trigger point. Try to remember it. This would also apply to people suffering from the "battered syndrome." Whether the person is young, as are battered children, or older, as are battered women, beaten at home or mugged in the streets, the results will be much the same someday.

Such trigger points in the *intercostals* may never be heard from until the person contracts a really bad cold or whooping cough. Suddenly during one bout there is a tearing wrench in the chest or upper-back area, and it may cause so much pain it is impossible to stand erect. Then *fear* of coughing amounts to sheer terror, and often enough, a cough suppressant will give you the reputation of a lush. What is the usual treatment? Taping, bed rest . . . "and a little something to make you sleep." If you are a movie star or, worse, acting in a show, you will be sent to the hospital, where you are apt to be told that a muscle has been torn from the rib! The diagnosis is probably wrong and the treatments don't work, other than the sedation, which works so well you can't.

The trigger points causing *intercostal* spasm are more honest than most; they are right *there*, where the pain is.

Have the subject sit on a chair with the painful side toward you, twisting away to put a slight stretch on the muscles and also to open up the ribs. Using a careful finger, or better yet a small bodo, slide carefully along between two ribs in the vicinity of the pain, until you elicit a gasp or a wince. The trigger point is there somewhere. Press gently on each tender place at half-inch intervals, and after every four or five, have the subject take a deep breath. If the pain changes in intensity or shifts even a little, you are on your way to clearing it out. Pay careful attention to any changes when the next coughing spell hits.

WARNING: Little old people, especially postmenopausal ladies, may have brittle bones. The condition is called *osteoporosis*. Be *very* gentle with their ribs, just about the same as you would be with a baby's face. It will still erase the points, and your gentle probing and caring will do more for that little person than all the

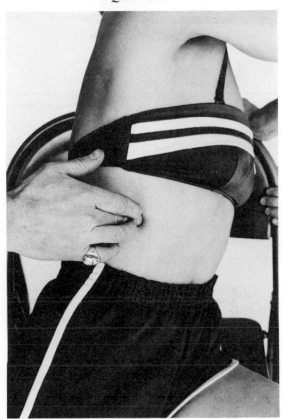

bed rest in the world. Incidentally, bed rest is easily overdone at any age.

Usually the posture anomalies, *round back* and *kyphosis* (which is an extreme form of round back), are put under *B*, for back. They belong under *C* for chest, because it is the chest muscles that pull the shoulders forward to round the back. It is the *pects*, not the poor, weak upper-back muscles that are at fault. Try to clear all the places in the chest muscles that could cause shortening spasm, and then do the following chest-stretching exercises.

Chest-Muscle Stretch: The Backstroke

The first chest-muscle stretch is the easier of the two. It is called the back-

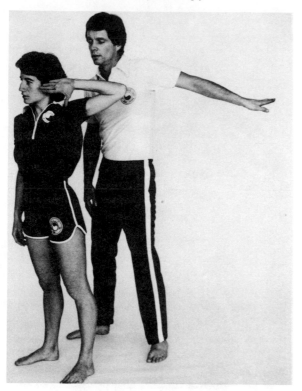

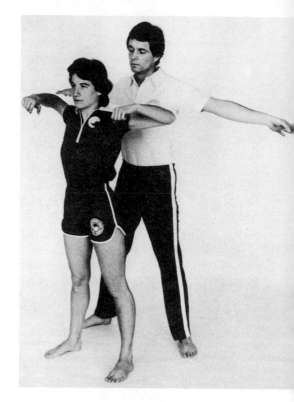

stroke. Stand with feet apart for balance, and place the back of one hand on the side of the cheek. Keeping the elbow pressed back as far as possible, carry the arm and hand around in a circle, allowing it to rest at the verticle while the other arm performs the same circling motion. If no pull is felt, then the elbow is not held back far enough. Alternate eight to a side.

Chest-Muscle Stretch: Snap-and-Stretch

Stand with feet apart and bent elbows held at chest level. Snap the elbows back on the count of one. Bring them back to the starting position on two and then fling arms wide and backward on three, finishing on the starting position on four. Do eight.

In addition to these, use the strengthening exercises in the *Self Center* section.

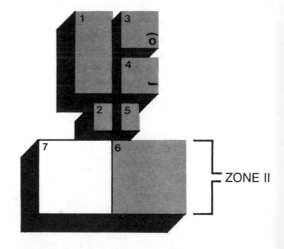

ZONE II, SEGMENT 7: UPPER BACK

The chest is in front, and the back of the front is made up of the shoulders and the upper back. Any trigger points active in those huge muscles can affect the chest and even the organs *inside* the chest, which is also referred to as the *thoracic*

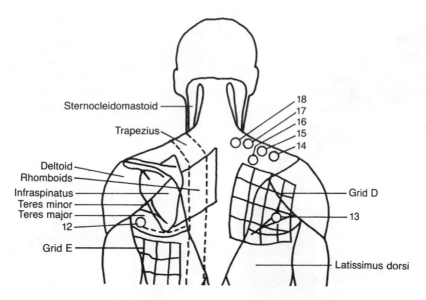

FIG. 5: UPPER BACK, POSTERIOR VIEW

cavity. The person with emphysema or asthma can suffer augmented pain and limitation in breathing when either the chest or the upper-back muscles are in spasm. Very often the sufferer feels as though the chest and back are strapped over with constricting bands. The person with emphysema, who can't get rid of all his used air, is also limited in what fresh air he can inhale. The asthmatic wheezes in both directions.

Often pain in muscles *under* the shoulder blade imitates a stab wound in severity.

The quick fix for the upper back would be easier if the subject were prone on the table, but in the absence of such luxury we have worked with subjects over filing cabinets, half-filled shelves, bales, boxes, the tires of semis and even on bars. Since the table is rarely available, but chairs are, we will continue using them as our supports.

One of the worst trigger points in the upper back (subjects will tell you it is *the* worst anywhere) is circle 13, on *Grid D.* It, like the *splenius capitis*, circle 66, at the back of the head, shares its area with other muscles. At circle 13 the edges of

the *deltoid*, the *trapezius, infraspinatus, latissimus dorsi* and both *teres major* and *teres minor* are in the picture. In addition, it is a part of the back that works most of the time. It takes part in the finest of small work such as that done by dentists, watchmakers, plastic surgeons and calligraphers. It also bears a share in all lifting and driving and in most sports.

The Scapula (Shoulder Blade)

Have the subject sit with legs apart, elbows on knees and head relaxed. Lean over and slip your arm under the subject's arm for stabilization and place your right elbow on circle 13 as shown on Figure 5. You will note that circle 13 is set inside *Grid D.* As with *Grid A*, on the forehead in Figure 2, *Grid D* will house many trigger points, but the area does not respond to the knuckles as used in the roller technique. Each square will have to be separately searched and, where trigger points are noted, the compass used thoroughly. So while 13 is apt to elicit pain (almost sure to), the other squares merit your attention as well.

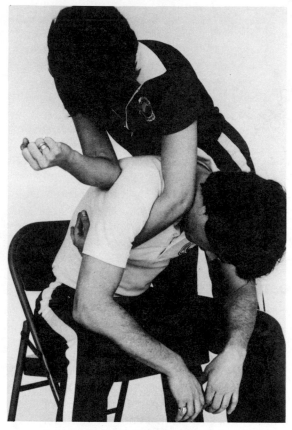

Scapula (shoulder blade)

Teres Major

The *teres major* rotates the arm, and we rotate our arms every day all day. It is circle 12 on Figure 5. Stand up straight and, placing the hands close together or even one on top of the other, lean down

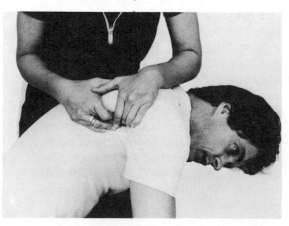

to grasp the *teres* (see Figure 6) and pull in and upward. If the muscle is strong and bunched, stand straight as you pull back. Use the front of your body to stabilize and as an anchor against which to work. Keep the pull steady and strong for seven seconds.

The Trapezius

There is another area in the upper back; it is the spot anyone who feels like helping a flagging co-worker will go for. It is made up of circles 13, 14, 15, 16 and 17, *on* the shoulders. Unfortunately, just rubbing the shoulders at those points brings no permanent relief. It is going to need something more. Circle 18 is also in that area, and we covered that one when we did the *splenius capitis*, in the back of the head. However, since you are now zeroing in on the upper back, with never a thought to headaches, we'll go over it again. A word about headaches and the upper back: Many of the former are caused by trigger points in the latter. Zone II abuts Zone I, and Segment 2 is next to Segment 7. They are co-workers, even relatives. While the name "neck" doesn't sound like the name "shoulder," here is a list of muscles that have feet in both camps and should be considered at least as in-laws.

> The trapezius
> The rhomboid minor
> The splenius capitis
> The splenius cervicis
> The levator scapulae
> The scalene

Have your subject sit sideways on a chair or on a box, leaning forward with elbows on knees and head relaxed. Stand to the rear and reach your free arm across the subject's chest to rest his back against your body. Start with circle 16, right in the center of the top of the shoulder, *midway* between the tip of the shoulder

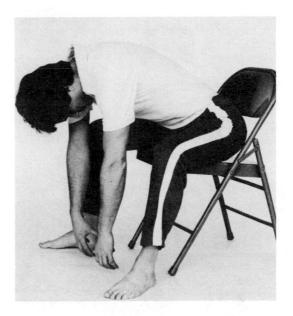

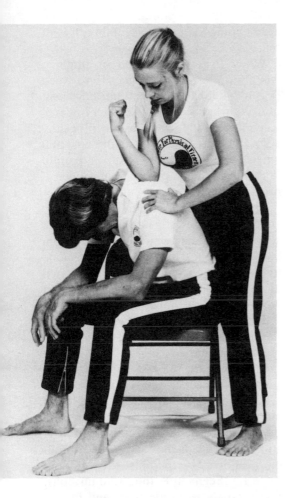

and the neck. Press down at the start and then use your compass technique. Keep in mind that the top of the shoulder is part of the upper back, which is usually overused but underexercised. Every one of those trigger points will be painful, whether there is pain in the area or not. Follow with the other circles on the shoulder and finish with circle 18.

Round-Back Stretches

The exercises for the upper back can and should be done often throughout the day. The round-back stretches are done by placing the feet flat on the floor and leaning forward to drop the arms between the knees while allowing the head to droop downward. Do eight *easy* bounces

downward. Then, keeping the arms straight, rotate them inward until the little fingers touch. Hold the stretch for a few seconds and then sit up straight. Press the shoulders back and then relax. Do at least three such stretches after trigger-point work. Try to tie the stretches in with your work. No cat leaves the hearth to go about its business before thoroughly stretching. Make it a point to stretch *gently* after every letter you write, phone call you finish or whatever your work calls for. It will take about a week before stretching becomes second nature. It is a potent weapon against tension.

The Door-Pull Stretches

Pulling against resistance is an excellent stretch. Pulling against a partner is more fun, but a door will do if you are alone. Set your chair far enough from an open door so you have to reach way forward to grasp both knobs. Pull back to stretch and hold the stretch for a few seconds, then release. Do five. If you are feeling strong, put your foot up on the edge of the door to give you extra pull.

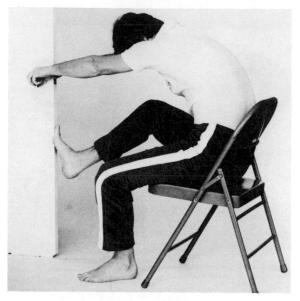

Door-pull stretch

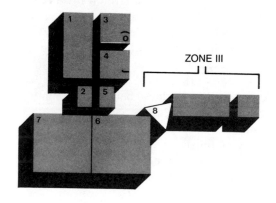

ZONE III

ZONE III, SEGMENT 8: THE AXILLA (ARMPIT)

It may be hard to believe, but your fingers begin in your shoulders, upper arms and armpits. Whether it seems to make sense or not, most chronic pain in fingers and hand has its origin far from the site of the cause. One of the reasons why soaking, splinting, rubbing and taping don't help much is that it is like looking for your lost cuff link under the light at the street corner although you distinctly heard it land in the gutter at midblock. There certainly is more light at the corner, but you aren't going to find your cuff link. It isn't there.

When fingers are numb or tingling, when one or another goes into such spasm that it bends sharply and stays bent to make what is called a "trigger finger," when fingers and hands lose their healthy color, when they are constantly cold and when they become so weak or painful that china and glassware are in danger of breakage, chances are you have trigger points in those three birthing centers the shoulders, upper arms and armpits. Not so long ago, a man who had suffered from daily headaches for twenty years came to the clinic in despair. He had tried everything but decapitation, saying that we were his last hope. There will come a day when Myotherapy will be among the first things tried, which will prevent much pain and save a lot of money, but for now we are the last hope for thousands of folks.

After a thorough search had been mounted in Zones I and II, he reported that although he felt generally better he still had his headache. The certified Bonnie Prudden Myotherapist then entered Zone III, Segment 8, the *axilla* (armpit). She tried the left side first, and in less then a minute the man clapped his hand to his head, saying, "The pain, the pain on the left side, it's *gone!*" The Myotherapist shifted her attention to the *axilla* on the right side, and in less than a minute the man sat right up. This time he was shouting. "It's *gone!* The whole headache is gone!" And he started to cry. He was pain free for the first time in twenty years.

The *axilla* is a hornet's nest of nasties. While, again, and especially in this case, supine would be easier, we are going to try to get rid of the trouble in a public place with no special supports. Have the subject clasp her hands back of her head. Reach your free hand around the back of the subject's shoulders for stabilization and place your knuckle in the *axilla*. There is no hard-and-fast rule as to where

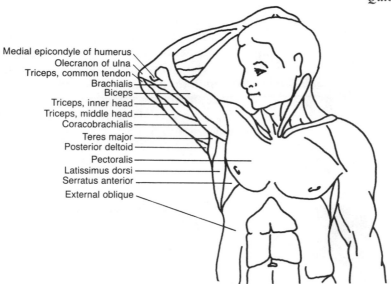

Medial epicondyle of humerus
Olecranon of ulna
Triceps, common tendon
Brachialis
Biceps
Triceps, inner head
Triceps, middle head
Coracobrachialis
Teres major
Posterior deltoid
Pectoralis
Latissimus dorsi
Serratus anterior
External oblique

FIG. 6: THE AXILLA

the trigger points are hiding; almost anywhere is apt to be sensitive, but the point where the *pectoralis* enters the arm is sure to be a good one. This is the spot that most troubles weight lifters, dentists and violinists.

The *axilla* is a bridge. It was the bridge from the overworked hands of the little lady who thought she had angina to the *pectoralis*, where she *felt* her pain. There are others, usually musicians (flutists, for

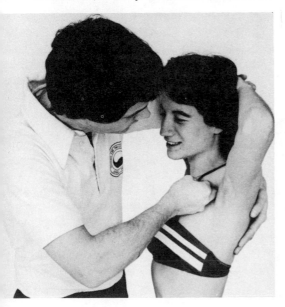

example) and crafts people, who suddenly lose the feeling in one or more fingers. They too think the trouble is in the fingers, but consider the strain in the shoulder, chest and upper back. A flute doesn't weigh much, but try holding your hands in front of your face for three hours!

Pianists, especially good ones, who practice hours and hours every day, are easy prey for trigger points in the chest, shoulders and *axilla*. The *axilla* will gladly start trouble in the upper arm, and from then on it's all downhill.

Axilla Stretch

After you have cleared the *axilla*, it will require the usual stretching in order to reeducate even such a lowly spot. Have the subject stand in front of you, feet apart and the arm you have just worked on straight up. Place your free hand flat between the shoulder blades. Grasp the raised arm at the wrist and pull slowly and steadily back to full stretch, or as close to full stretch as you can manage.

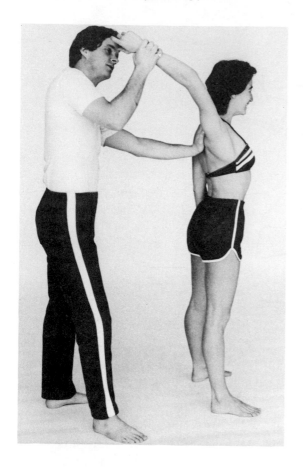

The range may be very limited at first, but that is one of the reasons for the pain: muscles shortened by spasm. Hold the stretch for a few seconds, pulling back a little in an even, slow rhythm. Then release to rest. Do several and do both sides.

Arm-Twist Exercises (Shoulder Rotations)

Drop the arm to the side and do the arm twists in *six* stages. Let the arm hang loose and turn it inward as far as possible so that the thumb can be made to point upward (male). Next rotate the arm outward so that the thumb points back (female). Do four with each arm and progress to the second stage, arms parallel or almost parallel with the floor. Then the third, with arms raised above shoulder level.

Repeat the whole series with the arms pointed forward.

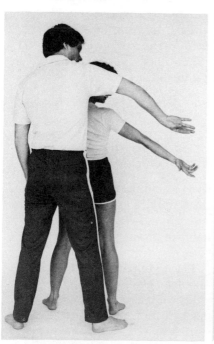
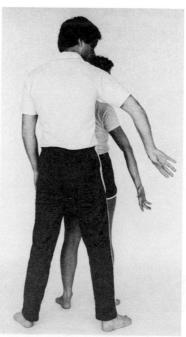
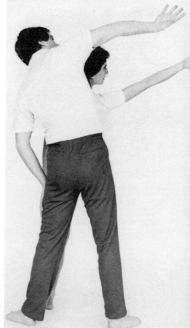

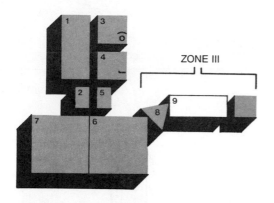

ZONE III

ZONE III, SEGMENT 9: THE ARM

Arm pain can range anywhere from the incredibly painful "bursitis" in the shoulder, down through the aching "tennis elbow," to the latest wonder, the "carpal tunnel syndrome" for pain in the wrist, hand and fingers. This last condition seems to plague musicians and dentists, and by this time you should know why: overuse of the muscles starting in the armpit.

"Bursitis" is rarely inflammation of the bursa in the shoulder. "Tennis elbow" happens far more frequently to electricians than to tennis players. The tennis player *may* develop the condition due to the vicious top spin he puts on the ball, but more than likely it is the result of aggravating an old injury. For the electrician the reason is all too clear: the constant, repetitive use of a screwdriver.

"Carpal tunnel syndrome" is one of the those things that are seldom what they seem. *Carpal* refers to the wrist, and the *carpal tunnel* is the osseofibrous passage for the median nerve and the flexor tendons formed by the *flexor retinaculum* (a network of cells) and the *carpal bones*. The pain in the wrist, hand and fingers is said to be caused by a tunnel that is too small or filled with debris. The *Journal of the American Medical Association*, in an article reporting on the operation, stated that if, after the end of a year, there was still pain, then it wasn't caused by

the carpal tunnel after all. It might be better to see if the pain is of muscular origin before using a knife. *All* knives leave scars, and scar tissue attracts trigger points. For the dentist or the musician, that could mean no career.

The quick fix for the arm might be needed anywhere: at the office, on the road, in the kitchen, before the concert, at the meeting, on the bus or in the air. Little children have arm and leg pain that is attributed to "growing," and oldsters have the same but attributed to "arthritis." Most of the time such pain is merely borne, or borne with the help of pills. If the arm aches too badly, a sling may be applied.

A sling immobilizes and in some instances might be helpful for a short time. Not too long ago the treatment for "bursitis" was *six weeks in a sling*. It would be far better to get rid of the trigger points and muscle spasm causing the pain than to try to keep it from moving. To begin with, when a limb is immobilized the muscles atrophy. They lose volume, strength, flexibility and coordination. Circulation slows and the nutrition to the entire limb is curtailed. That, in turn, slows healing.

If you are someplace where you can rest your arm in an outstretched position, say on a table or desk, the back of the car seat, a pantry shelf or even a railing, use it. Of course it would be best if the subject could lie flat, but you can't find that sort of accommodation at the office, in an air terminal or on the road, so learn to use what is at hand. With the subject's arm resting with the palm down, start at circle 76, up near the elbow at the edges of both the *brachioradialis* and the *extensor carpi radialis longus*. (The oftener you say those names the faster you will learn them.) This is the trigger point you first met back in the section on *Technique*. It is one of the key points for "tennis elbow." Follow the dotted line down the center of the arm at one-inch intervals, using your compass wherever

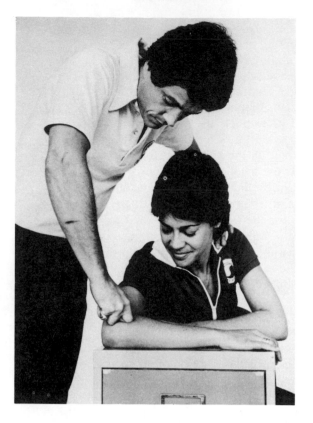

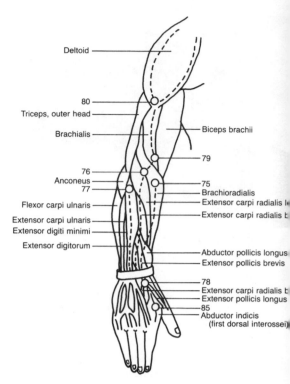

Deltoid

80
Triceps, outer head

Brachialis

Biceps brachii

79

76
Anconeus
77

75
Brachioradialis
Extensor carpi radialis l
Extensor carpi radialis b

Flexor carpi ulnaris

Extensor carpi ulnaris
Extensor digiti minimi

Extensor digitorum

Abductor pollicis longus
Extensor pollicis brevis

78
Extensor carpi radialis b
Extensor pollicis longus
85
Abductor indicis
(first dorsal interossei)

FIG. 7: POSTERIOR ARM (PRONATED)

there is sensitivity. Use your knuckle or elbow pressing straight down. Hold the pressure for the required seven seconds *only* on painful spots.

If you are faced with an aching arm in a place where there is no rest surface, stand facing the subject and place one thumb over circle 76 and cover that thumb with the other. You will find you have enough strength to erase most of the points.

When you have completed the line starting at 76, move outward to circle 77, the *extensor digitorum*. Follow the line down into the wrist. Don't waste time on painless spots. This of course requires the assistance of the subject, since he or she is the one who feels the pain and should say so.

Both of these muscles have a great deal to do with wrist action, and if they are in spasm they can cause carpal (wrist) pain, which may tell you that there is some-

thing to do for "carpal tunnel syndrome" besides soak it, splint it or ream it.

The work on the upper arm requires the subject to move back from the box or filing cabinet so the arm can be supported from elbow to armpit. Start at circle 79, the *brachialis*, which is a little above the elbow and usually as sensitive as circle 76 even in people with no arm discomfort. Press straight in at half-inch intervals until you reach circle 80. That is the start of the *deltoid* muscle, halfway up the upper arm. The *deltoid* resembles a small cape draped over the top of the arm. When you reach 80, work up the back edge of the *deltoid*, right into the shoulder. Then work your way up the forward edge. If the subject's arm is bony or painful, cushion it with a jacket or a sweater.

Return to circle 79 and work your way up to circle 80, but this time trap the trigger points by sliding off the line once the

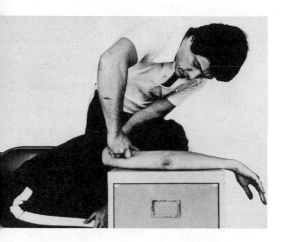

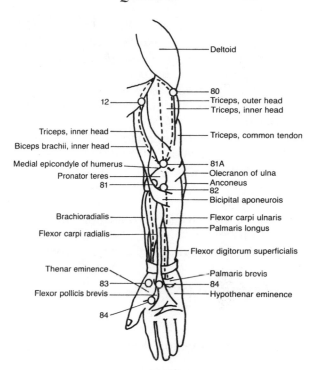

FIG. 8: ANTERIOR ARM

Labels on Fig. 8:

- Deltoid
- 80
- 12
- Triceps, outer head
- Triceps, inner head
- Triceps, inner head
- Biceps brachii, inner head
- Triceps, common tendon
- Medial epicondyle of humerus
- 81A
- Pronator teres
- Olecranon of ulna
- 81
- Anconeus
- 82
- Bicipital aponeurois
- Brachioradialis
- Flexor carpi ulnaris
- Palmaris longus
- Flexor carpi radialis
- Flexor digitorum superficialis
- Thenar eminence
- Palmaris brevis
- 83
- 84
- Flexor pollicis brevis
- Hypothenar eminence
- 84

pressure is on. Press into the *triceps* toward the back and then the *biceps* toward the front.

In order to get at the back of the arm, have the subject lean over to lay her shoulder on the table, cabinet, railing, whatever, palm up. Start at circle 82, just below the elbow. Work straight down the middle of the arm on the dotted line. As you do your compass left and right, you will cover the *bicipital aponeurosis*, the *flexor carpi ulnaris* and the *flexor digitorum superficialis*.

The second line starts at circle 81, right over the *pronator teres*. This is a "starter muscle"; it is responsible for getting other, larger muscles into action. Never miss circle 81 when you are hunting for the cause of pain anywhere in the fingers, hand, wrist, elbow *or jaw*. The *pronator teres* is a bad actor where TMJD is concerned, but so is the entire arm. The *pronator teres* is at great risk in anyone who must make small, repetitive movements with the hands. This is typically true of dental hygienists, who use a rotating motion as they scale teeth. The pain can travel up the arm, causing neck and facial pain and headaches.

To travel up the arm, start at 81A, one attachment of the *pronator teres*, at the *medial epicondyle of the humerus (funny bone)*. Move straight up to the shoulder at half-inch intervals over the middle head of the *triceps*. Then start again at 81A and

follow the inner line over the *inner head of the biceps brachii*. Lastly, starting at 81A, move up the third line along the edge of the *outer head of the triceps*. In this area we often find the causes of numbness and tingling in the hands.

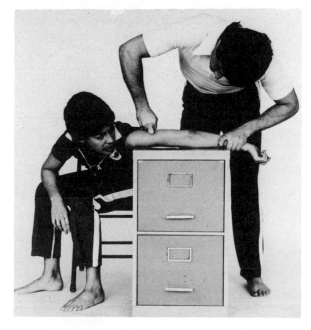

Starting at circles 81 and 82, go down the lower arm into the hand. The lines run over the *brachioradialis*, the *flexor carpi radialis*, the *flexor carpi ulnaris* and the *flexor digitorum superficialis*.

The exercises for the arm are the same as for the *axilla,* on page 75.

Shoulder pain is most often caused by a combination of upper-back spasm, chest-muscle spasm, and *axilla*, arm and hand spasm. To get rid of shoulder pain, *all* these areas should be covered, even the *sternocleidomastoids*, in the neck. The more muscles attaching to a joint, the greater the area that must be covered.

Arm-Rotation–Resistance Exercise

The same principle you followed for increased range in the neck is applicable to the shoulder. Grasp the subject's hand and have her rotate her hand first inward and then outward against your resistance. Start with very little resistance, but increase it as strength improves (see page 176).

Arm-Lowering Against Resistance

Place the injured hand over the healthy one at the wrist. Use the healthy arm to raise the injured one as high as possible *without pain or substitution.* Substitution in this case would be a hitched-up shoulder. Provide a little resistance with the healthy arm as the injured presses it down to the verticle. Repeat four or five times slowly, increasing the resistance and the range as much as possible *without pain.* At the close of the exercise check the range by having the subject raise the arm without assistance (see page 177). Repeat several times a day.

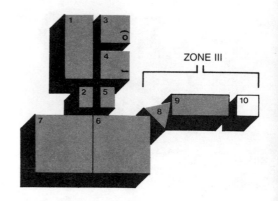

ZONE III, SEGEMENT 10: THE HAND

When it comes to the hand, unless the injury is acute, as in cuts, fractures or burns, do not begin to hunt for the trouble in the hand first. Start looking for the trigger points near the elbow and on the lines running up from the elbow to the shoulder, and that should include the edges of the *biceps*, in front, and the *triceps*, in back. You can find those lines very easily. Sit with your arm resting on your knee with the palm *up.* The elbow should be about near the knee. Make a fist and, keeping your elbow on your leg, bend the arm like a small boy showing off his "muscle." Grasp the muscle in your hand, thumb and fingers in opposition. Your thumb is on the right line. Slide it down to your elbow and press forward to slip under the *biceps* and then

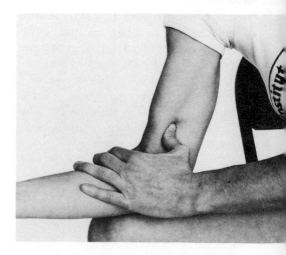

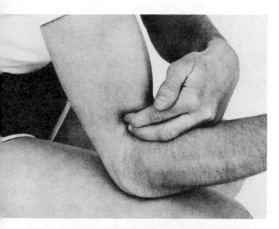

back against the edge of the *triceps*. Complete a compass with upward and downward pressure. Proceed at one-inch intervals up to the *axilla*.

Next, with two fingers of the working hand held stiff, press forward and then backward on the outside of the upper arm to pick up the edges of both *biceps* and *triceps*. Follow the line up to the shoulder.

The worst spot on the hand is usually circle 83, on Figure 8, but the two 84s can hold their own, as can circles 78 and 85, on Figure 7, if the hand has been overused or is plagued with arthritis.

This is another time you may need a small bodo, especially if you are working on your own hand. For one thing, both hands may hurt, and a painful hand isn't a good tool. In addition, the muscles of the hand are small and it is hard to hold a knuckle or even a finger at the right angle. The grip on the bodo provides better power and assists in direction.

The Finger-Squeeze Technique is excellent for aches, but also for swelling and weakness *after* you have done the *axilla*, arms and hands. Many people complain about one or the other giving trouble, and some fingers refuse to open or close all the way. Spasms in the arms, hands and fingers limit circulation and therefore nutrition. This prevents healing. The finger squeeze has nothing to do with the joints. Leaving out the knuckles, you have two joints in each finger, fourteen phalanges in each hand. The ones between the last joints and the tips of the fingers rarely complain if squeezed, but most of the others will. Lay your palm (or the subject's) flat and grasp the first phalange on both sides with your thumb and forefinger. Squeeze with considerable force, but be guided by the subject. If swelling or arthritis is present, the hand may be very sensitive. It will not be nearly as sensitive if you do them *after* you have done the arms. Even when you are reducing the swelling on a finger that has just been injured, do the arms as well. Any injury in Zone III will be a signal for all existing trigger points to light up, ignite and close all roads to and from the site of the crash.

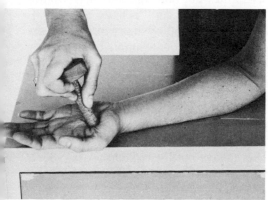

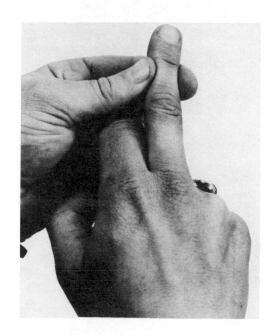

Squeeze each phalange on the sides and then move your thumb and forefinger to squeeze the back and front. Follow that by first making a fist and then opening the hand wide. You can include resistance for the hand by squeezing a ball, as everyone knows. This improves the grip muscles. Not so well known is the use of a rubber band for the muscles which open the hand and are the antagonists for the grip muscles. Bring the tips of the fingers together within the circle of a rubber band. Open your fingers wide against the band and then relax. Start with five. If that is impossible, the band is too thick; start with a thinner one. If it is very easy, then use two or even three bands.

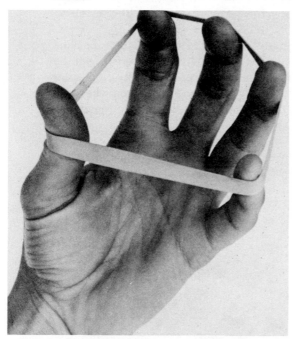

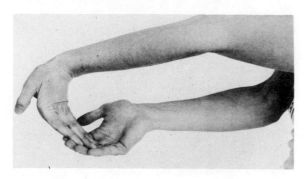

In order to stretch the palms, wrist and arm, lay the fingers of the right hand across the left while the elbow is in a bent position. Straighten both arms as you pull the fingers of the left hand back toward the body. Do three to a side.

The Back

At this point we come to one of the most important areas in the whole body, the lower back. True, if your lower back has never had a twinge but you do get pounding headaches, the former won't seem so terribly important, but let me tell you a little about back pain so you can be a better judge.

Like the other pains we have covered this far, most back pain comes not from disease, accidents of birth, or build, it comes from trigger points laid down in muscles through some often minor injury during life, *starting* in the womb and ending only with death. I have known oldsters to develop back pain, *for the first time in long lives*, when confined to bed in nursing homes. Some babies are born with painful backs. (Always check the back of a baby who cries when his back is exposed to cool air.)

Very few people are limited to one backache in a lifetime. Once the spasms begin, they are apt to continue at longer or shorter intervals depending on the physical and *emotional* stresses. They rarely decrease in severity, and even when they do, one cannot depend on the trend. A "bad back" is like a time bomb that can be set off by injury *anywhere* else in the body—from a simple tooth extraction to a sprained ankle. Any activity, from gardening to jogging, can set it going; the activity list includes making love, carrying a baby, lifting a child, a game of catch with the kids, sewing your daughter's wedding dress, et cetera. Don't leave out the twilight years, which here in America are bleak indeed for the incapacitated.

Now let's look at what a "simple" backache can do. A "simple" backache is one that comes on when you spend a long time over a desk or a drawing board. It could appear at monthly intervals with menstruation or be "picked up" in the delivery room from whatever it was that went on there.

If I walked into a board meeting to find twenty men seated around the table and said with assurance, "One of you will be dead by next Christmas," each would look at his neighbor and murmur, "Poor George, we'll miss him." Nobody ever believes the bullet has his name on it, which is one reason we have wars. But let's talk about back pain in America, and this we can do with every assurance in the world. Try this.

In your mind's eye, see those you love most. Line up five at the top of the list. Count off the first four in the line and ask them to lie down on the floor. Tell the one still standing to go into the next room and wait. Next, think of the people you would need if your family were to live comfortably and safely. Line up five farmers and follow the same routine, four on the floor and one in the next room. You will need someone to get the food to you, so line up five truckers and then five construction workers to build your house. You will need protection from fire and vandals, so follow those with five firemen and five policemen. Things will break down, so five repairmen. If you want variety in your meals, you will need five fishermen and five ranchers plus five butchers. If you are concerned that other nations may want what you have, you will need five soldiers, five sailors and five airmen. You will need five factory workers to make what you need. Should you have an accident or fall ill, you should consider five doctors, five nurses and five hospital technicians. You may want teachers for your children, so line up five for each age—elementary school, high school and college. Those are not all of the people we have grown accustomed

to counting on, but it's a start. Now take stock. There will be twenty representatives of these key groups walking about in the next room, but four out of every five, eighty to be exact, are lying all over the floor with agonizing back pain. That's what the statistics show, as does the show of hands in every audience I address except for a group of five hundred nurses who pushed that statistic up to over 90 percent. What the statistics do not show is the strain those damaged backs put on the few healthy backs.

Most backaches start out as "simple," but many, if not most, progress from mere ache to full-fledged incapacitating spasm, and that kind of pain demands a recumbent position. Just getting to the bathroom can be agonizing, and when it gets worse, the not so complicated act of getting on a bedpan is contemplated with terror, terror of ensuing spasm. Gradually (if you haven't already found your way to a hospital, traction, a myelogram, multiple medications or an operation) the pain recedes, but the sufferer is left with a fear. That kind of experience leaves even the most carefree (up to then) with a kind of sneaking, nagging anxiety about something known to the medical profession as "the next episode."

The "next episode" may start exactly like the first, but this time the sufferer's attitude is different. "Oh, my God! No, not again" is said in a variety of ways, but even those usually shy of Modern Medicine will find themselves calling a doctor, making an appointment and showing up in an office where sitting gingerly on the edge of a chair is de rigueur. A lot of back-pain sufferers stand, because they can't sit at all. The usual route is well known to almost anyone who has had a back that "goes out." Bed rest, heating pads, analgesics, "muscle relaxants" (which are really tranquilizers), X rays, myelograms, and if the pain doesn't go away but the patient goes to enough doctors, one of them will operate to find the cause of the pain. The operation will look grand on the X ray, but the patient usually has the pain he started with, plus a little or a lot more. In the past weeks we have seen five patients each with three or more back surgeries and *all* still suffering intractable pain. Now I think you should hear what a psychiatrist says about "intractable pain" patients.

There appear to be four stages of pain for patients with "chronic pain syndrome," where at least some psychiatrists are concerned. Thousands of back-pain sufferers are sent to psychiatrists every year because they don't respond to modern medicine's treatments for pain, and many develop an adversary attitude toward their doctors.

ZERO TO TWO MONTHS. This is the acute phase, during which there are no *personality changes*. (Italics mine. Did you know that more than your body is involved when you hurt all the time?)

TWO TO SIX MONTHS. This is the *subacute* phase. During this time the patient begins to wonder how long the pain will last, whether he will still have a job at the end of that time and what limitations will be imposed once the pain is gone. He has not yet begun to lose hope, but is irritable and has questions concerning the competence of his doctors.

SIX MONTHS TO EIGHT YEARS. (Don't think that years are not involved here or anyway used to be before Myotherapy. My back pain started when I was thirty and I went down with several "episodes" every year, was often totally incapacitated and sometimes landed in hospitals . . . until 1976, when we finally found Myotherapy. That's a total of forty-one years. President Kennedy hurt his back first in college and then in the South Pacific. He died wearing his brace. His brother Ted injured his back in a plane crash many years ago and still wears his brace.)

This is the chronic stage, during which the patient becomes depressed and has increased anxiety. *The suicide rate doubles.* Problems increase in all aspects of life: job, money, sex, sleep, interests, relationships with family and friends. Pain is the central theme, and everything and everyone must revolve around it.

THREE TO TWELVE YEARS. The subchronic phase. Most patients begin to accept the pain, and personality changes solidify. He or she learns to "function around it."

What does "learning to function around pain" mean to the patient, not necessarily the painless doctor who makes the pronouncement that he *has* learned? I have met three surgeons with back pain. All were good surgeons, none of them could stand up at an operating table to do the work they had studied for so long. One was sent to us three months after having had a disk operation which had not relieved the pain. Had we not been able to erase the muscle spasm, another disk operation was the next try. It took us one hour, and the operation was avoided. The second surgeon had the back pain, but not the operation, yet. One hour and that operation was avoided. The third was older and had been forced by pain to give up a flourishing practice. He had refused flatly to have an operation, preferring to retire. He too was rendered painless. But then there was our pediatrician in the fifties.

This doctor had been a college athlete, a skier after graduating from medical school and a pediatrician by specialization. He had had so many back fusions (five in all) that he walked around like a board and couldn't lift even his smallest patient. He was young, strong, handsome, bright, in constant pain and frustrated off the wall. Each year, he turned a little more sour, and the first to notice (out loud) were the babies, who screamed when he tried to minister to them. Today we could probably get rid of his pain and restore his popularity.

The psychiatrists talk about what happens to the emotions of people *in* pain, but how about the people whose emotions *cause* pain?

There *are* emotional conditions that

cause backache. My husband's backache came on the day he got a long white envelope from the government saying "Greetings." He had never had a backache before and, aside from playing soccer and tennis, falling off a horse two or three times, plus one minor auto crackup, no reason for a backache. The diagnosis was *spondylolisthesis*, a condition in which there is a forward displacement of one vertebra over another, usually involving the fourth and fifth lumbars. He was terrified of war but even more terrified of a knife, so the surgeons were unable to convince him that he needed an operation. He was deferred, of course, but the back spasms continued exactly as long as the war. When it was over, his back ceased to bother him. The spasms subsided and the vertebra slipped back where it belonged. But, if he had had the operation, he might still have the back pain.

I escaped surgery because a doctor I knew and trusted said, "Bonnie, you'll never get a better back than you have, with surgery." That was after one of the top orthopedic surgeons had said, "Well, you have unstable fourth and fifth lumbar vertebrae and sooner or later you will need an operation. You might as well have it now, while you are young." I escaped because I trusted one doctor more than another. I did have to wait until Myotherapy, however, to get rid of my recurrent back pain. So, while both doctors were right according to their own experience, people no longer have to make such a choice. Myotherapy can erase the pain most of the time.

Why am I so all-fired sure most Americans will develop back pain? Because my audiences by the thousands tell me they have back pain, because the greatest number of complaints in all of our clinics are about back pain, and for another reason that brooks no dispute.

In the early fifties, I was in Austria testing one thousand school children with the Kraus-Weber minimum muscular fitness test for key posture muscles (page 131). In those days it didn't even have a name. It had been developed at Columbia Presbyterian Hospital's Posture Clinic, in New York City. It was used for children with posture anomalies. I had borrowed the test some years before to test the children coming into my exercise school, and while using it I had discovered that the average American youngster was in terrible shape: 58 percent of them could not pass a test the doctors who had designed it said any healthy person could pass. Now we had come to Austria to see what European children were like. We had already tested a thousand Italian children and would soon test a thousand Swiss.

The director of the Health Department asked us why we wanted to test his children, and we told him we felt that children who failed to develop at least a minimum of strength and flexibility in key posture muscles (abdominals, psoai, back and hamstrings) would suffer with back pain as adults. In America 58 percent of our children failed to achieve those minimums, and about 60 percent of the adult population had back pain.

"Well then," he said, "if you are right in your thinking, then 10 percent of our children will fail your test, because 10 percent of our adults report back pain." When we had completed our testing we reported to him that indeed, yes, the failure rates were close. The Austrian children had a 9.5 percent failure.

The health director had assigned a young medical student to assist us in the testing; he was horrified when we told him just how many American youngsters failed to pass a test over 90 percent of the children in his country passed with ease. No Austrian child failed two tests, but 32 percent of the Americans had, *and some had failed all six*. "Why? Such a great country. You even won the war. What is wrong?" We told him about our cars, our

school buses, our poor physical education, especially in elementary school,
where it really counts. Even the poorest
school in Austria had *some* kind of gym,
well-trained physical education teachers,
and equipment (not merely balls). As a
medical student, he had been required to
know a great deal about physical education, and in Austria those two words
mean *physical education*, not the bastar-
dized version we have here called games
and sports. In summer he worked at it at
the ''camp'' we were testing. He looked
it too: slender, tanned and fit. It was hard
for him to believe that 91 percent of our
American elementary schools didn't even
have a gym, let alone teachers.

His interest was sparked then, and over
the years while he remained in Austria
he continued to give the test to the children. He found that as the deprivations
of the terrible war years receded, the
children did have higher failure rates, but
not within light-years of ours, which
continued to rise. In 1954, American
children *entering first grade*, *at age six*,
had a 54 percent failure in the minimum
test. The failure matched the year; today
it ranges between 85 percent and 100
percent failure for our little people. Since
physical education has in no way improved, we can only surmise that the
state of older children is now even worse,
since the starting failure rate assures it.
The young medical student doesn't have
to surmise, he has the facts. He finished
medical school and came to America. He
is Dr. Willibald Nagler, chief physiatrist
(physical medicine) at the prestigious
New York Hospital. What has he to say
now that he has been face to face with
the fact of back pain, rather than the pre-
diction? ''Four out of five Americans will
at some time be incapacitated by agonizing pain in their backs.'' That's 80 percent, a rise of 20 percentage points since
the plight of American children was discovered and the President's various
councils formed.

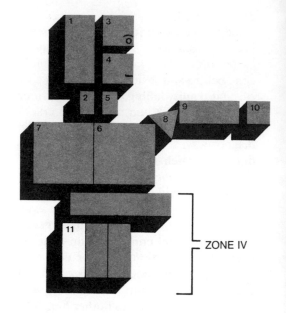

ZONE IV

ZONE IV, SEGMENT 11: THE BACK

Every muscle in the body has its job to
do, and every occupation, sport or way
of life will use those muscles differently
. . . sometimes overusing, sometimes
underusing, and sometimes, as in *substitution*, misusing them. All three ways
that depart from the normal can and often
do cause spasm and pain. Just consider
the posture in which the fetus lies tightly
curled for months before birth. It should
make us wonder whether trigger points
don't take up residence in small backs
even before the birth contractions add
their own share.

Future back pain can begin early, as
can posture anomalies, as any mother
who has a baby born with twisted feet,
torticollis or scoliosis (which usually
doesn't show up till later) will discover.
What is not so well known is that there
is something to do about it.

The quick fix for back pain usually
takes about five minutes, but you have
to remember, a quick fix is successful
mostly on people who can function even

though in pain. Also, it is an emergency measure allowing the sufferer to get through the workday, go dancing on that special evening, drive to the country over the weekend, perform on the stage or in the orchestra, teach in the classroom or make a speech. It is *not* a permanent fix. The pain may be erased temporarily but could return in a short or longer time. A quick fix is for now, not tomorrow. Please understand that the same trigger points that cause low-back pain can also cause upper-back pain, shoulder-girdle pain, stiff neck, sciatica, leg cramps, trick knees and ankles, and even painful feet, not to mention what looks like pain from hiatus hernia, vaginal pain and the pro-verbial pain in the after section. You must know there is no easy way of doing away with all of that, for one very special reason. Every one of those pains is in a muscle that is a two-way street. Whatever structures the lower back can affect are able to turn the tables and affect the lower back. All that means is there's more than one trigger point lurking. Don't think you flunk if you don't find every one of those points the first try.

For a trigger-point search going after low-back pain, we begin in the *gluteals*, the seat muscles. You will need a space where the subject can stretch out at least partially. We *have* used the floor, but aside from the fact that it may not be

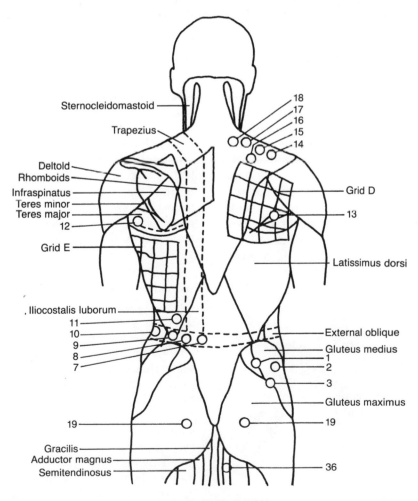

FIG. 9: THE BACK

suitable for lying on (dirty or too public), achieving the right angle with your elbow is very difficult. When we do many backs at a time in a gymnasiumlike setting as part of a Pain-Erasure Clinic^{SM}, we do have the subjects lying in lines on the floor; one *can* do the job there, but then the person doing the work has to be fairly agile, and enough of such strain can easily transfer the back pain from subject to operator. Not a fair exchange.

Look around you and see what is available that will present a hard surface. In the past year I have done backs in bookstores, on the edges of rickety crates and card tables, even in Texas, where the aches come six feet six. Perhaps you will find a low wall, a railing or a piano bench. Ideal of course would be a massage table, but we are not talking *ideal* in quick fix. The right word is adaptability, a quick fix *anywhere*. Most of the time, you can find two chairs.

Have the subject lie across the chairs placed next to each other, with the side you intend to work on *first* toward the chair backs. That is the side that must be supported. The other leg may hang off and the knee may even rest on the floor. Keep about six inches of space between the subject and the chair backs. Check with Figure 9, and you will find circles 1, 2 and 3, where the seat pockets of the blue jeans would be were the subject wearing them. If not, use your imagina-

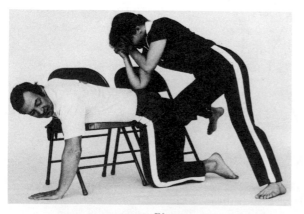

Pain-Erasure Clinic^{SM} is a service mark of Bonnie Prudden, Inc.

tion and *see* those pockets. Then wrap your mind around the following: *While pain may be anywhere in the back, the three major trigger points are in the gluteals, or seat muscles, at three points, labeled 1, 2 and 3*. That's a lot to believe when you have heard all your life (and so has the subject) that a "pinched nerve" is the cause of low-back pain. More of that later.

Next, lean across the body to work on the side *away* from you. In emergency you *could* press in from the near side, but the angle will be wrong and the leverage poor. It's a little like trying to shoot pool while standing on a two-foot box. Place your elbow in the seat pocket at the site of circle 2 and, using the cut-back-under that you learned in the *Technique* section, press down toward the chair seat and then cut back under the muscle toward the median line. In all probability you will catch a villainous trigger point under your elbow your first try. It is to be hoped that you told your subject to tell you what pain was felt on a scale of one to ten. Be sure to ease back a *little* if there is a howl signifying the upper limits of what the subject is willing to stand, and remember, macho bearing of too much pain is counterproductive. It tends to draw other muscles into spasm. Hold for seven seconds and then, *without altering the pressure, move your elbow in all four compass directions*. Hold for the full seven seconds wherever you find a trigger point. Release slowly and move on to circle 1, a little higher and about two inches inward, toward the spine. Note how far away from the spine you are and know that you are not even close to the sacrum, which is a triangular bone formed by the *fusion* of the sacral vertebrae. It has the shape and consistency of a shovel. Certified Bonnie Prudden Myotherapists have no truck with the spine, and although there are disciplines that base their whole work on the spine, we do not. I believe that the spine is like a well-ordered cemetery. There are all those lovely carved stones in a line, each with its name and place. Headstones don't "go" anywhere on their own. Neither do vertebrae. If one day the keeper of the cemetery finds a headstone pulled over on its side, he knows the *stone* didn't do it. A vandal did. Spinal columns have their vandals too, in the form of muscles in spasm, which when activated by trigger points are quite capable of pulling one or more vertebrae out of line. The cemetery keeper knows that if he doesn't get rid of the vandals by whatever means at his disposal, other stones will be pulled over. The certified Bonnie Prudden Myotherapist knows that righting the vertebrae is not the answer. A search for the vandal must be instituted; the trigger point (another word for vandal) must be found and deactivated. Then the headstone/vertebra will nestle happily in its appointed place *unless the vandal returns.* The certified Bonnie Prudden Myotherapist knows, and hopes the backache sufferer can be convinced, that safety from further depredations is assured only by exercise.

Finish the trigger-point work in that area by using the compass on circle 1 and then do the same to circle 3. Be kind to the subject, by using a kneading type of massage to the just-worked-over area. Have your subject get up and face the other way while you repeat this process to the other side. Next comes the vandal-insurance exercise.

Side-Lying Stretch Exercise for the Back

Have the subject lie on his side and draw the top knee up to his chest. You may have to help at first, as many people have no connection with exercise, thinking the word means push-ups or jogging. Then extend the leg straight down above the other leg. Finally, bring the leg to rest *on* the other and count slowly to three. That is to allow the muscles to relax, an-

other word having little meaning for Americans. The word relaxation usually means a weekend in the country or sharing a class in which someone tells them to lie on the floor while they *tell* their muscles to let go, starting at the head and progressing to the toes.

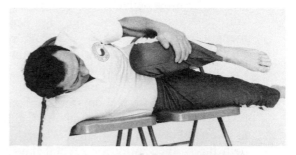

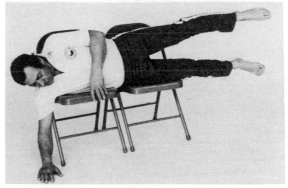

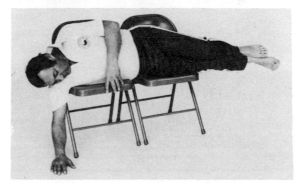

Do four of the side-lying stretches on each side and then ask your subject to sit up and tell you where the pain has moved to. *Don't ask if it is gone. Usually* the subject will put his hands on his back, twist the upper body at the waist and arch a little. Then two things are possible. He will say, "It's gone," usually followed with "I don't believe it." Or "I can't really tell till I stand up.'' So you tell him to stand up and find out where it is *now*. Then two things are possible: "It's gone; I don't believe it.'' Or "There's still a little over here,'' while pointing somewhere else. In the first instance, as in the headache found on the first try, you know where the most active trigger points are, and until you can get the time for permanent fix you can probably control further pain with those spots you just uncovered *if* he will continue with the exercises. The side-lying exercise should be done several times a day for the next few days, always morning and night and as often in between as possible. When the pain has stayed away for several days, cut back to doing them morning and night *forever*. It appears that major trigger points are forever too, and one must always be on guard against them. Whenever the subject has to stand for a long time or walk on cement, as on hospital or factory floors, there is an emergency alternative that can be done almost anywhere. Stand next to a table or desk and place your *right* hand on the surface for support. Pull your bent right knee up to meet your chest as you lean over. Use your *left* hand for this purpose. This increases the oblique pull on the muscles. Then stand straight to *relax*. Alternate four to a side. Lying is better than standing, but the latter is almost always possible. In case the pain did not go away, you have a next step.

Have the subject lie down as before while you check out three circles on either side of the back. One is circle 11, midway between the hipbone and the rib cage, about three inches out from the spine just above the belt line. You will find it on Figure 9. If your subject plays or ever played tennis, golf, basketball or baseball or had a whiplash injury (ever), there will be one or more in that area.

Lean across as before and, placing

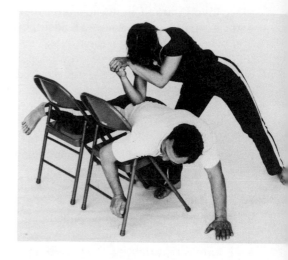

your elbow over circle 11, press down, then cut back to pull in. Hold for the usual seven seconds. While you are there, check out circles 8 and 7 in that order. If you arch your own back, you will find that the muscles running up either side of the spine are very strong, that they bulge and form two sides of the ditch in which the spine lies. You want to find the ridge on each side. Reach across to the outside of the ridge right on the belt line and press down and then toward you for circle 8. For circle 7 you can move your elbow *over* the ridge and press outward into the muscle. It is one of the few times outward pressure can be used. Hold for seven if you find sensitivity. Do a few more side-lying exercises and go through the same questions: "Where is the pain now?'' and so on. By this time you have probably done the best you can with quick fix. You may want to add circle 36, in the back of the upper leg, if your friend has spent the weekend jogging. Check the section on legs for that one. If your friend also has menstrual cramps, you will need to do the groin and abdominal work. Quick fix for the lower back should take no more than five or six minutes. Adding the groin will take another five.

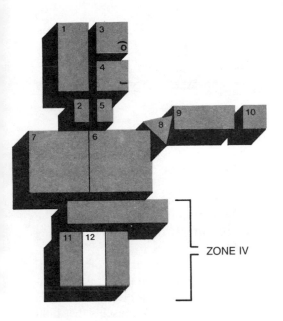

ZONE IV

These trigger points lie just under the outer side seam of your slacks between your waistband and the hem of your briefs. Check with Figure 10.

Have the subject lie on his side facing either way. Place your elbow over circle 5, the circle in the middle. Press down and hold and then execute your compass. Move on to the other two. Do both sides and then have the subject stretch by lying on one side and dropping the top leg down toward the floor in front for a few seconds.

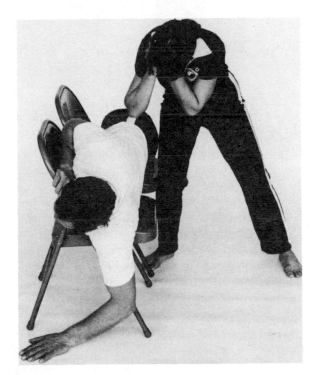

ZONE IV, SEGMENT 12: THE SIDES OF THE PELVIS

The *gluteus medius* stabilizes standing posture, and as most of us do a good deal of standing and mostly on ungiving surfaces, there are apt to be some very sensitive trigger points in that muscle. Any change of direction in sports will use the *gluteus* muscles, and anyone who is overweight is just asking for gluteal trouble.

There are three quick-fix trigger points in this area; if the subject who has already been treated to pressure on circles 1, 2 and 3 still has pain, you may well find the cause under 5, 4 and 6, in that order.

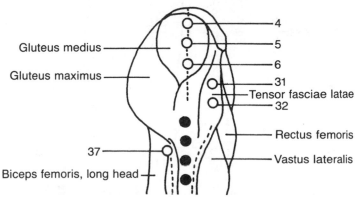

Gluteus medius —
Gluteus maximus —

4
5
6
31
Tensor fasciae latae
32

Rectus femoris

Vastus lateralis

37 —
Biceps femoris, long head —

FIG. 10: PELVIS, SIDE VIEW

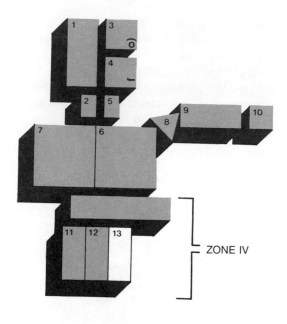

ZONE IV

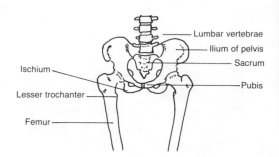

FIG. 11: BONES OF GROIN AND MID-TORSO

ZONE IV, SEGMENT 13: THE GROIN

The groin is the front of the back, just as the gluteal area is the back and sides of the front. No search for *back* pain is complete without a groin check, and the reverse is true: no search for the cause of abdominal pain is complete unless it is followed by the work you have just completed in Segments 11 and 12 in Zone IV.

When people have pain in the abdominal area, they think the same way as the headache sufferer thinks: "What's going on *inside*?"

Sometimes something *is* going on inside, but many more times, as with menstrual cramps, for example, something is going on *outside*, in the muscles that hold the insides inside. If you are one of those who must give up at least twelve days a year to such cramps, and for some the cost can run as high as thirty-six days a year, here is some good news. Such cramps are often caused by trigger points in the *abdominal muscles*, aided and abetted of course by trigger points in the *gluteals*. This is true also of the conditions labeled spastic colon and nervous stomach. Something else few have suspected: abdominal spasm pulls on the groin, which is adjacent to the thigh mus-

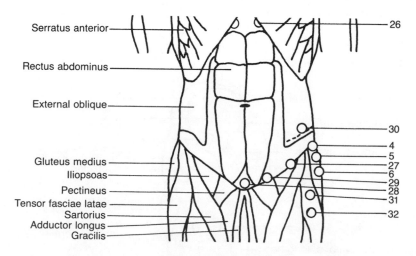

FIG. 12: ABDOMEN AND GROIN

cles, and the two affect each other to pull runners up lame. Even more ominous is the fact that the floor of the pelvis connects the front with the back, and a lot of structures important to health and happiness are in the floor of the pelvis.

The groin is another place where you can work both sides of the body from one position; you can start with circle 30 on the near side. Easiest for both subject and operator would be a supine position on a table, but pain is not that accommodating, and although abdominal cramping could start at home, it is just as likely to start in the office or the classroom or on the athletic field. Again, use what you have around, and what's around is usually a couple of chairs. Have the subject lie supine over two chairs (three would be more comfortable).

Look first at the bones of the pelvis in Figure 11, and note the *ilium*, the rim of the pelvis, where it juts forward to form the hipbone before it descends to the *pubis*. That point is known as the *iliac crest*. The abdominals tie into the pelvic structure, and very often you will find troublesome trigger points at the attachment where the tie-in is made. The athlete, dancer or heavy worker will lay in a supply through activity. The sedentary person will collect them because the muscles are too weak to handle everyday living without undue strain.

Place the fingers of both hands on the *iliac crest*, and using the wraparound you learned in the *Technique* section, push the skin over the edge and into the pelvic basin. Trap the trigger points by pulling back against the bone. Hold for the usual seven seconds, and without lessening the pressure use your compass left and right. There is room on the crest for two or sometimes three spots where trigger points might hide. Find everything you can.

To reach the area on the other side, stretch across the abdomen and place your fingers flat along the outside of the pelvis and your *thumbs* on the *iliac crest*.

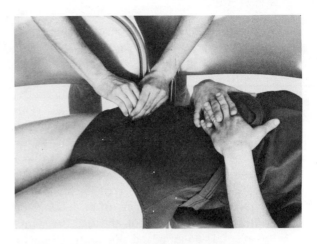

Push into the pelvis and wrap around as you did on the near side and hold for seven. Use the compass and be sure to clear any resident trigger points. If you miss one, you may be a smashing success right away but have your success marred by a return of the cramps later in the day.

The next target is the *symphysis pubis*, that spot where the pelvic bones come together at the base of the groin, the lower attachment for the abdominals. *Symphysis* denotes a cartilaginous joint in which the apposed bony surfaces are firmly united. For what it's worth, this is one of the most sensitive spots the trigger-point hunter has to contend with. *Always* found in women who have had babies and almost always found in athletes, truck drivers and others who sustain groin strain through physical activity whether it be work or play. All the people we have seen with arthritic hips have them, as do dancers and gymnasts.

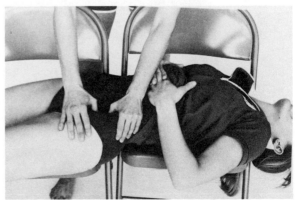

Check first with Figure 11, noting the *symphysis pubis*, where the bones are joined at the cartilaginous joint, and then with circle 28 on Figure 12. Place your elbow in the exact center of circle 28, where the bones come together. This "bridge" is not very wide, so try not to slip off to either side. Use a very gentle pressure and keep a watchful eye on your subject for signs of distress. After erasing the trigger point on top of the *symphysis pubis*, place the fingers of both hands on top of the same spot and use the wrap-around, pushing the skin into the pelvic basin and pulling back against the bone. Use the same technique for circles 29, which are on the same line but about one inch farther out on both sides.

Circle 27 has to do with the *iliopsoas*, a compound muscle made up of the *iliacus* and the *psoas*. Most people have never heard of it. The *iliopsoas* has its upper attachment in the lumbar vertebrae, which is an enormously important bit of information if you are looking for "vandals" that pull headstones out of line. It attaches to the lesser trochanter, in the leg (see Figure 11). The *iliopsoas* plays a considerable part in low-back pain, especially for those who were taught in school or the armed forces to do straight-leg sit-ups. When the legs are extended, the sit-ups are executed with a great deal of help from the *iliopsoas*, which uses the spine as the anchor against which to pull. Check with Figure 12 and note the size of the muscle, the little you can see, and try to imagine what it can do to the spine and therefore your entire back. If the knees are bent, the muscle is collapsed and cannot pull against the lumbar spine. This not only protects the back but forces the abdominals to do the work for which they were intended. We are *still* hearing of male P.E. teachers who flunk students who refuse to endanger their backs with straight-leg sit-ups.

Place your elbow on circle 27 and press straight down. You will have to take your cues from the subject, so be attentive to expression. With the pressure steady, use a very slow compass to locate the most sensitive spot, then hold for seven seconds.

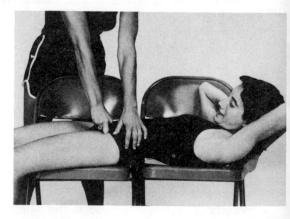

Groin Stretch

When you have checked out the seven points in the groin, you will want to use the stretch. Have the subject lie supine with the near leg bent. Pull the leg back to stretch the groin muscles. If the subject is very tight, just letting the leg hang off the chair or a table will be enough. Pull back or press the leg down, depending on the flexibility, in *gentle*, easy bounces to a rhythm, and then relax. Do three to a side.

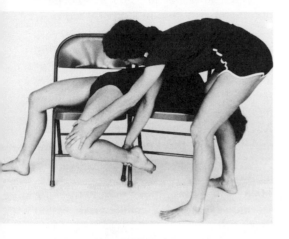

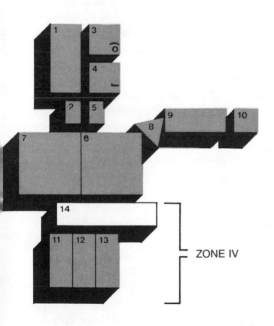

ZONE IV, SEGMENT 14: THE ABDOMINALS

When you checked out the groin for the cause of pain, you worked on the lower attachments of the abdominals in the pubic area and on the iliac crests. Now you need the upper attachments, cartilages of the ribs and the *xiphoid process*. This last is the little sword-shaped bone at the end of the sternum. It is the point known more popularly as the *solar plexus* (see Figure 46, on page 188).

Employ the wraparound technique you learned on yourself. Place your fingers *on* the edges of the ribs and press the skin over and up *under* the ribs. Don't be afraid. There is nothing frightening in there. Start at the *xiphoid process* and work outward along the arch of the ribs to the side where the rib cage starts curving .back. Use the one-inch-interval gauge. Do both sides.

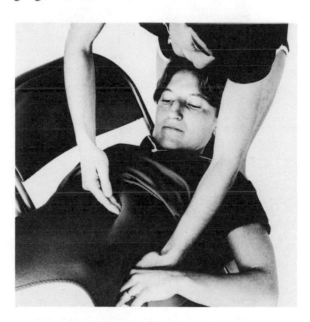

Abdominal Stretch

To stretch the abdominals, use the same position as in the groin stretch, but put a pillow under the hips. Stretch the leg back if the subject is flexible enough, and have her take five slow deep breaths into her *chest*. No abdominal breathing at this moment. Have her reverse her position on the chairs so the other leg is over the side and repeat.

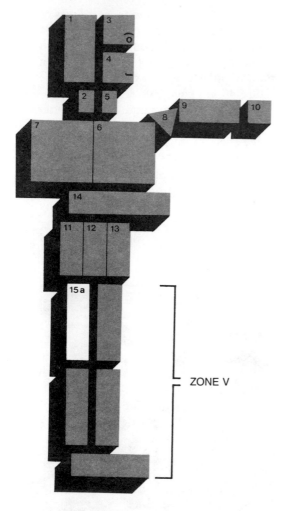

ZONE V

ZONE V, SEGMENT 15A: UPPER LEG, POSTERIOR VIEW

Few people appreciate their legs until for one reason or another they are denied their cooperation. Very few know about the delights legs *could* provide. Still fewer know anything about their intricate workings. Lastly, almost nobody knows about the care and feeding of legs, the preservation of legs, or that *legs* make a difference when it comes to the heart, lungs and *brain*.

We are still hugging the cardiovascular craze called "aerobics," in the name of which we have ruined millions of legs and through them millions of backs; also, contrary to expectation, reduced the aid needed by hearts in the form of auxiliary

pumps—a job for which *healthy* legs were designed. Using the fear of death by heart attack plus the American penchant for following anyone with a loud mouth and connections with Madison Avenue, uninformed and misinformed people have put an entire nation in jeopardy *via their legs*.

If you ask most Americans to describe a leg you will be told, "It is a means of locomotion." Right, but that's no description. "The leg is a long appendage that attaches to the body at the hip joint." And then? "It has another joint in the middle called the knee and one at the bottom called the ankle." All that is perfectly correct, but there must be more. Then will come the usual scratching around, eyes turned ceilingward, which to me means, "I wonder what she wants to hear?" It rarely means, "What do *I* know about this subject?" That's the way we raise students. Some will be able to add, "It has two bones in the lower leg and one in the upper. . . ." But most people have never really thought about it. Some may even know that there is such a thing as a *sciatic nerve*, which, when "pinched," affects the leg. Others may have the words *Achilles* and *quads* in their lexicons, but most of those are varsity. Some people speak of calf muscles, but few are on a first-name or any-name basis with any muscles, and although jogging has been with us for several years, few are interested in *what makes Sammy run*. They don't even really know what makes Sammy stop running either, even when they *are* Sammy, or Samantha. It's time we all looked into it.

Once upon a time America was an isolationist country. We felt (or our leaders felt) we didn't need to cooperate with anybody. Let Europe and everybody else destroy each other and themselves, they couldn't touch us. But they could and they did, and we began to find out how interdependent the world really is. And that was *before* the atomic bomb.

Then, too, like unseeing children, we overlooked the fact that there actually are a balance and interdependence in nature, so we destroyed our forests and the land blew away. We were surprised. Until very recently we didn't have the slightest idea that the parts of the human body are in *any* way interdependent, let alone *totally*. Doctors treated ankles and never wondered about the feet under them or the knees above. Psychiatrists treated minds and ignored the body entirely (as well as their own bodies). Only now are we beginning to see that if you damage a foot, the leg will suffer. Damage the leg (an auxiliary pump for the heart everyone seems so interested in saving) and the heart will suffer. Damage the heart and the brain will suffer. Treat all with consideration and respect and nothing needs to suffer.

The legs are profoundly affected by conditions in the pelvis, just as the reverse is true. Sciatic pain starts in the pelvic region as a rule, but the pain associated with hemorrhoids often appears after a long period of standing.

Before we start work on the all-important legs, there is some imagery that should be cleared up, if not out. For a long time we have been told (for sure, the average citizen didn't make it up) that back pain and sciatica (a pain that runs from the back down the legs) was caused by a "pinched nerve." *Pinched is the wrong word.* It scares folks to be told *something is pinching a nerve.* They imagine the poor suffering nerve being ground between the edges of two ragged bones and gradually fraying to pieces like an electric wire between two granite millstones. Since their education has not taught them otherwise, they fall prey to misinformation.

Nerves are rarely *pinched*, they are *squeezed.* When a muscle is thrown into spasm by a trigger point reacting to stress of some kind, the nerve traveling through it is apt to be squeezed in the spasm. It is much like the tail of a small dog that

has gotten caught in a crack. The tail (the nerve) will hurt where it is squeezed, but in addition the bark or the bite (referred pain) will be accomplished by the other end. The grab on the sciatic nerve, which stretches down through the legs, can refer pain all the way down through the ankle and foot to the toes. Such a *squeeze* can cause pain, tingling, numbness and even weakness anywhere along the way. *If the pain is in the leg but the nerve is being squeezed in the seat or thigh*, applications of ice, cortisone shots, taping, elevation, a cast, crutches and admonishments to "stay off of it" can hardly be counted on to get rid of the pain. Nor will arch supports, orthotics, special shoes, wedges and drugs. Giving up the sport that precipitated it isn't the answer either. The problem may go to sleep for a while, but it won't go away, and one day something as unathletic as walking to the mailbox could reactivate the resident trigger points in the *gluteals*, and there the pain is again. There *is* an answer, however: erase any trigger points you can find and reeducate the muscles with the right exercises.

Anytime anyone reports low-back, groin or knee pain, the muscles of the legs should be held suspect . . . especially the muscles in the backs of the thighs (Figure 13). Just knowing that the sciatic nerve runs down the middle of the back of the leg should warn you. When it reaches the mid-thigh, it splits into the *tibial nerve* and the *common peroneal nerve*, and both divisions proceed on down carrying whatever messages they have picked up along the way.

Have the subject lie prone over two chairs or, in this instance, the office files. For the quick fix, start at circle 36. Circle 36 is the start of the most troublesome line in the back of the upper leg. The *adductor magnus* appears to start at that point, but if we could lift away the huge *gluteus maximus*, we would see that the *adductor magnus* reaches right up into the pelvis and ties into the *ischium* and

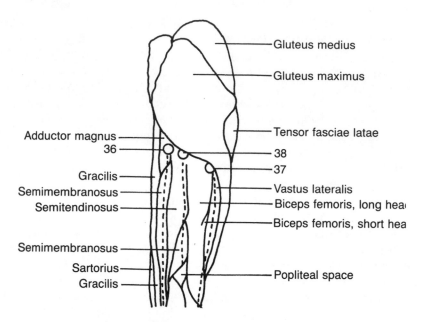

FIG. 13: UPPER LEG, POSTERIOR VIEW

the *pubis*. Athletes and dancers who suffer from dysmenorrhea may now understand why, just prior to menstruation and during the first day, it may feel as though the bottom is about to fall out. The overworked *adductor* muscles, often nests of latent if not active trigger points, could well be the cause. A thorough check of the pelvic muscles and also of the trigger-point-loaded legs could most probably prevent loss of performance, rehearsal, practice and competition time. Indeed, in addition, this precaution might well improve performance and endurance.

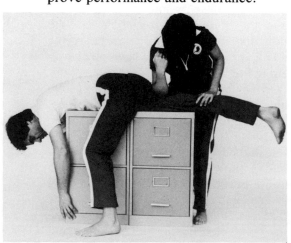

The line starting at circle 36 runs down the inner aspect of the leg on the *semimembranosus* and between the *semitendinosus* and the *gracilis*. The *semimembranosus* runs from the *ischium* to the *tibia*, the larger of the two bones in the lower leg. That should tell you that trouble even in the lower leg can easily refer pain up to the groin and lower back. The *semitendinosus* also attaches to the *ischium* and the *tibia*, with the same potential for troublemaking. *And both cross the knee joint.* As you can see, they are both large, powerful muscles; the larger and more powerful the greater the potential for harm, as strong muscles are very good at substitution. The *gracilis* attaches to the *pubis* and the *tibia* and is not to be forgotten when it comes to abdominal cramps, menstrual cramps, spastic colon, nervous stomach and the pain connected with hemorrhoids, or even a "trick knee."

Reach across the leg just below the buttock and try to feel your way *between* the muscles. Once you are set, press down and then pull toward you. Use part of the compass, the east and west directions, *across* the leg. The worst trigger point is usually about three inches down from the start, and it is always at least latent in the legs of athletes and dancers, who are athletes par excellence.

In quick fix for back pain, we check that one line only. Of course, if you are doing work on the legs for anything from arthritis of the knees to a pulled hamstring or even "heel spurs" (bony growths), you would be more thorough. See *Permanent Fix*.

Flexibility Bounce for Back and Hamstring Stretch

The stretch exercise for the backs of the thighs, lower legs and back is a combination exercise which follows after your trigger-point work has warmed the muscles. It is also done as a regular exercise after warm up or at the end of the warm-up series. This is a series of *gentle* bounces. Start with feet well apart and hands clasped behind your back, lean forward from the hips *with your head up*. Bounce the upper body down eight times. As long as your head is *up* you will feel the pull just behind the knees, in the *hamstrings*. Turn the upper body to the right as you bounce for eight and you will feel the pull on the inner aspect of the thigh near the attachments. Do eight to the left. Those three directions make up *one set*.

Next, let the upper body fall forward from the hips. Allow the head and arms to drop down, totally relaxed, for eight bounces. Do the same movement for eight to each side. This makes up one set for the back. After a trigger-point job on the backs of the legs, do three sets, but try to remember to do one set of each *every* time you go into your bathroom after some waist-twist exercises (see the *Self Center* section).

This is as good a place as any to talk about another fad: stretch. There is no question that stretch is important, since strength *plus* flexibility in the proper tim-

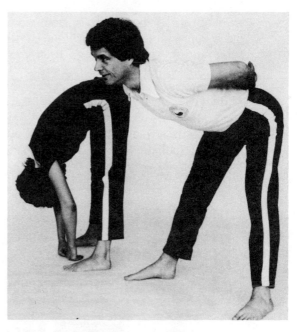

ing and intensity yield coordination. The question is *when* to stretch and *how* to stretch. Heaven knows that in America there is little enough solid information, but about stretch there is both myth and plain dangerous direction.

The first thing to remember is that when you really stretch for anything other than a test like the minimum muscular fitness test, on page 131, you warm up first. Trigger-point work warms muscles, as once the spasm is relaxed the circulation and therefore warmth improve markedly. Still, any stretching done following Myotherapy is very mild indeed. A warm muscle is 20 percent more efficient and has 20 percent more protection against injury. Hard stretching of cold muscle increases the chance for injury to at least a few fibers. If you are emotionally tense you may well injure more. *Do your serious stretching at the end of your exercise session,* whatever it is.

Next, right now there are two forms of stretch in America: *ballistic stretch,* which means gentle bouncing, usually to rhythm and preferably to music . . . and *static stretch.* In the latter you assume the stretch position and stretch the muscle as far as it will go and hold the stretch from twenty to sixty seconds. Both work, but if you want to know which one is both safer and more efficient, go to a good dance class, where ballistic stretch is used, and note the ease and extent of the stretch. Then go to a gym class where static stretch is used and note the difference. Static stretch sets up its own opposition; ballistic stretch bypasses the opposition.

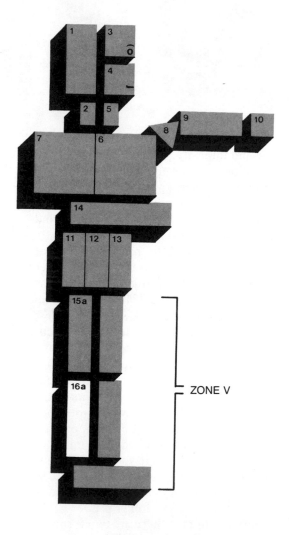

ZONE V, SEGMENT 16A: LOWER LEG, POSTERIOR VIEW

The lower leg *seems* to be far removed from the lower back, but if you realize that if you were a runner your heel would strike the ungiving cement surface of the road about a thousand times every mile of the way and that heel would be catching the equivalent of between two and three times your own weight with every strike . . . that would give you a different idea. Multiply your weight by three and that by a thousand foot strikes per mile and you will have a good idea as to what that one leg is absorbing. Three times the weight of an average man of 175 pounds would be 525 pounds on each foot. That times a thousand strikes is 525,000 pounds *on one foot per mile*. Now push that up to a "fun run" of six miles and you begin to understand about injuries. True, there is a tribe of Mexican Indians whose members can run up to a hundred miles a day, racking up over thirty million pounds per leg per run, but those men are not running on cement *and* they have been running all their lives.

If you are a 125-pound woman, the kind the physical educators branded as a weakling, unable to do an honest-to-god pushup a decade ago, you will hit that pavement to the tune of two and a quarter million pounds during your "fun run." If, God forbid, you are using running to lose weight because you really *are* overweight, you may be catching two and a quarter million pounds with a frame built to take, *safely*, far less.

Add to the above that heels refer pounding to the *tibia*, which is the long bone in the lower leg making up a part of the knee, and that the *tibia* and the knee refer the pounding to the great bone in the thigh, the *femur*, which is also a part of the knee, which refers to the hip joint in the pelvis, which refers to the spine, and that a great many runners believed the "expert" who told them to run on their heels. Add that all up and you have a nightmare on your hands. Just wait ten years.

Nor do you have to go to extremes; just try something as unathletic as the profession of nursing. Those shining halls in hospitals provide exactly the same ungiving surface as does the cement highway, because under the gleaming tile there is road-surface cement. Clock the miles covered by the nurse as she goes her rounds in the hospital, or the supermarket (same surface), or while she takes her "aerobic" dance class (same surface), or stands at the nurse's station, in the pharmacy or next to the patient's bed, and you have the same resistance to leg muscles and bones. There are miles of corridors and hours of standing, all on cement. And she doesn't even have the questionable advantage of orthotics—those expensive inserts supposed to improve gait—and running shoes. If she is overweight she is in double jeopardy. And how about her boss, the surgeon? He too stands on cement under tile in the operating room, and the same in his patients' rooms and the hospital corridors. He stands on cement if he goes to the Sports Medicine Center for his bum knee, on cement at the weight-training center, and he runs on cement if he jogs.

There are usually five reasons for doing a quick fix on the lower leg. The most prevalent is the *calf cramp*, and the second is called a "*shin splint*," which is actually a cramp in the front of the *tibialis anterior*, the muscle running down the front of the leg toward the outside. The third reason is a deep ache anywhere in the lower leg (often attributed to varicose veins and treated with elastic stockings).

The fourth is a sprained ankle. There is a fifth, but it is usually accepted as a heel spur. That is to say, it hurts in the foot and would be called a foot problem. But most of the time the *cause* is in the calf, a muscle in spasm pulling on the heel. A typical example of the little dog with his tail *squeezed* in a crack. His bite on the heel has ruined athletic careers. Daytime spasms in the legs usually occur after some form of athletic endeavor and, like low back attack, often show up on Monday morning after either a physically or sexually active weekend. The latter is, after all, very physical and very active, or should be. Heel spurs are *usually* associated with running but can easily accompany a condition called "The Classic Greek Foot," so named by Dr. Janet Travell, who has enormous powers of observation and a most unusual talent: the ability to put two and two together. It is also called Morton's Toe or "LST," for long second toe. Dr. Morton has written in his book about it and Dr. Travell observed that *all* the marvelous Greek statues of incredibly beautiful Greek models had such a toe.

Then there is the deep ache that usually occurs in legs forced by occupation to stand for many hours each day on hard surfaces. It is often attributed to varicose veins. Nighttime calf spasms, a frequent complaint of the elderly, usually follow the deep ache phase, probably years later.

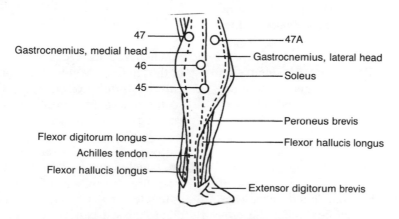

FIG. 14: LOWER LEG, POSTERIOR VIEW

There is one other complaint concerning the lower leg, and it deserves a separate section, not because it more often concerns the ankle and the foot than the lower leg, but because it bears with it a danger: surgery. The condition is called "tarsal tunnel syndrome."

Tarsal tunnel syndrome is a name that is fairly new, and while the condition is said to be "once rare," it is being diagnosed ever more often today. The symptoms presented are, of course, pain and also burning. It is said to be caused by *nerve compression or entrapment of the posterior tibial nerve as it passes along the inside of the ankle through the bony, unyielding tarsal tunnel on the bottom of the foot. The tunnel is formed by several of the bones of the foot and by a layer of tough fibrous tissue. The neurovascular bundle containing the posterior tibial nerve and blood vessels pass through this tunnel en route to the distal part of the foot. Swelling from repeated trauma causes the pain.*

This sounds like the little dog to me, and in our experience the crack *squeezing* his tail is *not* in the tarsal tunnel, but higher up, usually in the calf muscles.

Treatment varies depending on the doctor's training. It usually starts with rest and ice, and for the elderly, medication. For the elderly, almost *always* medication. While these may work while the leg is at rest, the pain usually returns when the leg is stressed again. That kind of treatment, which is palliative, does nothing about the cause: the trigger points. Those remain as before, either active or on silent alert. Provided with the slightest encouragement from an ungiving floor or road, they will return to attack.

For quick fix of the lower leg we are concerned with two lines. They are the mid-line, which bisects the *gastrocnemius*, the observable bunch muscle at mid-calf, and the inside line over the edge of the *soleus*, which lies under the *gastrocnemius* (called "gastrocs" for short).

The *soleus* is a stranger to just about everyone, including the average trainer, coach or doctor. However, the *soleus* is more than *a* key in lower-leg pain, it is *the* key.

Have the subject lie over two chairs, the filing cabinets, the side of a desk or any available surface that will support him. Place your elbow on circle 45 and press straight down, and if the subject registers pain, hold for seven seconds and then execute a compass. Move down the leg to the heel at one-inch intervals. Then, starting an inch above circle 45, move up the leg at one-inch intervals to the *popliteal* (back of the knee). Runners will squirm the whole way. When you reach the Achilles tendon on your way down to the heel, use your knuckle or a bodo laid sideways across the tendon. Elbows slip. Most people don't have many trigger points *on* the *Achilles*, but wait till you get to the usually ignored *soleus*!

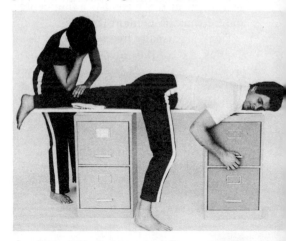

When you have covered the mid-line of the leg from heel to knee, use the *calf muscle stretch exercise*: Bend the knee so the heel approaches the buttocks as you press *down* on the ball of the foot. Few heels will make contact with the buttocks as a well-stretched leg should do, which should tell you that there are other trigger points marring the efficiency of that leg. You already know that trigger points missed can excite and reactivate those you found and erased, so while you may be able to make your subject pain free for the moment, you should arrange another session for permanent fix. If the subject is an athlete, an exercise program should be designed and every effort made to provide a "seeking massage" (see page 229) before competition.

As you press down on the ball of the foot and bend the knee, do so in short, *easy* bounces to avoid causing the spasm that could follow static stretch when it is applied to a less than healthy muscle. After about three bounces, release. Do this four times, then ask the subject to stand and place both feet close together. Flexing the knees in *easy* bounces five or six times is the solo way of stretching the calf muscles. Your subject should do them at intervals all day long, starting in the shower in the morning. Now you need to look at the *soleus*.

Even if the calf pain was gone after the above, don't overlook it. With your subject again on the working surface, check the inner line on the back of the leg.

The *soleus*, the mystery muscle, is even more important than the *gastrocnemius*, since it seems to cause even more pain but is rarely recognized as being of any importance at all. In addition, more and other trouble is overlooked through ignorance of the *soleus* and its environs. On the inner side of the back of the leg, lying under the edge of

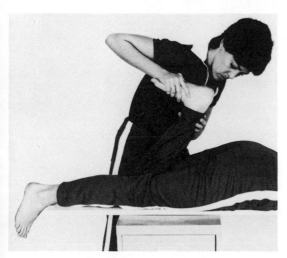

the *soleus,* is the *flexor digitorum longus*, which attaches to the *distal phalanges* of the four outside toes, which it flexes. Its other job is to extend the foot. You don't go anywhere limpless without help from that muscle. And you don't walk, run or jump on cement for any length of time without injuring it. Now let's see how badly.

Have your subject roll a little to the outside, thus exposing the inner edge of the *soleus* (circle 47). Bad as the gastrocs may have been, the *soleus* will be worse, so be gentle. Start down the line at one-inch intervals right into the ankle, following the initial pressure with your compass.

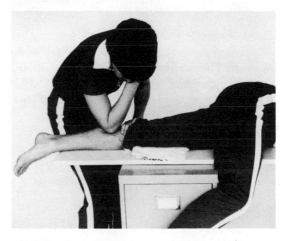

The soleus stretch exercise requires a knee bend as for the heel-cord stretch exercise, but this time turn the foot outward as you press down on the ball of the foot. Do four stretch-and-releases and then have the subject stand, flex the knee a few times and walk around. The pain will probably be gone. If it isn't, run down the outside line of the back of the leg on Figure 14. Start at circle 47A. The stretch for that line is done with the foot turned inward.

Such a quick fix done on each and every member of the Friday Night Bridge Club at the Senior Center, would guarantee sleep undisturbed by leg cramps and, in addition, remove the necessity for adding one more "just in case" medi-

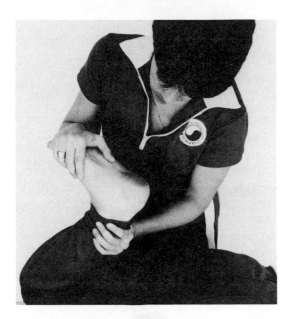

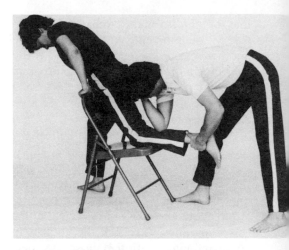

cation someone could do very well with-out. Those elderly friends of yours should be thinking as Suzanne Arms suggests in her book *Immaculate Deception* that "just in case" medicine isn't for me, I won't take it. Naturally that doesn't go for really needed medication, but, rather, those taken as prevention for something you *might* get at some future date. *If* you get the condition, that's time enough to take the medication. You may never be so favored. Remember my fourth and fifth lumbar vertebrae that "would some day need an operation, so why not now, while you are young?" Why not indeed?

I never needed it, not then or now. If you take out your trigger points and do your exercises, chances are you won't ever need such medication. If those elderly friends of yours won't pay attention for their health and their life's sakes, try this one on them. Medication often has a way of making the skin look like it was de-signed for an alligator with hives.

If it is impossible to find a surface where the subject can lie prone, you *can* do a quick fix with her kneeling on a chair. Place the knee toward the forward edge of the seat and the groin pressed against the back of the chair as you hold the ankle for support. It isn't too com-fortable and your work may be hampered a little if the seat gets in your way, but it does work and it can be done almost anywhere.

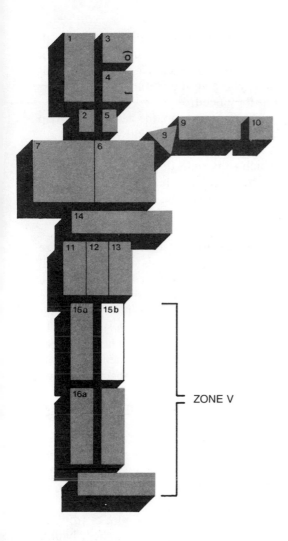

ZONE V

ZONE V, SEGMENT 15B: UPPER LEG, ANTERIOR VIEW

By this time you know that, yes, the fronts of the thighs may well have something to do with low-back pain and groin pain as well as pain in the thigh itself and the knee.

Only in the past few years have doctors, trainers and coaches found this out. Now of course, after racking up the backs of several generations of athletes with straight-leg sit-ups, bent-knee sit-ups have finally been accepted. Keep this in mind when *anyone* suggests you do *anything* that strains you *anywhere*.

The *pectineus* runs from the *femur* to the *pubis*. Most people have heard the

word sacroiliac in connection with back pain. But who ever heard the word *pubis* with back pain? It is a word mainly used by Ob-Gyn men when discussing "women's troubles." Men have pubic bones too, and many are injured during work or sport. It is called "groin pain."

The *adductor longus* also runs from the *pubis* to the *femur*, and it too contributes to groin pain. An elbow applied to the groin will send pins and needles to the *adductor*.

The *vastus medialis* is another knee-killer/groin-grabber. It runs from the *patella* up the *femur* and ties in at the pelvis. It is one of the two *main* concerns in knee pain, the other being the *vastus lateralis*.

The *gracilis* runs all the way up from the *tibia* to the *pubis*. If you check that one out and understand that while many cases of impotence and frigidity are due to spasm in the pelvic-floor muscles, the *gracilis* too takes part and must be cleared. That goes for the pain attributed to hemorrhoids, vaginal pain, anal spasm and the need to sit on a doughnut pillow. One more thing: the word "frigidity" is a poor appellation when used for sexual disorders in women. It implies an "I don't want to" attitude, which of course is the case sometimes, often with good reason.

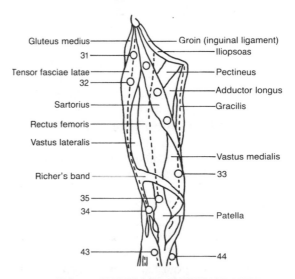

FIG. 15: UPPER LEG, ANTERIOR VIEW

But the word also implies a cold nature or a cold something, and that may be far from the truth. No psychiatrist is ever going to be able to clear up the "frigidity" in a woman who has a spastic vagina due not to her mother's early training but to a fall on the ice at age twelve.

The *sartorius*, the longest muscle in the body, runs from the *tibia*, or shinbone, below the knee, up to the *ilium*, in the pelvis. It is quite capable of pulling upward on the inside of the leg, thus throwing the knee out of kilter. Running on a leg that is out of balance will bring on pain quickly; walking on it will take longer, but longer isn't forever.

The *tensor fasciae latae* is a band running down the leg from the *ilium* to the *tibia*. It is the *iliotibial tract*, under which lies the all-important *vastus lateralis*. Pressing on the band and trapping the trigger points put into the side of the leg by participation in sports, involvement in accidents or sometimes a simple turning motion, can bring on some of the most exquisite pain around. The *vastus lateralis* runs up from the *patella* (kneecap) to the hip joint and the side of the *femur* (the thighbone). It was spasm in this muscle and the *rectus femoris*, in the front of the thigh, that made my first total hip replacement necessary, eleven years before we discovered Myotherapy.

The *rectus femoris* starts at the *acetabulum* (the bony cup that holds the ball of the hip joint) and the front of the *ilium*. It runs down to the *patella* and the *tibia*. Nor are we finished with the front of the thigh, which looks so trouble free in a bikini. Check with Figure 15 and note the *iliopsoas*, a compound muscle. The *iliac* part starts in the *ilium* and attaches to the *lesser trochanter*, part of the thighbone. It also takes in the *sacrum*, at the back of the pelvis. The *psoas* part starts in the *lumbar vertebrae* and runs to the *lesser trochanter*. Sound complicated? Think of it this way: When you do a straight-leg sit-up with your hands behind your head, you pull unmercifully on the *lumbar vertebrae*. If you bend your knees, you collapse that compound muscle, making it impossible to strain your back. In addition, you give the abdominals the workout they need.

The *femoris* bears the name for a group of *four* muscles called the *femoris quadriceps*: other than the *rectus femoris*, which runs right down the center of the thigh, there are the *vastus lateralis*, on the outer front and side of the leg, the *vastus intermedialis*, in the middle under the *rectus femoris*, and the *vastus medialis,* toward the inner side. They are referred to by athletes as "*the quads.*" The *quads* are the four horsemen of the knee for athletes; they account for more operations and misery than any other group of muscles, even those in the back. But they aren't innocent when it comes to the average person either. And it is trouble in one or more of them that often causes the problem called "growing pains," Osgood-Schlatter's disease, chondromalacia patellae and arthritis. All in the knee. A good many injuries labeled ligament tears are really the sins of the *quads*, and it is they that are contributing to the current flurry about the operation called arthroscopy.

The *quads* may cause a lot of trouble, but that is because we use them badly, overuse them, often underuse them and do not understand the connection between them and the long second toe. They are (as all muscles) very important, but these are more than just very important, they are indispensable. You can't climb up or down stairs without them, but now when you can't, at least you know where to start to make things right. If the *quads* are weak, you will have the devil's own time getting into or out of chairs, into and out of cars, and you will look old even if you aren't. There is an element in our society (it was never absent but sometimes, in history, controlled) that preys on weak, ill or damaged elderly people. These conditions show up first in the walk. But I know an elderly lady, well over sixty-five, who does one thousand *deep* knee bends a day, every day. She wears "sensible" rubber-soled, laced shoes. They look like ordinary shoes, but the toe boxes are weighted and of steel. So is part of the heel. She takes karate lessons twice a week, rides her stationary bike ten miles a day and uses weight bags for her exercises. I wonder what will happen to some unsuspecting piece of lawless element who believes what the government says about oldsters: that they are helpless.

The groin is the upper reach of the front of the thigh, and the knee is the bottom, and the work for the thigh muscles and the knee is the same. Why? Because spasm in any *one* of those muscles pulls at *both* ends, and those are the ends. Notice that the upper ends of all the muscles attach variously to the *hip joint*, the *ilium*, the *femur* and the *acetabulum* . . . but all four converge on the knee through the common tendon attaching to the *patella*.

For a quick fix of the front of the thigh, start with the *rectus femoris*. Look at circle 35 on Figure 15, just above the kneecap (*patella*), and reaching over the near leg, place your elbow in the center of the thigh of the far leg. Stabilize yourself by laying your free arm across the pelvis, with your hand over the hipbone. When you have pressed straight in, do your north and south compass moves, stopping for seven seconds if you locate any trigger points. Then do the east-west parts of the compass, and as you come to each edge, try to get your elbow in under the edge of the muscle. You may find that you can do the inner edge of the *rectus femoris* with more control if you attack from the other side of the body. In any case, advance to the groin at one-inch intervals.

The knee is called an inefficiently designed joint, but actually it can be very efficient if it is properly exercised in early childhood. By that we mean encouraged to walk everywhere, play out of doors, run, skip, hop, jump and climb hills and

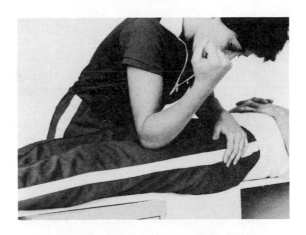

stairs. It is important to run on uneven ground and especially downhill. Packs should be carried on little shoulders. Little packs with light loads carried on *both* shoulders, with the weight evenly distributed, are right for a starter. As strength improves, add a little weight at a time.

It isn't the joint that is at fault, it is our way of life and our sports plus our way of handling those sports in relation to preparing for them. Our way of life is soft from start to finish, and we put soft bodies into sports like football, gymnastics, basketball . . . I can hear you now. *Soft!* Those guys! Everything is relative, and the knee isn't up to that kind of work and I'm not sure *any* human knee is for football. Of them all, of course, football is the worst because of "leverage." When a leg lies prone across a huge lump of muscle in a pileup and two hundred pounds of muscle and bone lands on the lower half, the knee has had it. It may recover, but it can never be the same again. In basketball it is usually a rotation that does the job. The rubber-soled shoe stays put and the body rotates around it much as in skiing when the ski goes into heavy snow called "mashed potatoes" and the body, unhampered, completes the turn. Suffice it to say here that Myotherapy works most of the time for chronic knee pain and for the knee pains we have already mentioned, and very well for strains and sprains as described in "Immediate Mobilization and Myotherapy," page 231.

When you were a little kid there was always some neighbor kid who was bigger than you, or even a favorite uncle who would grab your knee and squeeze hard, grinning and saying, "Horse bite!" You jumped sky-high and then went around the neighborhood to find a littler kid to "horse-bite." Those two points, the thumb on one side and the fingers on the other side, are the start of the lines for the *vastus lateralis* and the *vastus medialis*.

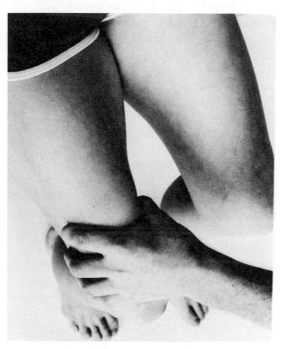

Vastus Lateralis

Have your subject lie on his side on a flat surface, in this instance a bookshelf laid over two filing cabinets, but two chairs would do. If you can find a jacket or a cushion, thrust it between the subject's knees for stability. If not, bend the top knee slightly. Start at the "horse-bite" spot, on the outside of the leg just above the knee, and on the outside seam of his trousers and circle 34 on Figure 15. Go up the leg at two-inch intervals,

slowly and patiently. These trigger points are usually bad even when latent and giving no trouble at all. You will find the worst one about one third of the way up. End your search at the hip bone.

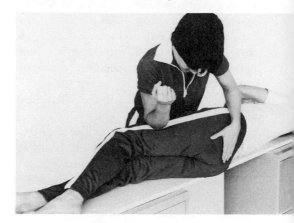

Vastus Medialis

Now for the inside line, which starts at the knee on the inside seam of the trousers at circle 33. With the subject lying supine and the knee slightly bent, move slowly at two-inch intervals up to the groin. Hold these spots, as always, for seven seconds. Don't forget the compass.

There is a way to do the knee while sitting side by side with the subject; this is the way we teach it to people who come to Pain-Erasure Seminars[SM] for a full

Pain-Erasure Seminars[SM] is a service mark of Bonnie Prudden, Inc.

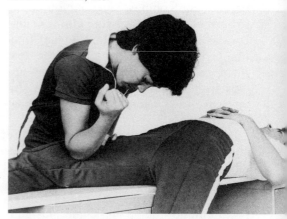

day of learning the techniques. The "hands-on" experience is very new to America; many people have never learned to help anyone in any way, physically. We have let others do for us for so long that many of us have no faith in our own hands. This is a mistake, because the hands are a reflection of the heart, and Americans are some of the most generous and caring people in the world.

This is one of the quickest of the quick fixes. Sit next to the subject and draw her near leg over yours. Place the elbow *nearer her body* at circle 33, near the knee. Hold for seven and execute the compass. Move up on the same line and repeat. The third trigger point should be about four inches down from the groin. None of them will be easy, but the middle one will be the worst. Pay attention to the reactions of the subject, especially if the knee has been giving trouble for a long time, as with "arthritis."

(and it is worst by any standards) is a third of the way up the leg. Stay on the line where the stripe or seam would be even if your subject is a small elderly person who wouldn't be caught dead in slacks or warm-up pants. Try to remember that knee pain has the same muscles pulling whether the sufferer is a football player, a housewife, an executive or a ten-year-old complaining of "growing pains." There is only one model of us, and we are not nearly so individualistic as we think. True, our accidents differ, but our muscles do not. And while acute injury demands specialized treatment according to what happened and what was damaged, chronic pain is something else again. Once the doctor says you have no anatomical pathology (fracture, tumor, etc.), think muscle spasm.

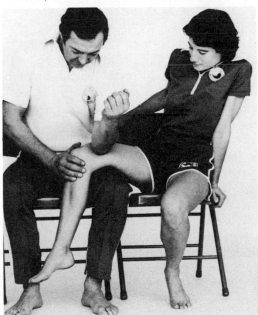

To do the outside of the leg, have the subject cross his leg over both his knee and yours. Again use the elbow nearer his body and start at circle 34, near the knee. Plan to make three stops for trigger points. Four at the most. The worst one

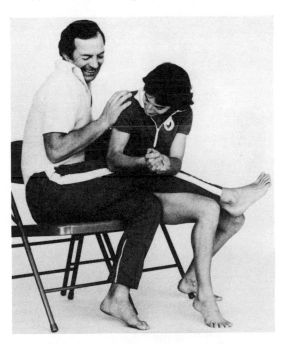

When you have finished with both the inside and the outside of the leg, have the subject stand and place both feet close together, then have him or her do two or three *half* knee bends, *keeping the heels on the floor.* Be careful! There are people who don't realize that *half* a knee bend means exactly that, not all the way to the floor. Usually the pain will either be much reduced or be gone altogether. But keep in mind and tell your subject also that a permanent fix will be needed to ensure that the pain stays away.

Then too, if your friend is a runner or other-sport enthusiast, he or she will need to be checked out from time to time even when there is no pain, just so there will be no pain. It won't take a lot of work, but enough to prevent or to undo the spasm that will assuredly follow extreme exertion.

To stretch the quads farther than just the half knee bends, have the subject lie prone and bend the knee while pressing down on the ball of the foot. If there is *pain* in the front of the thigh, you missed something. Look a little further. Do the same series of gentle bounces as you did for the calf muscle stretch exercise and do them often to relax and lengthen those muscles and keep them strong, flexible and youthful. What you don't use *fully* you will lose by imperceptible amounts until your loss will be perceptible indeed and usually by others first. Start watching the limited walking range of other people and determine *now* that this will not happen to you.

ZONE V

ZONE V, SEGMENT 16B: LOWER LEG, ANTERIOR VIEW

The *tibia*, the shinbone, is your guide in the lower leg. As in the back of the lower leg, one side usually houses more trigger points than the other. The more numerous, as well as more painful, will be on the line running down the outside front of the leg on the *extensor digitorum longus* but picking up the edges of the *peroneus longus* and the *tibialis anterior*. The *extensor digitorum longus* starts up in the front of the *fibula*, the smaller of the two lower leg bones on the side of the leg. It extends down into the first metatarsal, in the foot, the joint just back of the big toe. It has the job of flexing and inverting the foot. The *peroneus longus* attaches to the *fibula* and the first *metatarsal* as well, and when in spasm can do a real number on that slender leg bone. The *tibialis anterior* attaches to the tibia, the larger bone in the lower leg, and to the first *metatarsal*.

The *tibialis anterior* and the *extensor digitorum longus* play a large part in the action of the foot and lower leg caused by the long second toe. If you have this problem, check with "long second toe,"

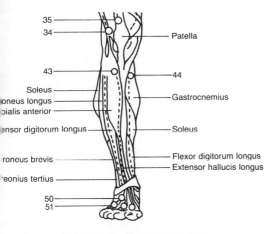

35
34
Patella
43
44
Soleus
ioneus longus
oialis anterior
ensor digitorum longus
Gastrocnemius
Soleus
roneus brevis
eonius tertius
Flexor digitorum longus
Extensor hallucis longus
50
51

FIG. 16: LOWER LEG, ANTERIOR VIEW

page 202, and pay close attention to the work that *must* be done on the outside line in the lower leg.

With the subject lying supine on the shelf laid over two filing cabinets or even just sitting in a chair with his calf flat on another chair, begin your search at the top of the outside line. Go down the leg at one-inch intervals into the ankle. Don't forget the compass and the seven-second hold *where there is pain*.

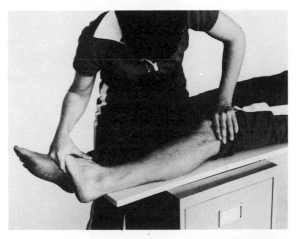

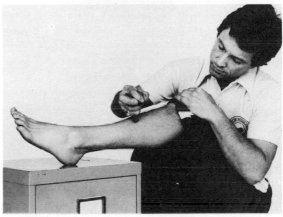

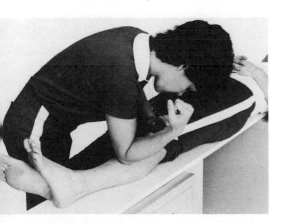

To stretch the muscles you have just freed of trigger points, rotate the foot inward and, while the rotation is held, draw the foot upward and then down to make the toes point first north and then south under the stretch. Relax and then repeat. Do four such stretches.

Doing Myotherapy on one's own legs is difficult because of the angle, except

with the bodo, when it is quite easy. If you have a tendency to leg cramps or "shin splints," you should have a bodo at home, one in the office and one in your locker at the club. If you run or hike alone and exercise your legs into cramps quite often, tie one to your belt or keep one in your pack or enjoy both of those sports with a knowledgeable friend. If you drive any distance at all, keep one in the glove compartment.

Most of the time, lower-leg ache responds to work and stretch for the muscles of the outer line, but should the ache remain, run down the line on the inner side of the front of the leg. Start at circle 44 after you have rotated the foot outward. The knuckle is the best tool here, as you will be pressing against the shinbone, the *tibia*.

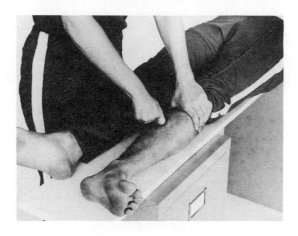

You will be passing over the edge of the *gastrocnemius*, whereas up till now

you have only gone down the belly, or full part, of the muscle. Then the *soleus* will come under your pressure and finally the *flexor digitorum longus*. Just knowing that the *gastrocnemius* plantar flexes the ankle (plantar pertains to the sole of the foot), that the *soleus* does the same thing and that the *flexor digitorum longus* flexes the distal phalanges of the four lateral toes and flexes the foot should warn you that there *has* to be trouble in those muscles for anyone who runs or stands a lot or is overweight.

To stretch this area, rotate the foot outward and pull the toes upward to full stretch and then relax. Do four.

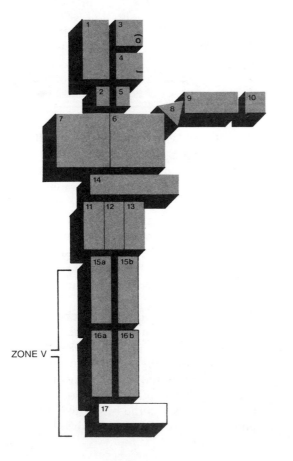

ZONE V, SEGMENT 17: THE FEET

If you have foot pain called anything from "age" to "arthritis," if you have a long second toe even without foot or leg pain . . . yet, if you run or engage in "spike sports" such as tennis or basketball, football, handball or volleyball, you may well have trigger points in your feet. Any activity with quick starts and stops or constant pounding or jumping about, as in "aerobic" dance, modern, jazz, tap or ballet, or any occupation that requires long hours of standing will garner a goodly crop. These trigger points can affect the feet, ankles, knees, hips and lower back, the groin, the floor of the pelvis and the abdominal wall.

In the foot, the trigger points on top of the instep just back of the second toe will be the most sensitive. After that, the best line to explore starts at circle 51, on Figure 17. The entire top of the foot may well be sensitive, and if the ankle has ever

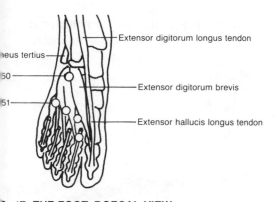

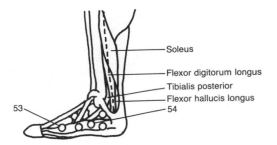

Extensor digitorum longus tendon

neus tertius

50

51

Extensor digitorum brevis

Extensor hallucis longus tendon

3. 17: THE FOOT, DORSAL VIEW

Soleus

Flexor digitorum longus

Tibialis posterior

Flexor hallucis longus

53

54

FIG. 18: THE FOOT, INSIDE VIEW

been injured, circle 50 will be a block-buster.

The small bodo can be of considerable help when working on trigger points in the foot. As in the hand, the spaces between the bones of the foot are very narrow; due to the shaft of the handle, the bodo can be controlled better than fingers or knuckles.

Sit opposite the subject and place the foot to be worked on your knee. Stabilize with your free hand. Using knuckles, fingers or bodo, then press straight down into the top of the foot for those trigger points on top of the instep.

To work with the trigger points on the inside of the foot, take the subject's entire leg onto your lap, as in the stretch exercises that follow. You will note on Fig-

ure 18, starting with circle 53, that the circles are not on a straight line. Instead of going straight up or down a muscle line, do your work on a zigzag. Use your compass wherever you can.

For the next step, the outside of the foot, place the leg across your lap and turn the foot inward to expose the whole side. Put a little pressure on to keep the foot inverted as you weave your way across the foot from ankle to toes, as in Figure 19. Circle 49, behind the ankle, should also be explored, with the foot held inverted but with the toes pulled slightly upward (dorsiflexion).

The sole of the foot is a minefield of trigger points. Also, everybody has them there. Even when they don't cause pain, they can cause both weakness and fatigue. "My feet are tired" is heard at least as often as "My feet hurt." Tired today, aching next year . . . or the next, or the next. Soaking the feet or elevating them may ease for the moment, but those are merely palliative measures and no real answer. The resident trigger points will

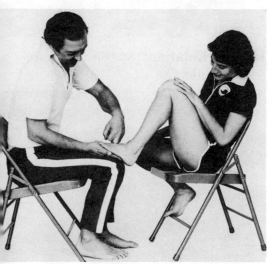

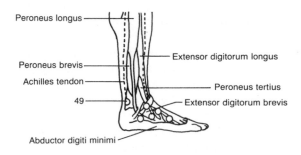

Peroneus longus

Peroneus brevis

Achilles tendon

49

Abductor digiti minimi

Extensor digitorum longus

Peroneus tertius

Extensor digitorum brevis

FIG. 19: THE FOOT, OUTSIDE VIEW

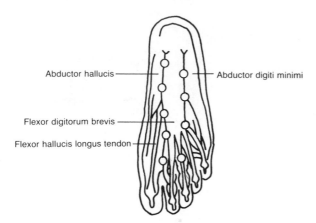

FIG. 20: THE FOOT, PLANTAR VIEW (SOLE)

Abductor hallucis

Abductor digiti minimi

Flexor digitorum brevis

Flexor hallucis longus tendon

Plantar Flexion, or Pronation: Stabilize the knee and press the instep and toes down as far as is comfortable.

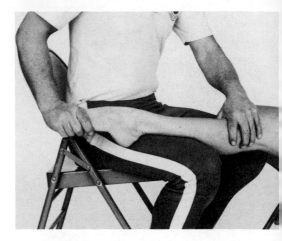

Supination: Stabilize the knee and press upward on the ball of the foot.

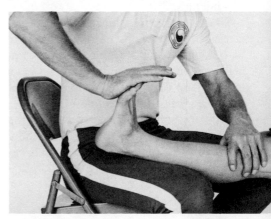

Inward Rotation: Stabilize the knee and invert the foot.

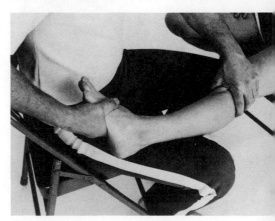

go to work when the feet do: the next day. The next night it will be the same old weariness again until the youthful spring is gone and the shuffle mistakenly attributed to age takes over as a habit. Painless folks bounce right along, enjoying the walk, the weather (rain or shine), the field, the hill, the trail and Fifth Avenue. The painful look terrible and should have Myotherapy.

The best way to position the subject for the sole of the foot is prone over a couple of chairs while you sit on a third at his feet. Put a pillow, jacket, sweater (any cushion) under the ankle and go to work. The small bodo is the best tool. Don't try to be exact, but remember where the worst trigger points live.

Passive stretch for the foot, ankle and lower leg is very important and is done with the subject sitting opposite. Do not overstretch; a trigger might go off and throw a muscle into spasm. If that should happen, be of good cheer, you will know exactly where the problem lies. Press along the muscle and stretch more gently. Lori's foot, in the picture, probably has more flexibility than yours, but you can always improve and should. Flexible ankles are slender, free of fluid, strong and useful. Be *sure* to check yourself for long second toes, on page 202, and if you find the condition is yours, take the appropriate measures.

Outward Rotation: Stabilize the knee and evert the foot.

Do several stretch sessions during the day and you will soon notice flexibility as well as strength and coordination improving. Others will see it in your walk. Do these with a friend after sports.

Do the entire series three or four times. If pain shows up anywhere in the leg, make a trigger-point search *in that area*. If you are using this series for *immediate mobilization*, use it every two hours after injury. If the leg is needed the following day, you may want to continue every two hours all night.

Active stretch is resorted to when people live alone. The Myotherapy can be done with the help of a small bodo, and when it comes to the sole of the foot place the bodo on the floor and apply the sole of the foot to the bodo, rather than the bodo to the foot.

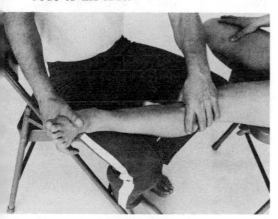

Plantar Flexion (Pronation): Sit comfortably and, laying the instep on the floor, slide the foot back until the weight is on the toes and instep. Press down *gently* in three easy presses, and relax.

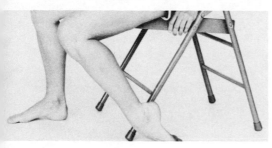

Supination: Place the ball of the foot on the rung of the opposite chair and, holding on to the seat for leverage, press the heel down in three easy presses, and relax.

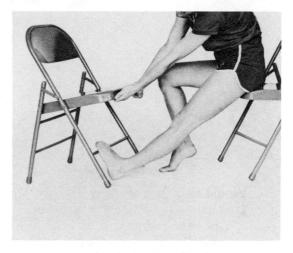

Inward Rotation: Lay the foot on its side and press the knee outward and down to put pressure on the outside of the foot. Three presses and rest.

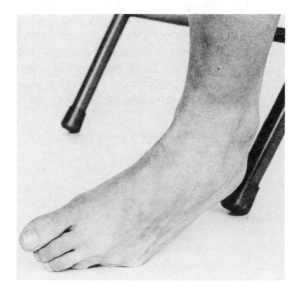

Outward Rotation: Push the foot backward as in Pronation but turned on its inside edge. Press down with the knee for three presses and rest.

Active stretches for the feet and ankles

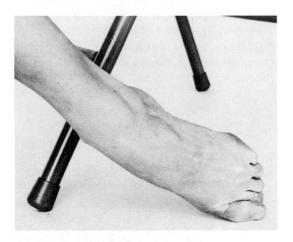

should be a part of every exercise program and a finish to every workout.

You have just gone from head to toe with quick fix; most people who can walk around, albeit miserably, will respond to it. It isn't magical, although a lot of people will think *you* are. It's very basic and understandable. A trigger point has thrown a muscle or muscles into spasm. The spasm causes pain, which tells the autonomic nervous system that there is trouble. The nervous system responds in the only way it knows and sends more spasm, which hurts more. Pretty soon you have a pain-spasm-pain cycle in effect, and it isn't going to stop until some-

thing (let's hope, your skill) interrupts it. When you *have* interrupted it, you must stretch the muscle to get the kinks out of it and set up exercises that will teach the muscle that there is a better way of doing things.

If you get rid of your friend's pain, great! At least you now know that you can do the same thing again and, if necessary, again and again. But that's not the final answer. You can get rid of the same pain on a permanent basis. That is the next step. It should be taken, as soon as you have time, with the help of the section on *Permanent Fix*.

Permanent fix is also used for more difficult problems: the people with long-term pain, people with serious afflictions, people who have been terribly hurt or grown old *in* pain. Don't start off with serious problems. Get your feet wet and your sword blooded and try your wings on easy things: back pain, headaches, "tennis elbow," "bursitis," "trick knees" and "carpal/tarsal tunnel syndrome," menstrual cramps and leg cramps. When you have had ten successes, you will be ready to try some tough stuff. If you take on too much too soon, you may get discouraged, and this is no time for discouragement. Not with what *you* know.

Permanent Fix

The permanent fix is an extension of the quick fix. The latter is first aid for pain, something to be done quickly and on the spot to alleviate the pain of the moment. The quick fix is like knowing where to walk in a minefield. Permanent fix gets rid of the minefield *and the enemy*.

In permanent fix you work as though dealing with a distant foe who can best be wiped out through isolation. You try to cut his supply lines before he can launch a major assault. In other words, you don't charge into the middle of his line, where his forces are strongest. Rather, you surround him from a safe distance, slowly clearing the area of snipers, sappers and roving patrols. Trapped in his command post (where the pain is most active) and unable to rally support on the outside, he can be finished off at leisure. Then, with vigilant attention given to mopping up the contaminated area (and any other area under his influence), you are able to end the war and keep unlawful elements under surveillance. *If*—and that if is the key to future painlessness—you can convince your subject to do the specific exercises you set up for his or her own particular problem, the pain need not return.

A good example of the permanent fix is help for a long-standing chronic pain in the shoulder. Shoulder pain, like TMJD (temporomandibular joint dysfunction, a pain in the jaw), is hard to eradicate. Both

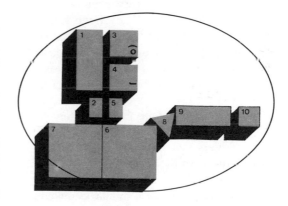

seem to sit in the center of things. They are surrounded by muscles that pull against the painful joint from all directions. Trigger points can hide anywhere, even very far afield, and though you wipe out a whole division on one front, you will still have to contend with others on the three fronts that have escaped your attention. Often, when you think you have neutralized one sector, moles, planted long ago in some other area, come to life and throw the whole front into flame again.

The periphery for the shoulder would include the hands and arms, the upper back, chest and neck, and the *axilla*. That would be an overlapping of Zones I, II and III. Conventional treatment today includes muscle relaxants, analgesics, ultrasound and injections of procaine or cortisone. There would also be some form of immobilization, usually a sling. Immobilization, even when needed, limits circulation and nutrition to the damaged area. In time the muscles atrophy. Even when the spasm-pain-spasm cycle has been broken by one of the foregoing modalities, the trigger points remain in the muscles like fifth columnists, just biding their time until some physical or emotional stress fires them up again. Relief is at best only temporary, and if the agony recurs often enough, an operation may be suggested. By that time it may even be necessary.

Permanent fix is resorted to when people begin to have higher expectations with regard to their lives. They have finally understood that pain is not a natural result of aging, old wounds and disease. The understanding that erasing pain is a skill, and that it is theirs to command, takes away a lot of anxiety and even terror. The not so simple fact that they no longer have to be afraid of pain, lowers stress levels, which in turn helps with pain control and erasure.

Permanent fix is also used when pain has gone beyond what a human being can bear and still cope with daily living. People in that kind of pain cannot go to work. They cannot support themselves or their families. Even when finances are not strained, they have emotional stresses that contribute handsomely to suffering. Once pain takes over, the circumference of their lives closes in and closes out everything and everyone they once enjoyed. They become the center of their very small world, and often, though unwillingly, the center of their family's life as well. They become a burden to everyone, but, most of all, to themselves. In a nutshell, it's a lousy way to live. This is doubly tragic when you consider that a few trigger points caught long ago might have prevented all the misery.

When the doctor is satisfied that there is no anatomic pathology, quick fix is in order. If there is *any* improvement or even any change, there is a good chance that Myotherapy is an answer; as soon as

possible, take the time to do a thorough job with permanent fix.

There are some things that may not respond. If you find *no* change after a thorough search, then the subject should go back to the doctor. Something unnoticed may be at work.

There are some elements that will militate against you if they are present; one is a desire on the part of the subject to put your results to the test *immediately*. She hadn't been pain free for months, until you cleared her back and legs of trigger points, but the very next day dashes out to do three months' worth of shopping, or he hasn't bent over even to tie his shoelaces since Halloween and the snowstorm has him trapped. Since he feels so good, he can't see why he shouldn't shovel just a little (which turns out to be the whole driveway). And then of course there's the athlete who was sidelined during September practice and the very last game of the season is next weekend. They'll do it every time. I know, because I've done all three. And then I'd end up back in bed thinking the treatment didn't work. The doctor used to be too exasperated for calm discussion and would shout at me, "Don't you know that's my back you are risking?" In a way it *was* his. He had taken it over for a while, as you will have to do with the muscles of overenergetic, overenthusiastic subjects. They are people whose motors are too big for their chassis and should not be criticized, just loved and fixed and encouraged to give their bodies the same chance *they* would give those of *other* people to heal.

Before you start your work with permanent fix, play detective. One of the things that makes Dr. Janet Travell so successful is that she is a medical sleuth. Find out what your subject knows about the past as it applies to today's pain, and just about anything could. If you have children (or intend to) you could provide them help with any pain problems they might encounter later in life by keeping track of what happens during the childhood years they will forget. Myotherapy^{SM} will be much more widely used when they are grown than it is now, and what they know about the history of their own bodies may speed up their search of themselves.

YOUR HISTORY . . . FOR YOURSELF

How Were You Born?

Find out if you had a normal birth. A normal birth is not to be confused with "natural childbirth." The word *natural* should always make you skeptical. It is *the* buzzword of the eighties and is usually applied to something for sale (whether you know it is for sale or not). *Normal* means the pregnant woman goes into labor and presently delivers a baby. As a rule, this can occur only outside of a hospital. An *ab*normal birth means one in which there is interference in the form of Demerol (which slows delivery) or Pitocin (which hurries it). Were forceps applied? Does anyone know why? Was the labor spontaneous, stimulated or induced? Was the labor long, hard or short? Were you brought in by C-section? What condition were *you* in? Was your head battered or out of shape? Were you in need of resuscitation? What else can you find out? Every one of those questions applies to you and to your children and theirs.

Induced labor and stimulated labor often batter a baby's head. These, as well as the use of forceps, can cause headaches right after birth as well as later on. Judging by the percentage of people suffering chronic headaches in America, we may well be The Forceps Generation. Analgesics interfere with *normal* labor, and anesthesia knocks the mother out, making forceps delivery necessary. Drugs cross the placenta to threaten the baby. Birth is the time when many problems start.

What Did You Look Like?

Were you battered and bloody? Was your head dented or out of shape? Were you blue? Were you pigeon-footed? Was your neck bent to one side? Did you have colic? Did you scream when you nursed? Somebody knows. Ask. If forceps were used, you may have sustained damage to your face, head or neck. If your birth was induced or stimulated, the battering may well have elongated your skull into a "pixie pate." This does straighten out after a while, but the pressure that caused it may also have laid down the trigger points that are causing your headache *today*. It may well be the reason your baby cried for weeks and weeks and was called colicky. Such birth injury may be the reason you have a tendency toward stiff neck and why cousin Andy never won a footrace. It may also be the reason your neighbor's little girl has been labeled minimally brain-damaged and why tiny Elizabeth won't leave her corner in the nursery school.

What Accidents Can Your Mother Remember?

Did you fall out of your high chair or off the bed? Did you put your teeth through your lower lip when you bounced your chin off the table? It was probably frightening enough to remember, because of all the blood and noise, even though a stitch or two put things to rights. Not quite. You now probably have trigger points in the *sternocleidomastoid* (SCM) muscles in your neck. And that may be the reason for the pain in your ear that nobody can explain, or for your dizziness, or even for your periodic bouts with laryngitis.

Of course you fell out of the tree, out of the swing and into the shallow end of the pool. Doesn't everybody? Let's hope everybody gets a chance to, but not that everybody gets hurt. Did you? Where was the damage and what kind? Many a case of "bursitis" is injected with cortisone, but a certified Bonnie Prudden Myotherapist who was told about a fall from a bucking horse as much as forty years ago would look for trigger points *on circle 13, on the scapula,* a spot often ignored when it comes to shoulder pain or arm pain, especially arm pain.

What Accidents Do You Remember?

You would be amazed at how easy it is to "forget" when it comes to accidents and injuries, especially if your sport, hobby or work lends itself to accident risk. Then too there is the "almost" accident. That's the one in which, through superhuman effort, you were able to prevent the worst from happening. Sad to say, you may have sustained more damage than had you fallen off the parallel bar or driven into the ditch. That accident you "avoided" may be the reason for the terrible pain in your upper back.

We had a young patient who was overly endowed when it came to her bosom—a condition not apt to be considered a minus in our society. She had been "doctoring" for upper-back pain for three years, and her doctor had finally sent her to a surgeon who was bent on cutting back on her breasts. Lest that sound callous, it's not always the worst idea when the bosom looks like a balcony, but this was not the case. You have to understand that this lady was very satisfied with the way she looked, and her husband was satisfied with the reason she was satisfied. They didn't want any drastic changes, even to ease her unremitting

pain, so as a last hope they tried Myotherapy. When I came to the question "Any auto accidents?" she said, "Oh, no . . . I was able to prevent one though. I just held on and steered for dear life." See if you can put your finger on the information you already have. Where was the pull during the "almost" accident? What muscles took most of the force? The trigger points were all over the pectorals, to begin with, and both arms. There was a "zinger" on circle 13, in the *scapula,* and in circles 1, 2 and 3, in the *gluteals.* Those last three are anchors for almost everything. It took an hour to prevent the surgery and the loss of an image. And we should always be wary when images are in danger; they are hard to replace . . . if indeed we *can* replace a lively self-image.

What Was Your Sports History?

A sports history, or the lack of one, can tell you a lot. Check with the *Sports* section and you will see how sports or no sports can set the stage for pain immediately or years later. This will apply whether you have given up the sport or all sports, taken up a sport or are reactivating an old one. The "trick knee" that bothered you in high school when you were on the football team can start to heat up again after the first set of tennis at the new club. Your serve could well aggravate the shoulder separation you suffered on the college team, and you may begin to hear from those old "heel spurs" after the town "fun run."

Of course if there is no sports history at all ("We never did anything in gym, I hated it"), that's something else again. We usually get that from girls and women. The male counterpart is "I was too short for basketball, too light for football and the baseball team were all graduates of Little League." What that describes is a sedentary way of life during the all-important formative years. Maybe your children or grandchildren are in those years now. The key to physical fitness in this country is choosing the right parents. If the parents are sports-minded, if they hike, canoe, sail, camp, play tennis or golf, swim, bike or enjoy *some* form of lifetime sports, the children usually get a good start. Once in a great while we can count on a teacher, but they usually come on the scene too late. There is the rare human being who rises to the top without help from anyone, but don't count on it for yours. The sad thing is that a great many more parents relax with TV than ever find their way into the sun.

Operations: What Were Yours?

There are all kinds of operations, which, leaving scars, set the stage for trigger-point activity. One wouldn't consider the extraction of a couple of wisdom teeth much of an operation, but it can set TMJD (jaw pain) in motion, with accompanying headache, earache, tooth pain, *tinnitus,* or eye, gum, face and neck pain as well as the pain in the jaw for which the condition is named.

Then there are the spinal operations, the disk excisions and fusions, which often leave the pain for which they were undertaken still pulsing. There are the carpal-tunnel and tarsal-tunnel operations and the operations done for sinus headache and hemorrhoids. There are also the "ectomies," which means cutoffs. There are many of those; here is a partial list. Does a part of you belong to the list?

Venectomy-
Splenectomy
Mastectomy
Cystectomy
Nephrectomy
. . . and ostectomy
can be done almost anywhere.

And there are

Sympathectomy

Hysterectomy
Orchidectomy
Oophorectomy
Ophthalmectomy
Appendectomy
Mastoidectomy
Hepatectomy
Pneumonectomy
. . . and tonsillectomy.

Let us not overlook cesareans and open-heart surgery. The latter causes all kinds of post-op pain in the chest, neck and shoulders and at every site from which the replacing veins have been removed.

Anytime you cut tissue you get a scar: from the littlest ones on your fingers, souvenirs of the first weeks in the kitchen, to the twisted cesarean scar that turns your nice, smooth tummy into the Maginot Line. Every scar, both those on the surface from your long-ago appendectomy, to the deep-lying scars from your vaginal hysterectomy or arthroscopy, have the potential for housing trigger points. If they are to be massive, as from a radical mastectomy (*still* done by less progressive surgeons), make sure you know which kind of operation is planned. They can cause pain in several directions. If the trigger points are near sensitive structures such as the eyes, nose, ears, throat, teeth or spine, they can keep you chasing to doctors for years.

So list your operations and stop turning purple with rage when it is suggested that you are a hysteric. You probably have a very legitimate cause for your chronic backache, nervous stomach, facial pain and what feels like a fallen uterus except that that's been gone these seven years. Check your scars and wonder about trigger points. That goes double if you have suffered an amputation and the missing foot, leg, hand or arm still aches, burns, tingles or screams with pain. It is called "phantom limb pain." The key is in the muscles that are left and in the scar tissue of the stump.

What Are or Have Been Your Medications?

The doctor usually prescribes medication, and woe to him or her who accepts medication from a relative or friend. Not that they don't mean well; they mostly do. But suppose that little white pill *their* doctor gave them is used for *your* sore throat and it happens to be penicillin. The doctor knows enough to ask about your allergies, but your friend may not. If you are allergic to penicillin it *could* mean the end of you. Although the doctor prescribes the pill, *you take it,* and medication has become more and more dangerous in recent years. And in this, as in other things about you, *you* are responsible. You will pay the bill no matter the price or who made the error.

The worst case of abdication from responsibility I've ever seen concerned a friend of mine who had lupus. She called to say she couldn't have lunch with me because she had developed a huge ulcer on her instep. On top of that, ten days before, the doctor had removed some tissue from the instep for a biopsy and now she had two ulcers and could scarcely walk. I went to see her and did Myotherapy on both legs from groin down to and including both feet. After a half hour per leg the angry redness around the sores was receding and the pain already gone. Her feet, which had been cold due to the spasms interfering with her circulation, were warm. In three days the better blood supply had brought increased nutrition to the area and cleared up the ulcers. I asked about her medication, and although she knew it was dangerous, she had never bothered to find out just *how* dangerous or what might come of taking it. The doctor too was evidently ignorant about that particular medication. Had he bothered to look into the PDR (Physician's Desk Reference), he would have saved himself the bother of doing a failed biopsy (they didn't find anything). It says quite clearly in the book, which is available in any library, that among many others, *ulcers are a side effect!*

Many drugs are a kind of trade-off. You take one for condition A, which may help with the symptoms of A but cause a miserable side effect called B. B has to be corrected with C and then later with D. All the while, the body, struggling desperately for some sort of homeostasis as it is attacked again and again by warring dollops of poison, gets sicker *and more painful*. No way to live, you would say, and so would I. Before you take *any* medication, find out what you are taking and what it could do to you. If you *must* take a given medication, read up on the stuff and know every possible side effect. At the *first* sign of one of them, stop the medication. If it's take it or die, that's one thing. If it's another kind of choice, say, take it or suffer pain, think Myotherapy followed by the right exercise for your condition. The patients I know who do best with lupus take nothing stronger than aspirin and work out daily.

You should also check with "Stress History Number 1," page 125 and "Stress History Number 2," page 290. Trigger points do their worst work when stress is present; now is a good time to check both your stresses and those of your subject.

When you start with your subject, keep good records showing where you locate trigger points and what the result of your search is. Make a tracing of the anatomical map showing the area of search and mark on it all the painful spots unearthed. We use blue ink to mark an *x* on the tracing the first time we work. If the spot is one of those "zingers," we circle the *x*. At the second session we switch to red ink. Thus, when there is no response where a blue *x* indicated a trigger point, we know we have cleared at least one. If there is a mild response, we know we got some of the problem but have a little more to do. If the response is just as acute as ever but the pain has left, then we know we have recorded one of those *matrix* areas that will just stay there waiting for an opportunity to flare. But we also know that should the ache return in the future, *there* is the culprit. The third time around, we use yellow. These records should be kept as guides to preventive measures when the subject might be under some kind of stress.

List What You Have Used in Your Search for Relief of Pain.

Before you embark on an effort to get rid of an old, old pain, one so long entrenched that it seems almost to be a part of you, make a list of all the things you have done to get rid of it. List the doctors you saw and when you saw them. If you can, find out what X rays were taken, how many and when. That means *all* of them, including the one that was taken because you thought you had fractured a wrist when skiing Mount Mansfield. You see, you'd forgotten that one, because you were only thirteen.

It isn't the one X ray the doctor wants to take for that sprained wrist that will give you cancer, it's the accumulation of rads over a lifetime. For me, thirteen is a long time and a lot of X rays ago, and although we weren't aware of the danger of rad accumulation then, we are now. *No* X ray should be taken routinely, and that means chest X rays and tooth X rays.

Not long ago a lady came to the clinic. She had been a patient with us for many years, a victim of "restless legs." That's a condition in which the patient goes to bed and an hour or so later wakes with the feeling that ants are crawling all over her legs, tingling, stinging, hurting and generally unpleasant. The only relief, until we tried Myotherapy, was getting out of bed and walking around until the sensations quieted, then back to bed for another hour, then walk, then rest. That would go on most of the night. Her legs had to be de-triggered on a regular basis,

and she knew what we could do for pain. But somehow she thought only of pain in her legs, not in any other part of her body. So when her neck and hand began to bother her, off she went for X rays. When I heard about it I was distressed, as I am all too often. *Twenty-six X rays for a pain in the shoulder and one in the hand!* I could and did eradicate both pains in less than half an hour. But how many unnecessary rads did she rack up? Too many, and for nothing. One of our boys totaled his car and very nearly himself. He had a six-inch head wound and multiple fractures of his *femur*, the thighbone. Including pre- and post-op X rays, all the CAT scans and those taken when, unconscious, he was admitted to the hospital, he was X-rayed twenty-six times, but his was a life-threatening situation. The mark of many X rays for minor complaints is both inefficiency and lack of education, or greed.

Another example seems to happen all the time. A woman had suffered what seemed to be a gallbladder attack, and the following day was sent for X rays after taking a medication, name unknown. She spent two hours being X-rayed on several machines, and when she stopped back at the desk before leaving she was told to take the medication again and report back the following day. They hadn't gotten what they wanted. The second day, she went through the same procedure, plus a session with a fluoroscope. Again at the desk she was told to return the next day. They *still* hadn't found what they wanted. The lady forgot her upbringing and how one was supposed (in the olden days) to receive medical orders. "I'd rather be sick and the hell with it!" she spat out and left, never to return. She never had another "gallbladder attack," either. It probably never entered the X-ray technician's mind that *there were no gallstones present* and that the complaint was the result of something altogether different: stress plus trigger points in the back and abdominal muscles. But something did come of the experience: the addition of innumerable rads.

Only once in my lifetime did any medical person ask me how many X rays I had already had in that lifetime. The question was asked last year by a medical *secretary*. You had better know about yours, and the next time someone says, "We'll just take an X ray to be sure," *you* be sure that it's unavoidable.

List All Your Occupations, from the Beginning to Right Now.

When you have listed them (my first was gardening for twenty-five cents an hour, aged nine), check with the section on occupations and find out what each one does to the human body and see if any of the pain sustained matches any of yours.

List Your Symptoms and Give the History of Your Present Complaint.

Where does it hurt? When does it hurt? Are some times worse than others? Is it continuous or intermittent? If intermittent, do you know what brings it on? Do you know what aggravates it? Where does it usually happen? Is there a progression? For example, if it starts in your neck does it spread to your chest, back or arm? Is there any pattern to the pain? Some headaches can be counted on to appear after a couple of drinks. Sometimes they accompany or precede menstruation, or appear on the day the payroll must be made up. Some headaches are called "mother-in-law headaches" and will show up over Christmas. Still others are connected with sex . . . when you'd rather not. Write down as much as you can about your pain before you tackle the next question.

Where Are the Stresses? (See also the section on *Aging*.)

Everyone has stress and there's no escape. Some stress can be handled all of the time and most stresses can be handled some of the time. *Where we get into trouble is when we try to handle all of the stresses all of the time.* There is an enormous amount of conceit there. Somewhere we have taken on the idea that we are iron people, invincible, indestructible, in charge of ourselves and our entire world. Not the whole world, of course, but ours, the one around each of us. Coupled with that idea is that *we* are responsible for just about everything and everyone in that world. Even when we *think* we are leaning on others, we don't give up the idea that we are responsible. *We* built this little world and we are damn well going to make it work. Hah! That's the stuff psychiatry is made of. Either way, we lose. If we keep plugging away day in and day out trying to make the world we made work, we may never look over the edge and see how small it is or how imperfect. If we turn to the wall, saying, "I can't go on," then we feel a sense of loss and terrible failure. In the one case we struggle harder to do what perhaps cannot be done and take on burdens that cannot be borne. In the second, we just plain give up. In either case the end is certain. The organism that is us begins to break down, crack up, fall apart and hurt. Soon after that, we lose the capacity to love, to enjoy and to live.

In *Pain Erasure the Bonnie Prudden Way*, the book on pain that actually works for the average human being, I wrote that my generation was told by our elders (who had been told by theirs), "You made your bed, now lie in it." That's terrible! I was six years old and in an orphanage. I had a bed-wetting problem. I was literally scared to death to go to sleep, because, if I wet the bed, *I had to stay in it all the next day.* Ah, you may think, I'll bet *that* cured you.

Not at all, but it did teach me self-reliance. I would discover that awful accident a couple of hours before the rising bell, while it was still pitch-dark. Shaking like a small leaf (six-year-olds are still very small and, in such circumstances, very frightened) I would slide out of bed quivering with cold and wet. I'd unmake my bed and drag the offending sheet down an endless almost black hall to the bathroom, where the dirty-laundry hamper was. There I would bury my sheet while extracting a dirty but dry one. The trip back was terrifying. The red votive light flickered in front of the statue of the Blessed Mother, who looked anything but motherly in that strange light, and I kept up a steady litany to her Son: "Jesus, please don't let Sister catch me" (He never did). Back in the dormitory I'd flip my soggy mattress and make up my cot and try to dry my nightie with the warmth of my body.

That's a pretty vivid picture of what we do to ourselves when we echo our elders with "You made your bed, now lie in it." Most of the time the crime is not ours, if crime there is. *I* could escape my bed because I took matters into my own hands and Sister was asleep. It's different when you are grown up. Then *you* are Sister and *you* never sleep. So you often stay trapped in your bed, confined in your imperfect world, straining and crying out to be free of the flickering red light, the displeased face, the long dark hall and somebody else's dirty sheet. When you fall victim to chronic pain, remember this story and wonder if maybe you are in the wrong place, with the wrong people and with a problem that would go away if you looked outside the walls *you* built, and then followed your eyes.

Emotional stress is a killer, the catalyst that makes much chronic pain possible. We know acute pain has a message, a warning. Either we are in danger of tissue destruction (your hand is on the hot radiator, get it off) or it tells of damage already sustained (your back is broken, don't move a muscle). But chronic pain also has a message: Chronic pain rarely surfaces unless there is a rising level of emotional stress. It says that the world we built is beginning to crumble. Of course, nobody wants to see this and many of us wear smoked glasses so we can't see it, not even when we fall over it. Sooner or later we *will* fall over it, and that's when chronic pain immobilizes us.

Acute pain rarely allows us to be stupid about our danger. Chronic pain doesn't either, but it takes longer to get its message across. At first it forces us to center our thinking on ourselves instead of everything and everyone else. Pain may even pull us out of the rat race for a time. If we don't listen, it steps up the pressure until there is little else in our lives. If we still turn a deaf ear, it may well take us out of the struggle altogether. Chronic pain tells us more than that we have a bad back, a spastic colon, heartburn, "bursitis," or cervical arthritis. Of course it tells us those things too, but they are to get our attention. It says much more. It says we are playing the game of Sisyphus, doing endless, toilsome tasks that will never be finished, and that *this* way at least, we cannot accomplish what we want. Sit down and fill out the following:

Stress History Number 1

Date today.
Age.
Where do I live?
Is this where I'd live if I had a choice?
What is my work at present?
Is this what I want to do?
What do I look like?
Is this how I want to look?
Who are my family?
Are these the people I want to be with?
Who are my friends?
What do we give each other?
What gives me pleasure?

Do I have opportunities to enjoy such things?

What do I get from life?

What do I give to life?

As it is right now, is it worth living?

How would I change it if I could?

Have I tried to make it different?

What didn't change no matter how hard I tried?

Am I sure that aspect *can* be changed?

Is it time to give up on *that* aspect?

What other choices do I have?

Given the way I am going now, what do I see ten years down the road?

Given my druthers, what would I like to see?

The Pain, or Any Pain.

WHEN DID I GET THE FIRST PAIN THAT WASN'T ACUTE? In other words, a pain that did not announce sudden damage such as a sprain, fracture, burn and so on.

WHERE WAS I AND WHAT WAS HAPPENING TO MY *LIFE* WHEN I STARTED THAT PAIN, WHICH WE WILL CALL CHRONIC? The first one I remember came on when I was six and in the orphanage. Granted the food was awful and there was never enough of it, but even I knew that when I was doubled up with stomach cramps, it wasn't what I'd eaten. Suddenly I'd feel this tightness in my stomach, and as it increased it would turn into very real pain. Then I'd be given ipecac to bring up the offending morsels. They never seemed to realize that we all ate the same pottage, but only I got sick. Well, hindsight being 20/20, I now know you can't cure loneliness, frustration and heartache with ipecac. In the two years I was there, I ran away six times. You can't say *I* didn't know deep inside what the disease was, and the cure.

WHAT KIND OF PAIN WAS IT THAT CAME TO ME, AND DID IT COME BACK LATER IN LIFE? Years later, after my marriage and the coming of children, there it was again, my stomachache. I finally went to a wise doctor, who examined me thoroughly and then said, "What do you do every day?" I went through the litany any housewife and mother could recite in her sleep. "And what do you want to do?" To my horror I was dissolved in tears. Presently I said, "Write, teach . . ." "Well then you must do those things," she said like some oracle while I scoffed inwardly. Where was the time coming from? Then she added the clincher: "You must tell your husband that either you will have part-time help to free you for what you are *driven* to do, or he can expect to have you in the hospital within six months." Now, *that* was an ultimatum, one I was incapable of making myself, for reasons of training. Women did women's work and if they couldn't they were failures. Failure wasn't in my programming, and how many of you are programmed to go down with colors flying thinking that is the *only* thing to do? Fewer now than there used to be, but make no mistake, there are still a lot of us around.

WHAT WAS GOING ON WHEN MY PAIN CAME BACK? Make a list of *all* the chronic disabilities you can remember, and that goes for hay fever, hives, rashes, eczema, dermatitis, boils, sties, stiff necks, tight shoulders, upper- or lower-back spasms, aching extremities, bad teeth, tics, stuttering, head colds, sore throats, laryngitis, TMJD, jaw subluxations (jaw goes *almost* out of joint and seems to lock), assorted or continuing aches and pains, "arthritis," dyspepsia, "heartburn," anorexia, bulimia, anemia and on and on.

NEXT TO EACH COMPLAINT, I NOTE WHEN THEY SHOWED UP FOR THE FIRST TIME AND THEN SEE IF I CAN TIE SUBSEQUENT BOUTS OF THEM TO EMOTIONAL STRESS OR A LIFE-STYLE CONDUCIVE TO STRESS.

WAS THERE A TIME WHEN I WAS FREE OF *ALL* CHRONIC DISABILITY? IF SO,

WHERE WAS I? WHAT WAS I DOING? WHO WAS (OR WAS NOT) IN MY LIFE AT THE TIME?

Don't be surprised if you can find only one summer in your entire life when you were free of everything stressful. Until the summer of 1976, when I was sixty-two, I could count on the fingers of two hands the number of *months* when absolutely nothing was wrong, when life was at least momentarily happy, peaceful and rewarding. There was a popular song that sums up how most people live at least part of the time and some live most of the time: "Stop the World, I Want to Get Off." That is a plea for surcease from pain, at least for a little while. We'll talk about ways to do that later on.

What has just been said may be totally outside your ken at the moment. That's all right. It may not apply to you at all. You may be the wonderful, fortunate exception. But then again, you may be blind when it comes to yourself. I refused to see myself for a long time, because I couldn't mesh what I saw with what I thought I *should* see. There's a word that contributes to stress: *should*. The *shoulds* and *ought tos* are deadly. They can range from "I guess I should take responsibility for that, my mother would have," to "Everybody else smokes, I guess I ought to." The latter is called peer pressure and can be just as demanding at sixty as at sixteen, and just as dumb.

If the above questions awakened an echo in your heart, are you ready for it? Nobody makes a move to do anything until the self is ready for the move. That's why nobody can give up smoking for you, or make a diet work for you. And nobody but you can answer the question "What do I really want from life?" Only you have that answer, but have you asked yourself the question?

So where does that leave us when it comes to permanent fix? You would not be reading this book unless *something*

was wrong, and with most chronic pain requiring permanent fix there are overtones of emotional stress. Stressful situations require change, but in order to make changes one needs both a strong, pain-free body and self-confidence. Of the two, the body comes first and then confidence riding in its wake. You don't even have to wonder; *it will be there*.

PERMANENT FIX AND REFERRED PAIN

You have already observed in *Quick Fix* how spots in various zones of the body can refer pain to neighboring areas and even distant zones. It is absolutely essential that you understand that; otherwise you may always stop short of a thorough job, a permanent fix, by overlooking some obscure key trigger point that seems to have nothing to do with anything at all. The following story is a rather dramatic way of bringing this home to you so you *cannot* forget it, but it describes an integral part of Myotherapy: *referred pain*.

I got my first never-to-be-forgotten lesson in referred pain while listening to a lecture by Dr. Janet Travell down in Washington. That was the subject of her lecture, and suddenly the lecture went from general to me. I heard her mention the "referred pain of toothache." Now, you know and I knew that an aching tooth is a signal to go to the dentist, who will tell you that, yes, there is another cavity. He will fill it and your tooth stops aching. Either that or, worse, there's an abscess and root-canal work is indicated. Well, I had the toothache and my dentist said the unthinkable: "I can't find anything, so we'll just watch it for a while." We'd been "watching it" for several months and I was tired of my aching tooth that had nothing wrong with it.

Dr. Travell had been discussing the *sternocleidomastoid* muscle in the neck, which could cause referred pain to the ears, forehead, teeth, etc. Then she said, "Even an old head injury can cause perfectly healthy teeth to ache." Well, I'd had a head injury all right. I tried to take out a tree along a ski trail many years before when my ski tip hit a rut and I dived straight into one of Vermont's famous sugar maples. It raised an egg-sized knot on the top of my head just right of center. At the time, I'd been absolutely delighted that I'd had the accident and survived and that the knot was precisely where it was, *just right of center*. Why? Because all my life I'd *known* I was going to have something *terrible* happen to the right side of the top of my head.

As a rock climber, one is allowed certain peculiarities and forebodings, at least in the presence of other climbers. No one ever questions a decision not to climb today or not that particular chimney or even with a particular person. Risking your life continuously seems to give climbers an edge, or they probably couldn't do what they do. My "edge" often made me edgy about falling rocks, and my climbing partner used to be quite annoyed with my worries that he might dislodge one. My premonition was almost realized one summer in the Dolomites when another party, high above us, sent an Idaho-potato-sized rock plummeting past my head. It tore through my parka hood and left me paralyzed with fright. But unhurt. "Well," he yelled up at me, "there went your accident. You can take it easy from now on." I did, because I believed him, but he was wrong and so was I. It was the following winter that I hit the tree. Surely that was it! Shortly after that, I went into business full time and lost the opportunity to make the really difficult climbs and was lulled into forgetting my fear and the caution I should have exercised.

My tooth had been treating me to a dull ache for a week when Dr. Travell said a head injury could cause such pain, and I reached up to the spot where the knot

had been and pressed my worry area. Zing! Right to the aching tooth like an electric shock! Wow! She's right. I sat there marveling at the intensity of the pain in my tooth activated by my own hand over six inches away. When I took my hand away, *the toothache was gone!* Instant dentistry! I could hardly wait to tell her, and that night at dinner she explained how she thought it worked. I found her explanation in a paper later, and here it is:

Recognition of the physical basis for the symptoms from myofascial trigger points is difficult because myofascial structures are not visualized by the usual radiological examination [which is why my dentist couldn't find anything wrong] and because no blood or urine test pinpoints the problem [which is why a lot of sufferers are told their pain is all in their heads]. The diagnosis can be established by objective signs on palpation of affected muscles and by the observation of restricted motion. The pattern of referred pain evoked by palpating a myofascial trigger point is a subjective phenomenon described by the patient. [The trouble with this is that you would have to know something about trigger points to make a diagnosis, and where is the average dentist going to learn about them?] However, that pattern for a given muscle is similar enough, from person to person, to be predictable. [If I had told Dr. Travell about my head injury when I came to her for a toothache that looked to her like a healthy tooth, she would have gone hunting for the trigger point under my scalp, as you will be able to do when you've finished this book.] When the patient's description of palpation-evoked pain matches the known pattern for that muscle, the accuracy of the reporting is verified.

I was tremendously excited with "my" discovery about myself, and after that, for years, any time my tooth complained, I cut the initiating factor off at the pockets by attacking the offending trigger point. It was in my scalp, and I knew just where. All it required was a few seconds of pressure. Then came the summer of '72, and my destiny, feared for so long, met me at dusk.

A friend of mine owned an English mastiff guard dog, a dog with headaches (he used to rub his head against trees constantly and even debark them) and a vicious disposition. He had already bitten six people, all friends who would not have reported him even if there had been anyone to report to. He weighed all of 263 pounds in his stocking feet and had never said a cross word to me in his life.

The old adage about letting sleeping dogs lie should be modified, especially if the sleeping dog is *large*. If for some reason you *have* to wake the dog, do it in easy stages, making sure the dog knows *you* are the person disturbing him and also why. What does he know from a blob in the dark? That terrible evening, I was going down the hall and looked at him sleeping so peacefully against the wall outside the plate-glass door. Then I saw the blood on his paw. Without thinking, I opened the door and stepped out. "Oh, James, did you hurt yourself?" I said as I stooped to examine the injury. There was the most ghastly roar and then incredible pain, and I jumped up dragging 263 pounds of mastiff attached to my head, but not for long. So explosive had been my reaction that I not only lifted him to a standing position, on his hind legs, but as I crashed backward through the glass door, I tore him off my head. I know I screamed, because I heard it as if from a great distance. I also know I told him to get the hell out of there, which he did. He hadn't known it was I, and it was my fault. Even in the most terrifying moments when blood was spraying over him, the wall, the door and me, I knew and was angry at myself, not the dog. I knew I'd been bitten, but not that I'd lost one third of my scalp *from the top of my head just right of center.*

First aid is a very handy thing to know, and I sent someone for Band-Aids and a wet tea towel. I couldn't understand their confusion when I said, "Pull the two edges together and stick a Band-Aid over it." The rug in my bathroom is white, so,

rather than bleed all over it, I remained in the hall, so I never saw the extent of the injury. We finally got things under control with a bath towel and headed for the hospital to get "stitched up." I never did see the injury until days later, after various skin grafts had taken and 270 stitches were removed. My premonition of disaster had been right all along, and number-three accident had finally happened. It didn't quite kill me, but I'm told it was right close.

For our purposes here, you will be interested to learn that I never had a toothache again. The muscle in which the irritated trigger point was lodged had become an hors d'oeuvre for a dog and was gone forever. It is not the sort of dentistry I would recommend, but it's a terrific example of how trigger points can cause referred pain and how, when the trigger point is not in existence, there is no referred pain. In Myotherapy we aren't that extreme, but we do deactivate the trigger points, and thereby we get rid of the pain.

Permanent fix means you are going to work toward getting rid of pain on a permanent basis. If quick fix worked temporarily, you can be sure permanent fix is not only the next step, but *the* step. If the subject will then cooperate by doing the specific exercises you line up for the troublesome areas *and* embark on a general exercise program such as the one found here *and* give some thought to a sensible diet, you will have success.

After the doctor has told your subject that there is no anatomic pathology causing the pain, then you are ready to start. First, you will need a table on which to work. You can work on a kitchen or dining table or a desk if the subject is small, but if not, then the subject will be uncomfortable, as parts will always be hanging over the edge somewhere. There are foldaway massage tables, which are perfect if you can swing it financially. If not, two sawhorses and an old door would do well enough. Pad with a couple of blankets.

Having taken the history as best you can (you will get better at it as time goes on), you now need to know what your subject weighs. Why? Because the person in pain who carries too much weight compounds the problem. Overweight interferes with good posture and puts extra stress on muscles not designed for either the weight or the off-balance position of the body. Exercise is the best weight reducer, but the person in pain cannot exercise properly, and often not at all. Once the pain is gone, exercise should become daily, as should the act of weighing in. As the physical image improves, so will the self-image. The starting weight, good

or bad, is just that: a start. Try to weigh at the same time each day and wearing as little as possible. Enter the weight on your chart, which should be near the scale and complete with a pencil. You would be amazed at the excuses the mind can make to avoid facing the truth.

After weighing in, get your subject's measurements. Why? Because the scale cannot give the true picture. For sure, 150 pounds of blubbery fat is one thing, but 150 pounds of bone and toned muscle, quite different. But, your subject says, "I don't want to weigh 150 pounds of *anything*, I want to weigh 130 pounds." Great. A nice goal, *but*, when you have erased all the pain caused by the muscles in spasm and your subject has started to

FIG. 21: WEIGHT CHART

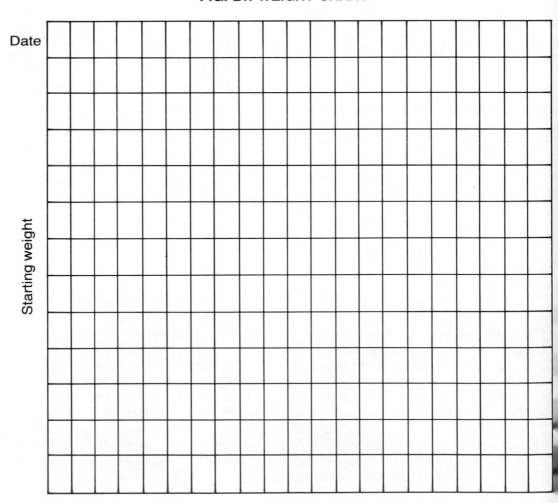

exercise (while using a sensible diet) fat will be replaced by smooth, attractive muscle, which looks good and is very useful, *but weighs more*. "I'm not losing anything" is the usual cry of woe. Oh yes she is, as her measurements will show, and that will keep her on her program.

Then there is the man who weighs 150 pounds of nothing much, due to pain over years. He too needs to measure, and that's because he should watch carefully to see where he adds the weight he wants; it should *not* be on his abdomen. If he does add it there, then his program and diet need checking.

One other thing: a tape measure is a lot easier to pack than a scale when you go on vacation, and on vacation is where getting in shape should be easy and fun. The tape measure hanging on the bathroom door reminds you that lunch may be lovely, sandwiched as it is between breakfast and dinner, but a slim waist is just right when it is between a tight seat and slender upper body.

The third test you and your subject should use is the Kraus-Weber minimum muscular fitness test for key posture muscles. This is the test we have used all over the world to check on minimum fitness levels. The *key* posture muscles are the upper- and lower-back muscles, the abdominals and the psoai. There are six tests in all, five for minimum strength and one for minimum flexibility. If one test is failed, the subject does not have that minimum needed for daily living.

Everyone should take the K-W test about every three months and always if there has been an illness or an injury or an operation or even a bout with emotional stress. If the test cannot be passed after some such event, the body is telling you it has been (or is being) severely

FIG. 22: MEASUREMENTS

Date								
R. arm								
L. arm								
Chest-bust								
Midriff								
Waist								
Abdominals								
Hips one								
Hips two								
R. thigh								
R. knee								
R. calf								
R. ankle								
L. thigh								
L. knee								
L. calf								
L. ankle								

FIG. 23: THE KRAUS-WEBER (K-W) TEST

Six tests for minimum muscular fitness.   Function and posture. Check often.

BOX A

Date			
A +			
A −			
P			
UB			
LB			
BHF			

BOX B

Substitution			
Leading elbow			
Arch			
Scoliosis			
Round shoulders			
Swayback			
Pigeon toes			
Turnout			

stressed and needs more physical outlets than it is getting. This is particularly true if there is a sudden failure of either test 2 or 6. Test 2 is A − and is for abdominal strength minus the help of the *psoas*; test 6 is for BHF, back and hamstring flexibility.

after a test, know that an illness or injury will move you into the danger of failure. You really need more than a bare minimum. If you can't sit up, you fail. Give yourself a *0* (zero) and check with the correctives right after the test.

A + (Abdominals plus Psoas)

Lie supine with feet held down and hands clasped behind head. Roll *slowly* up to a full sitting position. If you can do that, even though it is with a struggle, you pass. Give yourself a check next to A +, in Box A. If there *was* a struggle, then add a small *c*, which stands for "with difficulty." Whenever you have a small *c*

A − (Abdominals Minus Psoas)

Lie supine but with knees bent, feet held down and hands clasped behind head. Roll up slowly to the full sitting position. Mark, as for A + but next to A −, a check for pass, *c* for "with difficulty" and *0* for failure. Check with the correctives if the test is failed.

Box B: If the person being tested for minimum abdominal strength sits up with

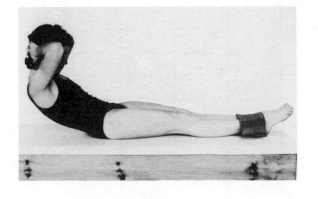

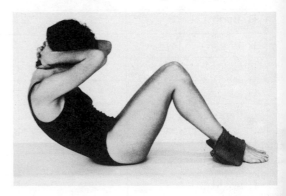

a jerky motion and a straight back, rather than *rolling* up smoothly, it means "*substitution.*" The muscles are weak, and muscles not meant to do the job are taking over. Enter a check next to *substitution* and use the correctives at the end of the testing. Use the roll-downs over and over, trying for a curled back, rather than a stiff, flat one.

If, when doing *either* a sit-up or a roll-down, the subject *leads* with either elbow, there is uneven muscle function. Enter *R* or *L* next to "Leading elbow," in Box B. Then, aside from hunting for trigger points that might cause such imbalance, we will need to strengthen the weaker side. Do the roll-*downs* described in the correctives, but with the opposite elbow leading.

P (Psoas)

Lie supine with hands behind head. Raise both legs at the same time to a height of about eight inches above the floor or table and hold for ten seconds. Count seconds by adding a three-syllable word such as "chimpanzee" to the number. If the legs come down before the allotted ten seconds, enter the second of descent next to P, in Box A. If passed, enter a check. If there was difficulty, add the small *c*.

Box B: People who have weak *psoas* muscles often give evidence of this condition by presenting a swayback, or *lordosis*. If, when the legs are lifted, there is a pronounced arch in the back (see page 183), enter a check next to "Arch" and give considerable time to the correctives for the *psoas* at the end of the testing.

UB (Upper Back)

Lie prone with feet held down and hands clasped behind head. Raise the upper body high enough so that the chest can clear the table. If the subject lacks the needed back flexibility or has large breasts, she would require more than the normal flexibility in order to clear the table. Put a pillow under the hips. That will also be the solution if the person has back pain and lacks even that minimum strength for painless hyperextension. Hold the lift for ten seconds. Enter a check for pass in Box A next to UB. Enter *0* for failure to hold the full ten seconds and a *c* if the pass is accomplished with difficulty. Few fail to pass this test unless there are trigger points causing spasm and pain. Once the back *and groin* are cleared of trigger points, it is usually easy. *No* European child failed to pass. Do the correctives if difficulty or failure was encountered.

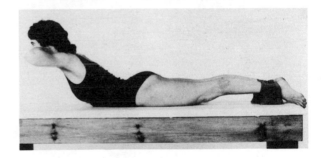

LB (Lower Back)

Lie prone with upper body held down, and raise both legs so that most of the thighs clear the table. Count a ten-second hold and then enter the score next to LB, in Box A. Do the correctives if needed.

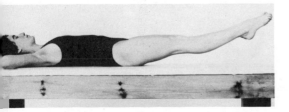

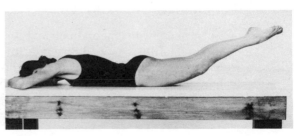

BHF (Back and Hamstring Flexibility)

Stand with feet together and knees held straight. Bend forward from the hips and try to touch the floor in front of the toes. Hold the reach for a slow count of three. If the floor is touched and the touch held for three seconds, enter *T* for touch next to BHF, in Box A. If the fingers cannot reach the floor, enter the number of minus inches between fingertips and floor. See correctives. If the hold is held with difficulty, any injury, illness, enforced bed rest or even emotional stress will cause failure in this test. Do the correctives often throughout the day and every day.

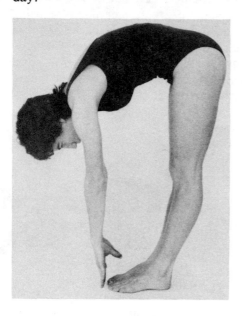

CORRECTIVES FOR THE KRAUS-WEBER TEST FOR MINIMUM MUSCULAR FITNESS

Abdominals (A + and A −)

Sit straight with knees bent and feet held down, arms stretched forward. Roll *slowly* down to the lying position, trying to feel each segment of the spine touch as you roll. When your back is flat on the floor, roll up to a sitting position again

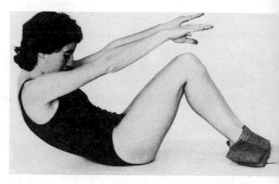

while throwing the arms forward to assist with the roll-up. Do five of those exercises night and morning, always remembering to take the descent as slowly as possible. At the end of a week, change to the next exercise.

Start at the top of the sit-up with arms folded in front of your chest, and roll *slowly* to the lying position. Then sit up with arms held the same way. It should be possible, but if it is still difficult, roll down with arms across the chest, but use the first exercise with arm-throw for your sit-up. Repeat five, night and morning, for a week. As soon as possible, sit up with arms across chest. The third week, roll down with hands clasped behind head and up with arms across the chest.

By the end of the third week you should be able to do five sit-ups morning and night with hands crossed behind your head; these should be made a part of your daily routine. To increase abdominal strength with little effort, carry a book behind your head for extra weight. See page 166 for weight bags, which are more convenient.

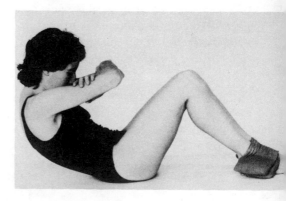

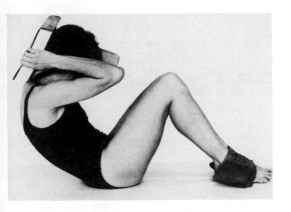

slowly, so that *all* parts of the muscles will be worked evenly. Bent-knee sit-ups are safe.

To strengthen the *psoas*, lie supine with knees bent above the torso. First, being sure your spine is tight to the table or floor, extend both legs overhead so that torso and legs form a right angle. Then lower the legs to the bent-knee rest position above the torso. Next, from the rest position extend the legs again, but a little closer to the support surface, *while being sure the spine is still down*. Retract to the rest position. Then extend and retract, each time a little lower, until you find you cannot keep the spine down. That means *substitution* is starting. Return to the angle of the last successful extension, when you could keep your spine down, and do five. Repeat five, morning and night, and very shortly you will find yourself able to go lower and lower as *psoas* strength improves. *Never* let any exercise person direct you to raise *straight* legs from the supine position to the right-angle position as an exercise. It will strain your back.

Psoas

The *psoas* is a very important muscle where the back is concerned. It attaches to the spine near the waist and also to the *lesser trochanter*, part of the *femur*, the thighbone. That means that when you do a sit-up with legs stretched, the *psoas* as well as the abdominals come into play. Fast straight-leg sit-ups with the hands clasped behind the neck (a favorite in boot camp and football practice) strain the back while doing little for the abdominals. *Never* do a straight-leg sit-up with the hands clasped behind the neck as an exercise, and when doing sit-ups, *do them*

Upper-Back Corrective

Lie prone and raise first the left arm and then the right. Alternate sides, being careful to keep the chest on the floor or table. Do not roll from side to side for greater lift. You want to strengthen the upper back and stretch the *pectorals*.

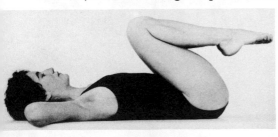

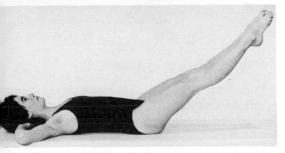

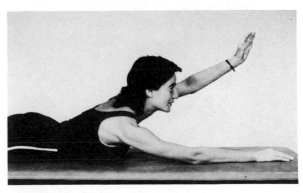

Lower-Back Corrective

Lie prone and lift first one straight leg and then the other from the hip. Alternate sides for eight; do three sets.

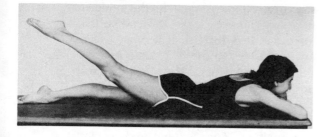

Flexibility-of-Back-and-Hamstrings Corrective

Stand with feet apart and hands clasped behind back. Lean forward from the hips while keeping the back level *and head up*. Bounce gently and rhythmically downward eight times. Then drop the arms and upper body downward and bounce again for eight counts. This makes up a set. Do three sets when you do your daily work on correctives, but also try to remember to do these bounces often during the day. Stress is daily and usually all day long. Stress shortens muscles, especially those of the back and hamstrings, and therefore working against this shortening should be made a part of every hour of the day.

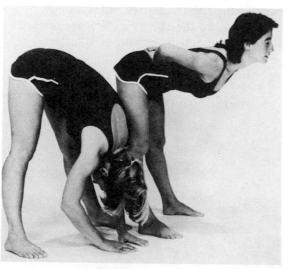

Scoliosis

A lateral curvature of the spine, scoliosis is easy to discover while you are testing for minimum strength and flexibility. It is covered later on in the book on page 167, but make a practice of looking for it in every test you make.

Scoliosis Test

Have the subject stand with back to you and feet apart. As he/she leans *slowly* downward as though to touch the floor, stoop over to watch the level of the back. If one side rises higher than the other at any time during the descent, a *scoliosis* is present. Enter the fact in Box B and check with the work to be done for the condition.

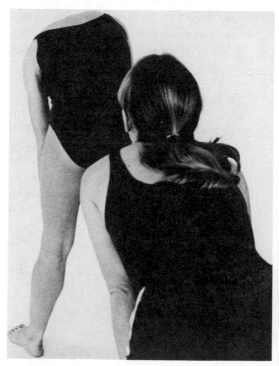

Round Back

Round back, or round shoulders, or in its extreme form, *kyphosis*, causes a great deal of discomfort, gives the sufferer a defeated look and even limits the action of the lungs. It usually begins either because an accident has put trigger points into the *pectoral* muscles, which cause spasm and shortening of those muscles and overstretch of the upper-back muscles, or because there is an excess of emotional stress. There are, of course, the problems some teenage girls have: inability to accept growing size, which is making them taller than any one of their peers, especially male peers, or growing breasts before such a phenomenon is acceptable. Then they develop the *habit* of rounding and pulling in.

Of course, either a sport (usually basketball, which requires a constant forward reach with both hands) or an occupation (any close work with the hands) can cause round shoulders, as can the disease known as *osteoporosis* (an abnormal rarefaction of the bone resulting in demineralization), but it is usually preventable with a little *attention to trigger points in the chest muscles*, exercises to stretch those muscles, weight work to strengthen the upper-back muscles . . . and diet.

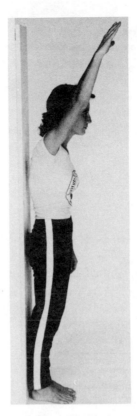

ficiency in minus inches, and aim with Myotherapy and exercise to obtain full stretch and touch with each wrist.

Kyphosis Test

The *kyphosis* test, or test for round shoulders, will show you where you are before you start your posture work, and later, how far you have progressed. Should you be in line for any chest operation, from open-heart surgery to mastectomy, the *kyphosis* test is a must, so you will know how to set your recovery goals. If you are not at *least* as flexible after you have rehabilitated yourself, you haven't completed the job, and *you*, not the operation, are at fault.

Stand with your feet together and your back to the wall. Press your heels, buttocks and shoulder blades against the wall and keep the contact. Raise first one straight arm and then the other, trying to see how close you can bring the back of your wrist to the wall. Measure the de-

Swayback

Swayback, or *lordosis*, is an abnormal curvature of the lumbar spine, which in itself can cause back pain, but the body's effort to substitute for impaired function can add pain in the upper back, the neck, the legs and the feet as well as the groin. Swayback is often seen in little girls and, oddly enough, in very active youngsters. They often develop the *habit* of a swaybacked stance in the playpen. When confined, active children try to better their condition by standing, but the bars provide a constant hold of regulation playpen height, and the "best" position for the baby's hold is one with the feet back from the bars but the chest in toward them, causing a swayed position. To correct swayback (lordosis), use the exer-

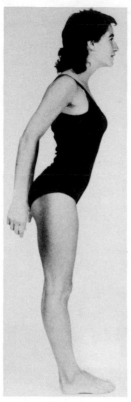

cises for the *psoas* in the correctives. In addition, do the cat-back exercise, page 143.

Pigeon Toes

Pigeon toes are easy to spot (and easy to fall over). They are *not* normal. Not long ago, an orthopedic surgeon told me, "All the good athletes have pigeon toes, and I used to try to imitate them when I was little. They really don't matter." But they do. A lot of athletes have a lot of problems, often resulting from old injuries, and pigeon toes can result from prenatal damage, so athletes substitute in order to accomplish what they want to do, and all the wrong muscles take over the jobs they were never designed for. This puts strain on them and additional strain on the muscles prevented from doing their allotted work by muscle spasm. This not only adds to the discomfort of the athlete but sets a whole generation of would-be athletes on the wrong track as they try to *imitate* the substitutions resorted to by their heroes.

If a child's feet (or anyone else's feet, for that matter) turn in, he or she needs Myotherapy to the insides of the legs from groin to ankle *and* a trigger-point search in the *gluteals* as well. Then the legs need to be stretched by turning them outward many times a day. Enter the fact of pigeon toes in Box B, and don't overlook them.

Turnout

Turned-out feet are another form of posture anomaly and, like pigeon toes, are usually due to muscles in spasm, but on the *outsides* of the legs. Check from hips to ankles, and stretch by turning in. Be sure to enter a check next to Turnout, in Box B, and while you are at it, check for flat feet, which often go with turnout.

Now you have a pretty good profile of your subject (and let's hope you took the same tests yourself, so that you know more about yourself than you did) and are ready to go to work charting a human body.

Make tracings of the following figures having to do with the head . . . and don't allow yourself to be intimidated by the names of muscles; they are no more complicated than Tiberius, Caligula, Claudius and Nero and even come from the same language, Latin.

From now on you will be mightily concerned with two facets of erasing pain: referred pain and the degree of pain felt and reported by the subject. *Pain erasure*, whether by quick fix or permanent fix, is a partnership. You *and the subject* have equal responsibility. You will contribute the objective part, and the subject will provide the subjective findings. *Before you start*, remind your friend that *you* don't know how much it hurts, and that far from distracting you with conversation, the more talk there is about the pain elicited, the easier and more efficient

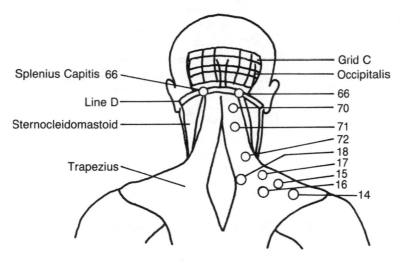

FIG. 24a: BACK OF HEAD, NECK AND UPPER BACK

your job will be. Also remind your friend that the pain is not supposed to be "unbearable," "agonizing," "frightful" or anything even close. If it is, then it's the subject's fault, because three little words, "Take it easy!" will lighten your pressure and keep any pain within bounds. When I work on little children, even as young as three, and I say, "I don't want you to *let* me hurt more than you can stand. Do you understand?" Yes, they understand and so do I. When a timid "Take it easy" or "Stop" is sounded or a little hand is raised, I ease off. They soon find, as your friend will, that *they* are in charge, and after that most of them will take a lot more discomfort than when tense and terrified. Also keep in mind that your friend may have been intimidated and hurt, as I was by someone who said scathingly, "Oh, you're just scared; keep quiet." Both you and the subject will be surprised to find that, after a few sessions, he or she may take over, saying, I think there's one a little to the left, or maybe a shade higher, farther in or out. Then, when you follow his or her directions, bull's-eye!

It is not necessary for the subject to be in pain in order to do permanent fix. Trigger points in residence will respond even when pain is absent.

The maps you are about to make are the responsibility of *both* of you. That's one way Dr. Travell took my mind off the trigger-point injections, which are far more painful than simple pressure. I knew I was *helping* when I told her what I felt. You not only want to know if the trigger point kept its pain to itself in the spot under pressure, but if it referred pain to another area, and exactly where the bell rang. In addition, you want to know how painful your pressure is on a scale of one to ten. Explain too that you will both save time and effort if the subject will respond with "Just pressure" when there is no responding pain but merely the feeling of pressure that any *healthy* muscle would feel if pressed.

In permanent fix you have time, privacy and a comfortable place to work. You also have your maps before you waiting to be filled in. Use a blue pen for the first mapping, red for the second and yellow for the third (then make a new map!) Have your subject strip to underwear, a bathing suit or a leotard. You don't need to see skin, but it helps. As in quick fix, where undressing is impossible you have to go by felt muscle outline. You are about to embark on the great adventure of our century: that of erasing pain.

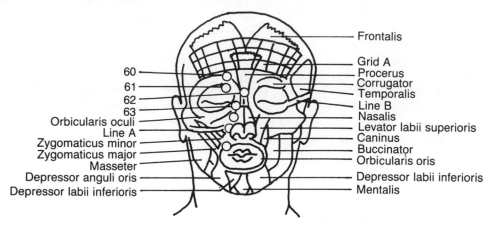

FIG. 24b: FRONT OF HEAD AND FACE

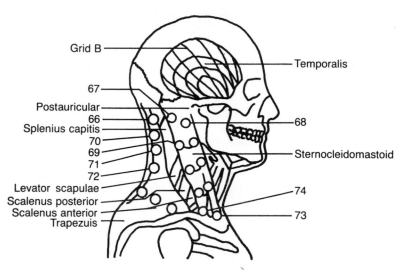

FIG. 24c: THE NECK

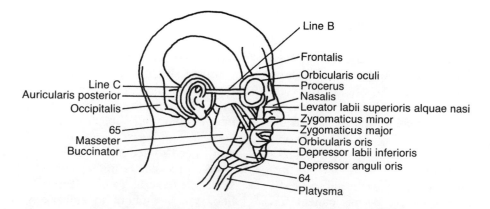

FIG. 24d: THE SIDE OF THE HEAD, FACE AND NECK

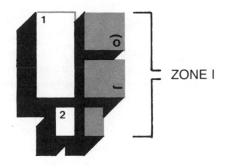

ZONE I

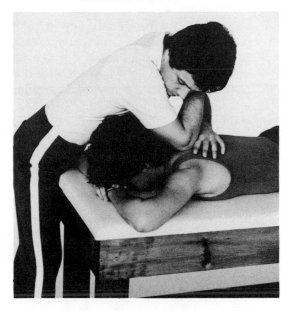

ZONE I, SEGMENTS 1 AND 2: THE BACK OF THE HEAD AND NECK.

Have your subject prone on the table and check with Figure 25. Start with circle 66, the *splenius capitis*, doing *both* sides, as usual. Follow that with the three circles down either side of the neck, just as you did in quick fix.

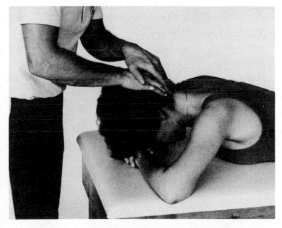

When you reach the fourth circle on that line, circle 18, the distal, or farther, end of the *splenius capitis*, change from fingers to elbow and lean across the body for better leverage and control. Be sure your compass technique is thorough and you miss none of the trigger points. Check the sprinkling of dots around circle 18, in Figure 25, and consider each one important. One of the reasons acupuncture, acupressure and even trigger-point-injection therapy often fail to achieve *permanent* relief is that there are infi-

nitely more trigger points than was at first suspected. The *matrix* points have been pretty well identified, but their children, the satellites, have not. Those satellites do not seem to conform to any map yet drawn, but are determined by the way each individual has lived, what his or her sports, accidents and occupations have been, and even by the personality of each individual. That is why you spent so much time on history.

Next look at Line D, on which you found the *splenius capitis*, circle 66. You will note the black dots all the way across, from ear to ear. Line D also covers the base of the *occipitalis*, the muscle covering the back of the head under Grid C. On page 36 you learned the *roller*

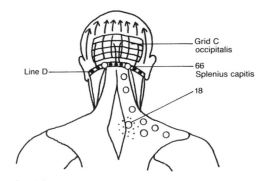

FIG. 25: BACK OF HEAD, NECK AND UPPER BACK

technique, and it is needed now. Use it, rolling the knuckles *slowly* over each square on the grid, halting for the required five seconds wherever you discover sensitivity. Carry your rolling technique as far to the side as the ears and right up to the top of the head. Keep in mind the trigger point at the top of my head just right of center that made a complaining invalid out of a perfectly healthy tooth.

When you have finished, place your fingertips in a slightly spread position and, using the thumb for stabilization, press against the scalp as you make small circles with the fingers, moving the scalp over the skull. The scalp is not supposed to be glued tight to the muscles that cover the bony cranium. If it is stiff and resistant you are dealing with muscle spasm, and the area will need more work. Not only does such spasm cause headache, it can make shampooing a most unpleasant event. Mothers may wonder why one or another of their babies screams like a banshee at bath time, especially when it comes to hair washing. Almost none know that it is neither fear of the water nor bad temper, but trigger points making what should be a fun time into a nerve-wracking chore. The baby may well grow up to hate the hairdresser more than the dentist, depending on where the trigger points are.

When you have what is usually called a colicky baby, go over the history just completed and write down all you can remember about the baby's birth and also what it looked like when you first saw it. A forceps delivery is often responsible. First comes the headache, which the baby protests and, while crying, swallows air. That brings on the colicky stomachache. Usually the formula or breast milk is blamed for the painful distress, but changing the formula or replacing the breast milk with formula rarely solves the problem; the headache continues and so does the noise.

To test for this condition, wait until the baby is *not* crying, and then press *lightly* on two or three points on the baby's face. If the first pressure elicits a grimace and the next two or three produce a wail, you have hit trigger points and probably erased three. Trigger points in the baby's facial muscles or those under the scalp require only a three-second hold. If you try for three points three times a day it won't be long before the pain is gone, the endless crying over and bath time a delight.

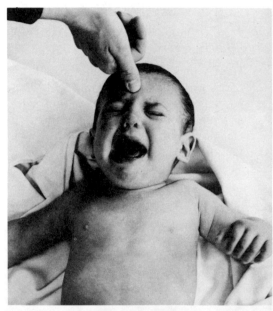

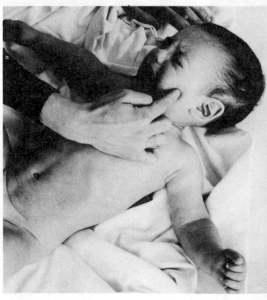

If vacuum extraction was used during the baby's birth or if Pitocin caused a very speedy birth, or if labor was induced by breaking the bag of waters, thus removing the protective cushion in the earlier stages of labor, you will probably find trigger points on the top of the head, the sides and the back. Do a little gentle massage from time to time to encourage healing through increased circulation.

When you have completed the back of the head, the neck and circle 18, have the subject do:

The Prone Neck-Stretch Exercise

Rise up on both elbows, allowing the head to hang loose to stretch the neck, *occipitalis* and the top of the upper back. Hold the hang for about three seconds and then, keeping the chin as close to the chest as possible, turn the face to the left and hold for three seconds, then three seconds to the right. Those three moves make up a set. Rest for a few seconds in between and then repeat. Do three sets.

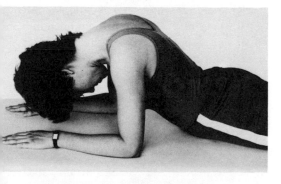

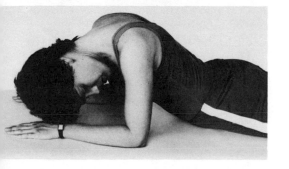

Angry-Cat and Old-Horse Exercise

Start in the hands-and-knees position with arms held straight. Press the entire back up into an arch and drop the head to stretch the muscles you have just freed and also neighboring muscles that might affect the newly relaxed muscles if they are also harboring trigger points.

Keeping the arms straight, allow the back to fall in like the sagging back of an old horse. If it will not arch down into a sag, suspect trigger points in the groin, *abdominals* and fronts of the thighs. Those areas need work. This is especially true if your subject has a "flat back" (having very little lumbar curve). Do this exercise eight times night and morning.

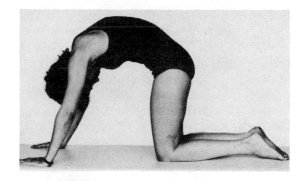

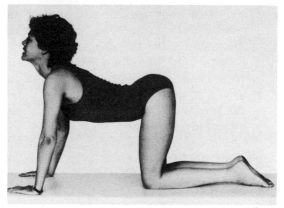

Thread-Needle Kneeling Exercise

Hands-and-knees position. Reach through between the supporting hand and the knees as far as possible to stretch the upper back, then carry the arm back through and upward, pointing to the ceiling. Follow the hand movement with your eyes. Do four on each side to make up a set. Do four sets daily.

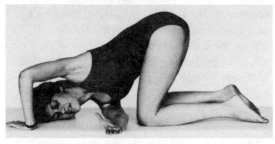

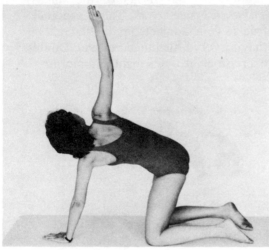

Follow your work on the back of the head with the sides, the *temporalis*, first on one side, then the other. Use the same roller technique. When you have completed your trigger-point work, press the area with the heel of your hand and move the muscles as far as they will go in every direction.

The *orbicularis oris* is indicated by the black dot just above the lip in Figure 26; it is involved in all lip movements. It is very like the *orbicularis oculi*, which circles the entire structure of the eye (page 57). The *orbicularis oris*, circling the mouth, is especially important to you if you have a baby who cries during or after sucking. The entire muscle is suspect when there is any interference with *any* lip movement.

Place your thumb on the spot signified by the dot and begin your search. You will be pressing the muscle against the *maxilla*, the bone of the upper jaw. Using the compass, search as far in all directions as the skin will allow from that first point of contact. Anyone who has had dental work in this area will probably have sensitive spots and be pleasantly surprised to find how relaxed the face feels once the search is complete.

Go around the *orbicularis oris* across the upper lip at finger-breadth intervals just as you did around the eye. At the corners of the mouth you will be pressing against clenched teeth, and as you press *back* you will encounter the leading edge of the *masseter*. There is almost always a sensitive spot there, which you will investigate thoroughly in a moment. As you come around under the lower lip you will be pressing on the *mandibula*, the horseshoe-shaped bone of the lower jaw, the largest and strongest bone in the face. The *mandibula*, which plays an important role in jaw pain (usually called TMJD, temporomandibular joint dysfunction), is very much like those tombstones we spoke of earlier, the vertebrae that are all set up in a line until some vandal pulls them out of line. If one of the powerful muscles attached to the *mandibula* houses a trigger point that throws it into spasm, the jaw *joint* may well respond with pain and the diagnosis be *malocclusion*. Too often that diagnosis is followed by grinding down teeth, fitting splints and retainers and even braces, which are designed to *urge* the jaw back into line and balance. One cannot *urge* a spasmed muscle anywhere, and the jaw muscles are incredibly powerful. Not long ago a dentist who worked for years to relieve TMJD watched a Myotherapist render his wife painless and bring the jaw muscles into equilibrium. "I can't believe it's all so simple," he said. "I've been doing this work for twenty years, and you've had such success in twenty minutes." It does seem unbelievable very often, but if you understand that a muscle in spasm will not respond to force other than to exert still more force or at the very least match that force, you can appreciate why TMJD is a hard nut to crack. But if you understand that a trigger point (at least one) is at work to keep the muscle in spasm and that erasing it will allow relaxation of the muscle, then it isn't so hard to appreciate. Increased force usually spreads the pain to include the teeth, the ears, the eyes, throat, head, mouth and shoulders. It may even bring on *tinnitus*, ringing in the ears.

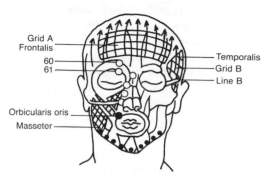

FIG. 26: FRONT OF HEAD AND FACE

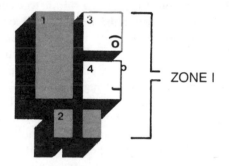

ZONE 1, SEGMENTS 3 AND 4: FRONT OF HEAD AND FACE

With the subject lying supine, stand at the head of the table and reach over the forehead to press on the *orbicularis oculi*, circles 60 and 61 on Figure 26. The *orbicularis oculi* is the muscle that circles the eye and is your takeoff point for the front of the face and head. Mark down any trigger points you uncover on your map and check out the *procerus*, between the eyes. Do the three circles running down the side of the nose from the corner of the eye to the nostril on both sides. Then do Line B, with its three sensitive spots between the corner of the eye and the ear. Stretch by pressing near the temple and moving the tissue under your fingers in every direction. Do both sides. You learned this in *Quick Fix*.

To stretch the area around the eyes,

keep them closed as you raise the eyebrows as high as possible. Then scrunch the face tight like a kid eating a lemon. Finally, relax, and with eyes closed, look left, right, up and down. That makes up a set. Do three with a few seconds rest in between.

After the eye-muscle stretch, apply the roller technique to Grid A, the *frontalis* muscle. Carry this work right up to and including the top of the head. Have the subject turn the head to the side the better to expose Grid B.

The black dots along the lower edge of the *mandibula* in Figure 26 have a matching row of spots just under the jaw. If you place your thumb on each of the spots you can see, and a curved forefinger *under* the jaw, you will trap any trigger points in the *platysma* muscle, underneath, and several other muscles in the face, of which the lower edge of the *masseter* is the most important in TMJD.

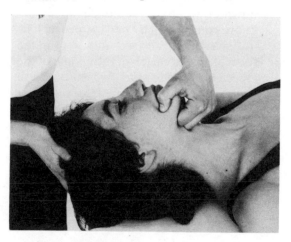

When this muscle is behaving, it closes the jaw smoothly and evenly, but often, as stress levels rise and trigger points come alive, it causes uneven jaw pressure and both grinding and clenching of teeth. It is exactly like those powerful thigh muscles, which, when they go into spasm, pull on the knee and cause pain in the joint. Conventional medicine usually looks for trouble in the knee *joint* and the jaw *joint*, but the question "What is *causing* the knee to lock or the jaw to run off the track?" is seldom asked. Usually the cause is a trigger point throwing the powerful muscles into spasm so that they cannot perform the functions for which they were designed. Not only is their own work curtailed, but they can cause trouble in the neighboring structures and in the face. That's a large order. What is needed most of the time is neither a brace nor a splint (same with the knee), but a trigger-point search and some stretching exercises.

The *masseter*'s action can be felt if you will place both hands on the sides of your face while your jaw is relaxed. Tighten the jaw muscles by clenching your teeth and you will feel them bulge against your fingers. This is the famous "frustration muscle" you are feeling. This is the muscle you tighten when you close your finger in the drawer or when the screen door slams *again*, right after you have said, "If that door slams again I'll kill somebody." It is the *masseter* that clamps down on what you would like to say but know you can't and keep the peace. The *masseter* houses masses of misery in the form of spasm smack in the middle of the face. One way to start that misery is to smack a child (or anyone else) on either side of that face. A slap stings for a moment, and even though the slapper is ashamed of having done such a thing in a fit of temper, he or she is not unduly worried. The kid probably deserved it. Not so. Whatever the youngster did, it can't be bad enough to deserve months and often years of TMJD facial pain as

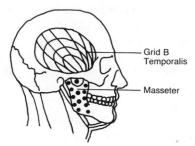

FIG. 27: SIDE OF HEAD AND FACE (JAW)

an adult. It may not surface for a long time, until the emotional climate around that person turns sour. *Any* blow to the face can lay down trigger points in the *masseter*, and *any* frustration, especially the kind you'd rather not admit to even to yourself, can light them up. If one morning you wake with jaw pain after a fight with You-know-who and the dentist says, "Malocclusion. Splints may help," think *masseter* and trigger points. Ask yourself whether there isn't some other "mal" in your life besides your jaw and whether setting it to rights shouldn't come first before expensive dentistry. You may be lucky if dentistry is all you'll be sent to find. Jaw pain can refer in all directions, and there's a specialist at the end of each directional arrow.

TMJD pain can take in the head, face, ears, eyes, throat, neck, chest, shoulders, upper back, arms, hands and *axilla*. Every one of those structures can *cause* TMJD.

Conventional medicine and dentistry handle the pain with injections, analgesics, splinting, grinding teeth down so the two sides of the jaw match, retainers and braces. Sometimes root-canal jobs are done on perfectly healthy teeth. Occasionally such teeth are extracted, but the pain continues. It hurts in the jaw, all right, and the jaw is certainly offside. Gadgets that are used to test the equilibration of the *mandible*, the lower jawbone, prove it all too convincingly, just like the X rays showing arthritis of the spine. X rays will have to be taken of the jaw, too, but muscles in spasm don't advertise that fact on X rays, and the dentist remembers only one word from dental school: *equilibrate*. I've said it before and I'll say it again: you can't *force* a muscle. Something is causing the *masseter*, the "frustration muscle," to spasm. The dentist usually grinds down the teeth on one side, gets a good equilibration test and shakes hands with a happy patient. A week, a month or two pass and the patient is back with the same pain and the same uneven jaw. This can't be repeated too often because teeth aren't tall enough for much grinding down. Next, splints, retainers and braces, but while such aids can direct teeth into straight lines and keep them there, they have little or no effect on muscles in spasm. Try to imagine that you have the little finger of the nastiest, meanest, most hateful person you know between your teeth. If you bit down as hard as you could, you would go right through that finger, not just to the bone, right through a knuckle, gristle and all. Now imagine that kind of power *out of control*. That's what the TMJD sufferer has to deal with, muscles that to some degree are out of control, and no piece of metal or plastic is going to do the job. We have to find the *cause* for the spasm, the trigger points in the muscle in spasm *and those at the other end of the line*.

When we deal with TMJD using Myotherapy, we start our hunt in the hands and arms; some dentists who have begun to use Myotherapy have now equipped their offices with treatment tables so that they can do a complete job from the soles of the feet to the top of the head. After all, a long second toe could start the imbalance, and so could a leg that is not quite as long as its mate.

The *axilla* is like a nest of hornets where the head, face and neck are concerned, and what joins the *axilla*? The chest. Women who do fine needlework, crochet or knit often set their muscles up for spasm. So do men who are jewelers, etchers or accountants with their files of

figures. Spasm in the hands signals the arms, the upper back and the chest. The resulting pain sometimes mimics heart attack, and all the reassurance in the world won't convince the person in the middle of the night that death isn't imminent. Only getting rid of the spasm will do that. But ask your patient what she/he does with the hands.

Starting trigger-point work for the jaw in the outlying districts does four things. It locates trigger points that either cause or contribute to spasm in the jaw muscles. Secondly, Myotherapy is like a warm-up exercise: it opens up constricted areas and allows the blood to circulate more freely. This in turn improves nutrition to the area and speeds healing. A warm muscle is even more flexible, and the jaw can be opened wider without causing subluxation (a partial dislocation). And something else: the patient relaxes. Many people after having Myotherapy say they feel spacey. Some, whose normal manner could be likened to a cup of Mexican jumping beans, crave a nap. It is thought that Myotherapy may activate endorphins, the brain's own, self-manufactured pain controllers. In any case, a dentist who uses Myotherapy as a tool will get far better results with TMJD than will the one who relies on the old methods.

Note in Figure 27 how the *masseter* covers the jaw joint and that there are black dots all along both leading and trailing edges. They can be randomly sprinkled in the middle as well. Have your subject relax her jaw by opening her mouth slightly (there are 4 million TMJD cases reported annually and 3,800,000 are women). You start your search on the leading edge by pressing into the cheek and then back. If the jaw is subluxated and you find the trigger points, it will slip back in. If you have a jaw that subluxates from time to time, take a good look at your life and also the circumstances you are under when it happens. There is a lot of truth in the title of the book *Who's the*

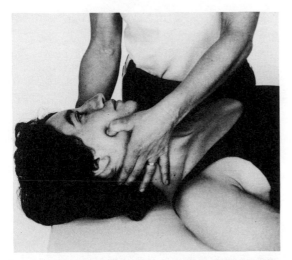

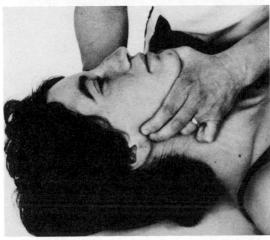

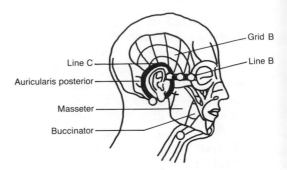

FIG. 28: SIDE OF JAW

on the outside of the cheek opposite the finger inside. Have the subject relax the jaw and you will find you have trapped some very mean trigger points between your two fingers. Clear out as many as you can find, always remembering that facial trigger points are especially painful and the subject may want some respite from time to time. While you are in the mouth, check every trigger point you can locate in the gums and both the floor and the roof of the mouth.

To stretch the jaw, open and close the mouth several times.

Check with Figure 26 and note the cross-hatchings on the face laterally to the nose. The *zygomaticus* muscles often house trigger points. See if you can unearth a few.

Matter with Me? You could replace the word *me* with *my jaw* and be close most of the time. To get the other edge of the *masseter*, start just below the ear and press forward.

Inside the mouth there is another minefield sown with trigger points. Ask your subject to open her mouth and, keeping your palm facing *inward*, press your forefinger as far back as you can between cheek and teeth. Then ask your subject to gently close her mouth so that her teeth come together next to the front of your finger. The tip of your finger will fit snugly in a pocket between the teeth and what will feel like a tight band. Then have her clench her teeth, and the *masseter* will grip about one third of your finger. Place the forefinger of your free hand

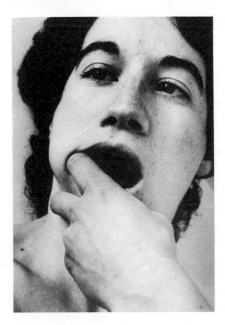

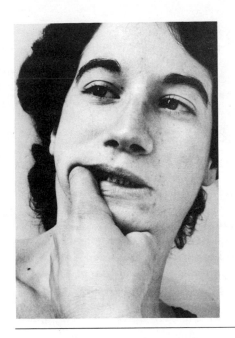

Turn the subject's head to the side and, using your fingers or knuckles, press at finger-breadth intervals all the way around Line C, which circles the ear, covering the *auricularis* and *temporalis* muscles. If you have not yet used the roller technique on Grid B, do so at this time. Stretch by using the heel of the hand to move the scalp in all directions.

Use the same technique for *tinnitus* (ringing, roaring, hissing, etc., in the ears). The problem is very rarely *in* the ear, but, rather, caused by spasms in the muscles somewhere in Zone I, II or even III. Remembering that neighboring structures often affect each other and that the mouth is very neighborly indeed to any structure in the head and neck, check out the entire area.

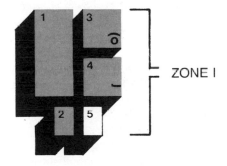

ZONE I

and bad, and appearance. A proud head depends on the cooperation of the neck muscles, and so does the hangdog look.

Air passes through the neck to the lungs and food to the stomach; the neck is a periscope that permits us to observe

ZONE I, SEGMENT 5: FRONT OF THE NECK

The neck is extremely vulnerable and houses some very important structures. It is the conduit through which passes the life's blood to and from the brain via the *carotid artery* and the *jugular vein*. The *larynx*, which makes instant communication possible, nests there, as does the *thyroid gland*. The neck depends on the seven fragile cervical vertebrae, which, when moved by powerful muscles of the neck, contribute to posture, both good

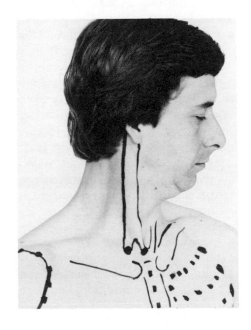

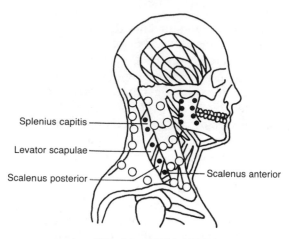

Splenius capitis

Levator scapulae

Scalenus posterior

Scalenus anterior

FIG. 29: NECK, SIDE VIEW

the world in every direction. It is a valuable piece of equipment and needs very special care, the more so since loss of function can be crippling. There are some very unpleasant injuries that can befall the neck; of these the most common is whiplash, but the most obvious is a condition called torticollis, Latin for twisted (tortus) neck (collis). This condition can start at or even before birth, from any one of a number of types of accidents and can even be the result of the limitation of movement imposed by an occupation, say playing the violin. One or more muscles go into spasm and pull the neck like those vandals in the graveyard and the neck takes on a life of its own. It may turn to one side only, and any attempt to bring the head to the forward position meets with failure. The head may even be pulled down so tight to the shoulder that it appears to be resting. Nothing could be further from the truth. The neck suffering with torticollis cannot relax; even when the rest of the body is asleep the spasm maintains that tortured position. Conventional treatment often includes being strung up in a head hammock to produce traction. Traction for any extended period (minutes can sometimes count as an extended period) can and often does cause additional damage to injured muscles.

Usually the muscle in trouble in torticollis is our old friend SCM, the *sternocleidomastoid*. You have already learned how to deal with that in *Quick Fix*. Another muscle that seems to be involved in torticollis is the *trapezius*, in the back of the neck. To those add the *levator scapulae*, which attaches to the upper four cervical vertebrae and to the *scapula*, or shoulder blade. Shrug your shoulders and you have activated those muscles. Now, the next time you look at a group of little children, watch for the one whose shoulders are pulled halfway up to his ears *as a habit*. Not only does he look inadequate and scared to death, he is setting his shoulders and neck up for lots of pain and stiffness. Look at the teenager who has those same shoulders and you will notice that what started there has now spread to the *pectorals*, which has given him a round-shouldered look. In time the head will jut forward to put even more pressure on the neck. This condition is called a "forward head." Imagine what all this strain can do to the jaw.

The cervical vertebrae are a continuation of the thoracic vertebrae, which the contracted chest muscles have been pulling into a deeper than normal curve since nursery-school days. As the neck follows the exaggerated curve, the head tips downward. Unless some substitution is made, all the subject can see is the ground in front of her feet. In order to see efficiently, the head must be raised. Try it yourself and notice the strain in the back of your neck. Besides, it looks awful. While a forward head involves all of the neck, upper-back and chest muscles, it starts with the *levator scapulae*.

Turn the subject's head a little to the side and press all four fingers into the neck back of the *sternocleidomastoid*. Hold the pressure for the usual five seconds and then stretch by turning the head as far as possible in the same direction. Continue down the line at half-inch intervals, and the next two or three pres-

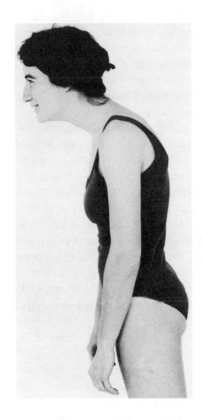

sures will trap trigger points in the *sca-lene* muscles, which attach to the sixth and seventh cervical vertebrae and raise the first and second ribs. Later, when you are trying to alleviate trouble in the chest, remember that it is not enough to check out the *sternum* (breastbone), the *clavi-*

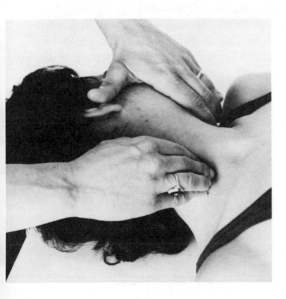

cles, the *pectoral* muscles and the *inter-costals*; the *scalene* and all the neck muscles may well play a part.

The neck muscles should be explored for *any* problem in Zone I, but also those in Zones II and III: asthma, emphysema, heartburn, shoulder and arm pain, upper-back spasms, angina, mock angina, chest pain from overwork or sports, aching after a fall, colds, flu, fever, posture anomalies, work-related pain and even disease such as arthritis, stroke, MS or lupus.

Cervical arthritis with spurs is a scary diagnosis, and there is no question that it can be seen on the X rays even though you may need a little help when you look, and *do look*. Be very sure those are *your* X rays you are looking at. Today's hospitals are not noted for efficiency. Sometimes they lose X rays altogether.

If the pain in your neck and the limited range of motion is so diagnosed, be aware that you have lots of company. Most middle-agers have some arthritis, but not all of them have pain. All the people who have come to us with that complaint improved their range of motion and had less pain within minutes. When trigger points were found and erased in neighboring muscles, the pain left. If they continued with their exercise programs, the muscles remained free of spasm and therefore of pain and they had good to excellent range of motion. *But* when they went for new X rays, the condition, including "spurs," was still there. In other words, while the arthritis may have contributed to the pain, especially at the start, the pain was basically muscular and therefore controllable with Myotherapy. So if your X ray says "arthritis," don't go into a tailspin. If you don't hurt, what does it matter if the X ray is a little cloudy?

Neck collars are like traction; they contribute more pain. Traction actually damages muscle fibers; neck collars immobilize. Years ago after a dive into a shallow pool, I developed one of those necks and I wasn't middle-aged yet either. The treatment was hanging daily in a head-traction gadget for half an hour and then a neck collar the rest of the time. These episodes used to come on about twice a year, and looking back now (how wonderful is hindsight) they occurred when life was just about unbearable, thus making it truly unbearable. Since we learned how to take the trigger points out of the muscles, I haven't had a neck or a back spasm, and there is no reason for you to have them either. So hang up your collar and check with *Quick Fix* and never, never string yourself up in a head halter again. Arthritis was never cause for a hanging.

Birth, accidents, sports and occupations twist and torture necks; so does age. Attend any meeting of senior citizens or go on a tour catering to the retired and you will see an assortment of rounded, often fibrositic (thickened) shoulders that would put the fear of God, aging and deformity into any intelligent person. No intelligent person should permit it to happen, and most of the time it is preventable *if* one has the necessary information. What rounds backs? Rogue muscles round backs. What turns a healthy, strong muscle into a destructive force? Spasm. What causes spasm? Usually trigger points. At the first sign of a rounding back *at any age*, but most especially at middle age, clear the trigger points from the head, neck, chest, upper back and arms. Exercise the affected muscles *and examine the life-style*. It won't get any better until *you* do something about it.

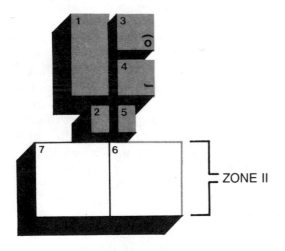

ZONE II, SEGMENTS 6 AND 7: CHEST AND BACK

The chest is like a basket stuffed with treasures. The basket part is made up of twelve pairs of ribs, an even dozen. They articulate with twelve thoracic vertebrae. That's twelve more neat little tombstones that are often blamed for upper-back pain. In front, the ribs are continued as cartilage. The upper seven are attached to the sternum and are called "true ribs." The lower five, which do not articulate with the sternum, are called "false ribs."

The treasures within are the heart and lungs, those organs of "aerobic" fame. Then of course there is the *thymus*, between the upper lobes of the lungs. Most people don't know what it is, where it is, or why it is. It reaches its maximum development in early childhood, and while it was once thought to be an endocrine gland, it is now considered part of the lymph system. So we don't just change our minds about surgical procedures like

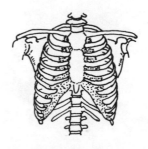

FIG. 30: BONES OF CHEST

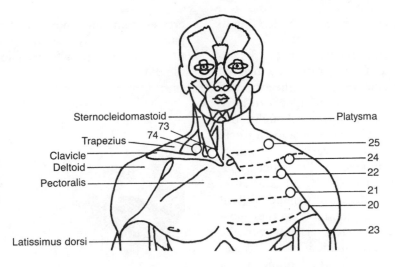

FIG. 31: THE TORSO, FRONT VIEW

tonsillectomies, we also change our opinions about internal organs.

There is also the *esophagus*, which comes from the Greek *oisophagos*, which breaks down to *oisein*, to carry, and *phagema*, food. It is the musculomembranous passage extending from the *pharynx*, in the throat, to the *stomach*.

The *trachea* is another treasure. It is the cartilaginous and membranous tube descending from the *larynx* to the left and

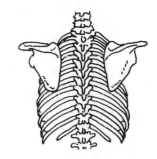

FIG. 32: THE BONES OF THE UPPER BACK

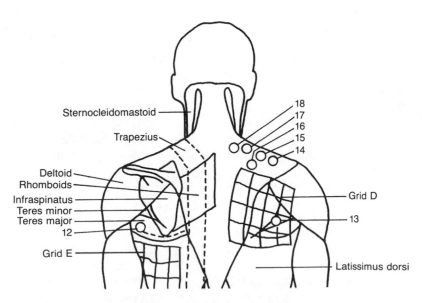

FIG. 33: THE UPPER BACK

right branches of the *bronchi*, leading to the lungs.

The back of the chest-basket looks unimpressive as far as bones go, just the twelve thoracic vertebrae, the ribs and the two *scapulae*, which appear to have been pasted on as an afterthought. But look closely at those ribs and those in front of the chest. Every single one of them is held in place and together by *intercostal* muscles. As the lungs attempt to fill with air, the chest expands fully if those intercostals (and a few other muscles) are free of spasm. If, however, the intercostals are loaded with trigger points, then there will be limiting spasm and sometimes pain. There will certainly be a limit on how much air you can take into your lungs (vital capacity).

If improving your *aerobic capacity* is the aim of your jogging program, you could jog from here to the Coast (if you could jog at all) and the improvement would be negligible. The same goes for the best athletes, but on a different level. If you want more air in your lungs, look to the *intercostals*.

Check with *Quick Fix* for the chest. You have already had some instruction in working over the *pectorals* and the *sternum*. What we have not yet covered is the muscle under the *pectoralis major*. It is the *pectoralis minor*.

The *pectoralis minor* attaches to the third, fourth and fifth ribs in front and the *scapula* in back. When, in an asthma attack, you feel pain in the front of your chest and also in back under the shoulder blade, the *pectoralis minor* may be at fault. When you fall on your back and it hurts *in front* when you try to take a deep breath, the injured *scapula* may be reaching through your chest to pull on your ribs via the *pectoralis minor*.

Slide your hand under the *pectoralis major* from the side and press on the ribs beneath. Hold any trigger point you find for the required seven seconds, then follow with the snap-and-stretch exercise, on page 70, in *Quick Fix*. Do those exercises night and morning, but if your pain is tied in any way to your occupation, make time for a few sessions during the day.

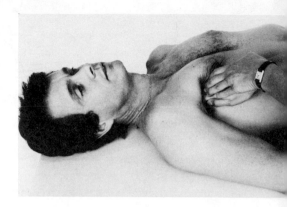

Broken or bruised ribs often come back to haunt with pain years after the event laid down a flock of trigger points in the *intercostals*. Nor did you have to break anything or manage a black-and-blue mark. Straining for breath in an asthma attack, coughing, sneezing, riding a bike, or bouncing on a snowmobile or a horse could do the same thing. Just accomplishing the serve of the year could also serve to prepare the *intercostals* for pain long after you have switched from tennis to golf. No one knows why Jim gets chest pain from pushing a lawn mower to make enough money to cover the gas bill for his jalopy, while a football player can have mayhem committed on him every Saturday and merely ruin his knees, but it happens.

Have the subject lie on his side over a folded pillow. This puts the *intercostals* on a slight stretch by opening the ribs. Use either your fingers or a small bodo to get at the trigger points between the ribs. Of course do both sides even if the pain is unilateral. It is helpful if you use a felt pen to mark each spot where a trigger point was unearthed, so you won't get lost. There are a lot of spaces between ribs, and the one you missed may be the granddaddy of the crowd.

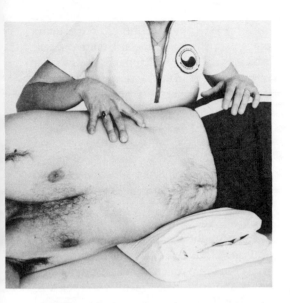

Intercostal Stretch

Take the same side-lying position over the pillow and take a weight bag or other fairly heavy object (an iron would do) in your free hand, allow the straight arm to move from above your head (preferably hanging over the table or bed) in a wide arc down to your side. As you raise the arm from side to overhead inhale fully. As you lower, exhale. Do eight to each side.

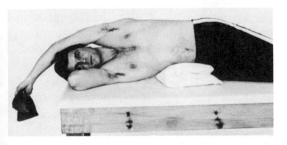

Asthma and Emphysema

If you are dealing with either of these conditions, start your trigger-point search on the *sternum*, as you did in *Quick Fix* on page 64, *then* add the *intercostals*. It is not necessary to wait for an attack; you can do the work anytime at all. There is a good chance you can make the next attack less exhausting. It is also possible

to abort an attack by doing a good job on the *sternum* and the *pectorales* major and minor at the first wheeze. Stress contributes greatly to asthma attacks, and the mere knowledge that one *can* be aborted is a huge help. It could go far toward lessening both the severity and the frequency of attacks.

Emphysema is a disease in which there is a pathological accumulation of air in the lungs that cannot be expelled. This limits the space that can make use of fresh air, with all the expected difficulties: breathlessness, fatigue and poor endurance. Myotherapy to the *intercostals* can help, as will the exercises made possible through improved flexibility and more efficient breathing.

Stitches

Stitches while running cause considerable pain in a sport that is supposed to be enjoyable. What causes them? Muscle spasm, and of course trigger points. Where do you look? In the *intercostals* and also in the *abdominals* (see page 154).

Heartburn

Heartburn is felt to start in the chest and rise from there, very often taking in the whole throat, and even the ears, with pain. It can be a very uncomfortable condition; some sufferers have to sleep propped up on pillows. It is said to be part and parcel of *hiatus hernia*, but it is very easy to eliminate. Start with the pectorals as you did in *Quick Fix* and add the back work to be presented in the next subsection of this section. Be sure to take in the *axilla*. One can only wonder if, when the only symptom of *hiatus hernia* is heartburn, the problem really is *hiatus hernia*. When you don't have the pain after doing Myotherapy to the suggested areas, maybe it wasn't hernia after all. If you still have the pain, then try including the work in Segment 14, in Zone IV, the *abdominals*.

Vital Capacity

One good way to see how well you have done with the *intercostals* is to test for vital capacity. *Before* you do the trigger-point work, put a tape measure around your chest and expel every bit of air you can. Really press down. Then fill your lungs completely and watch the tape measure for plus inches. Some people have as little as a half an inch expansion. Singers and mountain climbers can go as high as six inches. This is a quick way of checking aerobic improvement due to your exercise program or the efficacy of your Myotherapy attempts.

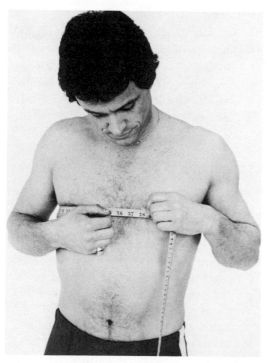

Breast Surgery

We have discussed what lies *in* the chest, but not what lies *outside*: the breasts. Some studies say that one woman in eleven in the U.S.A. will be stricken with breast cancer. Other studies report one in fourteen. It doesn't matter much which is right if you happen to be number one. What is true is that few doctors know of the exercises needed for post-mastectomy patients. That means that if a woman is to be really rehabilitated, she will have to find her own program. And going back to what we said in the beginning, since her physical *education* was so inadequate, what does she know that will help her to choose?

Before she chooses what exercises to do, she might want to choose what operation to have. There has been controversy raging over mastectomy these last years and, it appears, with good reason. One hundred years ago a very talented surgeon, Dr. William Halstead invented the operation called "radical mastectomy," one of the most mutilating operations we have. Often it leaves the chest sunken and the arm weakened and swollen. The "radical mastectomy" removes the entire breast, the muscles on the chest wall beneath it and the *axillary lymph nodes*, in the armpit.

Dr. Halstead's report on his first thirteen cases was buried in a long paper on the treatment of wounds, and subsequent reports were anecdotal and lacking in both statistical analysis and long-term follow-up. There was no firm evidence that his operation enhanced survival, yet *it* has survived since 1882. Why? Because he had a fine reputation. He was one of the founders of Johns Hopkins Medical School, in Baltimore, Maryland. He was the first surgeon to put his medical team into rubber gloves, and he developed regional anesthesia by injecting cocaine into nerves. He paid a heavy price for that one. First he became addicted to the cocaine and then to the morphine he used to help himself out of the cocaine addiction.

It wasn't until the late fifties, over seventy-five years later, that surgeons began experimenting with other therapies. Until then, if a woman experienced breast cancer, she was doomed to a "radical." Where did the first study to prove such mutilation unnecessary come from? Italy, the land that loves women and beauty. The study was done in the National Tumor Institute, in Milan. In that study seven hundred and one women took part, and while half were subjected to Halstead's "radical mastectomy," the other half had a very different procedure: only one fourth of the breast and *some* of the lymph nodes were removed. This was followed by six weeks of radiation therapy for both groups. After seven and a half years, the survival rate was the same for both groups. You can be assured, however, that neither the emotional nor the physical trauma was the same.

There is a new study going on today called "Lumpectomy." Dr. George Crile, Jr., in *Surgery, Our Choices and Alternatives* (New York: Delacorte Press, 1978), says that "Lumpectomy" plus the radiation treatment is just as effective as either the "radical" or "modified radical" mastectomy. Dr. Avram Cooperman, Professor of Clinical Surgery at Columbia University College of Physicians and Surgeons, says most women may not even need radiation after "Lumpectomy" and underarm-node removal.

We are getting smarter, it seems, and we are doing what I hope we will do more of. We are beginning to question. There has been a comparative study by Dr. Josef Vana at Roswell Park Memorial Institute, in Buffalo, New York. There were thirty thousand cases of breast cancer in 670 hospitals in the United States between 1972 and 1977. They have shown that there is a marked shift away from "radical mastectomy."

Studies like that should make us feel good about our own questioning and unwillingness to take anyone's word as gospel, *but* up pops something new. It is called "prophylactic mastectomy." That is breast removal "just in case." *The New England Journal of Medicine* reports that

it is being done *despite* the disagreement as to what constitutes "premalignant changes." No matter *what* your problem, question . . . *question* . . . QUESTION.

Whatever form of mastectomy you may have or have had, it is essential that you get back into condition, preferably better than the condition you were in before the operation. The arm and shoulder exercises on page 76 are good for starters, and the weights for the upper back will pull you into a proud, upright carriage. The snap-and-stretch and the backstroke will stretch the chest, *axilla* and arm muscles (*Quick Fix*, pages 69–70). Check your progress with the kyphosis test, page 137.

Pulley Exercises

The pulley exercises are ideal for starters after mastectomy or shoulder work. I invented the pulley for a friend who had had a "radical" over twenty years ago; no one could understand why she got back to full range and strength so quickly. The gadget makes use of a plastic pulley (don't buy a little or cheap one, they squeak and they don't *feel* good). You will need ten feet of quarter-inch nylon rope. Tie two dowel handles (four inches of broomstick for each handle will do) to the two ends of your rope after it has been threaded through the pulley. Then you will want about eight inches more of the nylon. Tie one end to the top of the pulley and make a good-sized knot at the other. Drop the knotted end over the top of the door and close it tight. Now you have a pulley for standing work. In the section called *Self Center* you will find a different way to attach the pulley for standing, sitting and even lying. If you wish to use the door for sitting or lying, just lengthen the piece of rope over the door to match the need.

If you are still in the hospital, ask for a support frame. When I was in the hospital for my second hip replacement, I used the frame for arms before I was allowed out of bed to try out the new hip. Two things are thus accomplished: Circulation is improved generally, and you never settle into any kind of acceptance of a hospital bed. Out is where you want to be, and *soon*.

Shorten the rope by wrapping it around the dowels, and use the "good" arm to stretch the painful arm gently to as full a stretch as possible. Then pull down with the painful one while giving a little resistance from the "good" arm. Set up a rhythm, preferably to music, and you will find the muscles responding with less and less discomfort and soon with both strength and range.

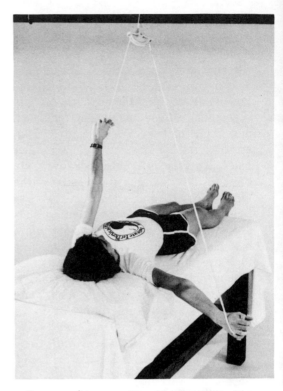

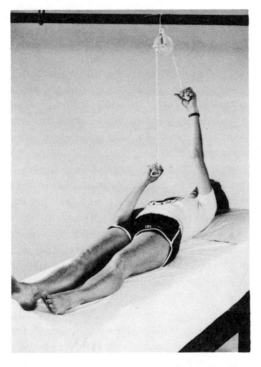

Next use a lateral pull by dropping first one arm to the side and then the other. Add to that a clock dial. Pretend your bed is the face of a clock, and as you drop the right arm to nine and the left to three, set up a rhythm. After a few pulls, press the right arm down to eight and the left up to two. Then move to seven and one and then reverse. Be sure to hold the rhythm.

Later, when considerable flexibility has been regained, "prone pully" can be used. The trick (and there is one) is pulling *down*. Each down pull paves the way for further stretch. Even if the lift is a fraction of an inch, that's a start. Eventually the lift increases. Lie prone with head resting on the support surface and pull down with first one arm and then the other. The arm being pulled up can offer any degree of resistance desired. Start with the arms parallel and gradually widen the distance between by reaching to the side.

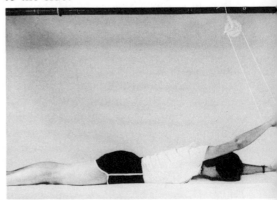

In time, shorten the rope so that the back arches and, when the arms are even, the chest is off the table. This causes the subject to "hang in" the ropes and the stretch will be more extreme. Always let your body tell you how much to do, and if the subject is a compulsive overdoer, monitor the exercises carefully. Overdoing usually sets one back and causes discouragement, not to mention pain.

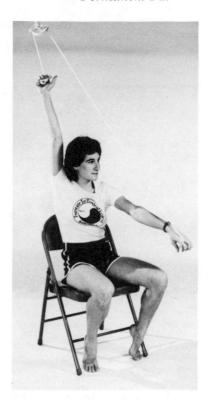

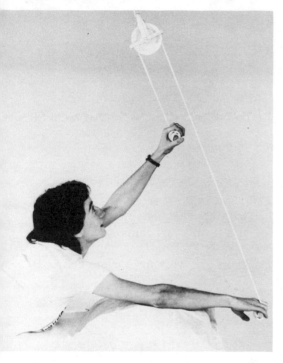

Using the pulley while sitting in a chair is good for both post-op patients and for those confined either temporarily or indefinitely to a wheelchair. Sitting encourages inflexibility not only in the legs, but in the arms, chest and shoulder girdle as well. Be sure to use music; the average popular tune runs from two and a half to three minutes. Start with *one* minute and work up to three, a complete band or record. You can increase the work load without increasing the time, by offering more resistance yourself.

Standing exercises with the pulley work the torso, arms and shoulder girdle from every angle. Start with feet apart facing the pulley and work free without

resistance for a few bars of music and then begin to add light resistance. When you are strong enough to desire really heavy resistance, check with the *Self Center* section, and use the weight bags.

To stretch the chest muscles, face away from the pulley with arms spread. Start in the upright position and gradually work down toward the floor.

To stretch and strengthen the sides, turn sideways to the pulley and pull the arm on the away side overhead. *Always* do both sides even though only one may *seem* to need it. As you work with the pulley you will find many ways to use it. The key to staying with it, however, is music.

Trigger Points and Scar Tissue

There are usually trigger points wherever there is scar tissue. As it is with other trigger points, which nest all over the body, they can be dormant for years or active from the first wounding. If they

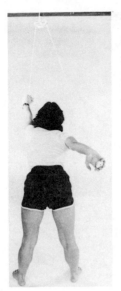
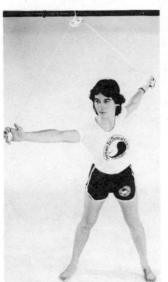
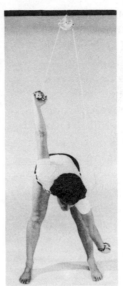
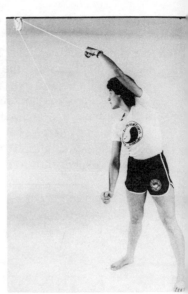

Standing exercises with pulley

are active you can't miss it, because you will hurt, but they do other things that are less attention-getting and which in a way are more damaging. One of these is to cause stiffness. "Well," you say, "you can expect stiffness after an operation." Of course you can, but not for long. The stiffness needs work, and unless you get after the trigger points the stiffness becomes permanent as muscles shorten. Another thing that trigger points do is cause weakness. "Well," you say (and so does just about everybody else), "you can expect weakness after an operation." True, but not for long. If weakness and stiffness persist, think *trigger points* and go to work on them.

Be very gentle at first, using searching fingertips along the scar edges. Keep track of where you hunted and just how bad the trigger points were, *from day to day*. If on Monday they were "screamers" but on Wednesday they were merely "grumblers," you have made progress.

If you are dealing with chest scars, keep in mind that the chest is the other side of the upper back, the bottom of the neck and the top of the *abdominals*.

Every one of those areas may be involved and most certainly the *axilla* and the arms as well. Don't just think "scar," think "neighbors." Consider all of those neighbors and work them over. You want your body back.

ZONE II, SEGMENT 7: UPPER BACK

The first thing to notice about the back is the line running down the middle, designating the spine. Certified Bonnie Prudden Myotherapists do not "manipulate" the spine; we never touch it.

Back in *Quick Fix*, in Figure 5 you cleared out the trigger points at the *teres major*, at circle 12. Then you did circle 13, over the *scapula*, and also the ones up in the shoulder area, circles 14 through 18. To do a really good job you will need to check out the entire upper back, starting with those two lines running down the back just left of the spine. When you have done the left side, you must then follow with the right.

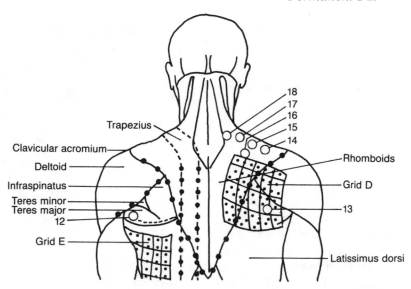

FIG. 34: THE UPPER BACK

You already know *why* the upper back runs into so much trouble. It is both underexercised and overworked. In older people, there is often so much spasm and so little elasticity that the upper back, mid-back and lower back seem to have coalesced into one solid mass.

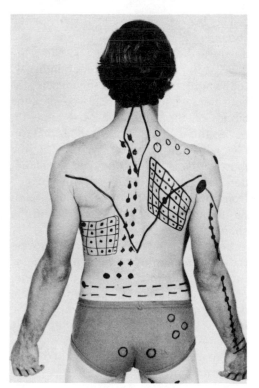

The cape-shaped *trapezius*, which we have already met in Zone I, Segment 1, the back of the head, and Segment 2, the back of the neck, attaches to the *occipital* bone on Line D and the spinous process of the seventh cervical vertebra, all twelve thoracic vertebrae and the *clavicular acromion*. It is one of the muscles you *must* strengthen if you want freedom from round back and poor posture. Imagine what multiple trigger points in the *trapezius* could do to augment pain in its associate and near neighbor the chest.

The *infraspinatus* attaches to the *scapula* and the *humerus*, the bone of the upper arm. So while the pain may be in the arm, the cause may be in the back, and vice versa.

The *rhomboid major* attaches to the second, third, fourth and fifth thoracic vertebrae and the *scapula*. The *rhomboid minor* also attaches to the *scapula* and to the seventh thoracic vertebra. Do you remember that the *pectoralis minor*, in the chest, also attaches to the *scapula*? You can have pull from front to back, *or* back to front.

The *latissimus dorsi*, which lies under Grid E, attaches to the spines of the lumbar vertebrae, the *thoracolumbar fascia*, the *iliac crest*, the lower ribs and the *scapula*. That's an enormous spread of influence.

The *erector spinae* are the erector muscles of the spine. That is the name given to the fibers of the more superficial muscles of the back. They attach to the spines of the lumbar vertebrae and also the eleventh and twelfth thoracic vertebrae and the *iliocostalis*, the *longissimus* and the *spinalis* muscles.

Permanent fix for the upper back will take time, so don't try to hurry. Check Figure 34 and note the double line of dots running up the back. The inside line is about an inch out from the spine and the second line is on the outside of the muscle's belly. Note in the picture the deep trough running from waist to neck in the back. It is right above the spine and flanked by the muscles you are about to work on. Notice that the muscles are full and wide at the waist, narrowing as they rise toward the shoulders.

With the subject prone and relaxed, reach across the body to place your elbow on the outside line of the muscle on the other side of the spine, press down and then pull in toward your own body. Cover the subject's body with your own and with your free arm. This stabilizes your body and also diffuses some of the pain that might be felt, since there is more

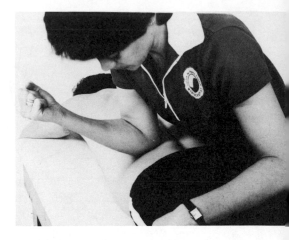

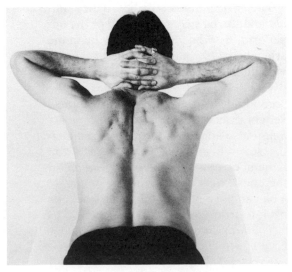

than one point of sensation. Hold for the usual seven seconds.

To get at the other side of the same muscle, place your elbow in the trough and press away against the inner side, the inner of the two lines on Figure 34. Proceed up the back at one-inch intervals. Then do the same to the other side of the back. If lying prone is uncomfortable for your subject, place a pillow under the chest or waist, depending on which feels better.

The *trapezius*. Start at the tip of the shoulder at the *acromion* and move downward at an oblique angle along the edge of the muscle at one-inch intervals to the point at the base of the muscle. Do both sides. You have already covered the circles on the shoulders, 14 through 18, but do them again. Do both sides and follow with the edge of the *deltoid*, the muscle that is like a cape over the shoulder. Check along the line of dots leading from the edge of the *trapezius* to a point on the arm a few inches down from the shoulder.

You now come to Grid D, which covers the *rhomboids*, *teres major*, *teres minor*, the *thoracolumbar fascia* and the *scapula*. Start at circle 13, on Figure 34, but don't stop there. Put your elbow into every square on the grid, spending a little compass time in each one. This is one of the most sensitive and overworked areas in the human body; trigger points in this

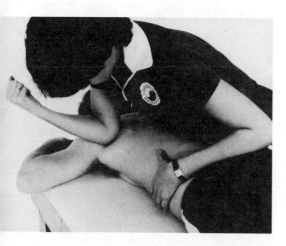

area refer pain in every direction, up the neck to the head, through the body into the chest, down the arms and the mid-back and into the lower back. There is no end to their mischief or their influence.

Follow Grid D with Grid E, which covers a good part of the *latissimus dorsi*. Have the subject on his or her side with the upper arm stretched overhead. Use the same search technique you just used for the *intercostals* (page 154). Do both sides and then use the same stretch for the *latissimus* as you did for the *intercostals*.

Follow with a standing exercise, lateral stretch (see picture on page 219, in the section on *Sports*). Stand with feet apart and reach straight up with the right hand. Next, slide the left down the outside of the left thigh to the knee. That brings your body into a lateral bend. Next, pull your reaching hand in to cover your ear and then reach out overhead as far as possible. Do four such reaches to one side and then the other to make up a set. Do three sets.

Problems in the upper back are myriad and can stem from as far back in time as birth, when tiny shoulders, like tiny heads, are so at risk as they battle their way down the birth canal. From then on the risk increases as we suffer from unforeseen accidents, and then in the sports field, sprains, strains, bruises and bashes. But it is to occupation that we must look

for certain-sure trauma, and while the trauma may be unforeseen by some (most) people, you won't have that excuse anymore. There is no escape from the damage we pick up on the job as we repeat the same motions over and over for years and years. Those injuries are in the province of permanent fix on a continuous basis, because most of us *have* to continue to work, and the field we have chosen will continue to hurt us even when we understand our peril.

Then there are the postural problems in the upper back, many of which do not *originate* in the upper back at all. Take one shoulder higher than the other. This is usually blamed on habitually carrying a brief case in one hand or a baby on one hip. Neither is normally the real reason. I found a very real and unsuspected reason when I was visiting Dr. Travell. We were sitting at opposite ends of the table and I was wearing a brown wool sheath with a high collar. There was a line of small gold buttons which ran from collar to hem at about half-inch intervals. "Bonnie, your buttons are crooked," remarked this latter-day Dr. Joseph Bell of Edinburgh, Scotland, on whom the character of Sherlock Holmes was modeled. I looked down and, sure enough, the line of my gold buttons took a sharp swerve to the right, coming back into line at the break in my lap. I had already noticed that one shoulder was lower than the other, but I'd put that down to carrying a heavy record case for thirty years. I tried sitting up straighter and the button line straightened at once, but one sitting bone rose about a half inch off the chair. Sit on your hands and you will feel the "sitting bones," the knobs of the *ischii*. I sat back down on the two bones and immediately my button line bent. What does that mean? There are at least two explanations. Either one side of me was smaller than the other, which is not at all uncommon, or the smashing blow to my pelvis in that long-ago ski accident had broken the bones in such a way as to give me a structural abnormality. Since one of the fractured bones was the *ischium* on the right side, which had healed in an overlapped position, chances were good that I was now rather imperfect and therefore uneven. There was of course that ever-present possibility and one you should consider if *your* sitting bones are uneven; somewhere in that powerful set of back muscles there could be a mighty spasm.

At the time, we didn't know that my deteriorating hip joint (posttraumatic arthritis) was sending signals in all directions. The ones going down the leg even curled my toes. The ones referring up included the entire back and neck. The "cure," which in this instance is a euphemism for "feel better at least for a while" has a name. We call it "the *Reader's Digest* cure." We got out a pile of *Reader's Digests* and tried each one for size. Summer editions are slimmer than Christmas editions, and we found September to be just right for my discrepancy in *ischii*. My buttons were straight, my shoulders even, and when I had to sit for hours at the typewriter there was less fatigue. It is a great *temporary* aid if your problem is spasm, rather than being unevenly made. For years I kept copies of *The Reader's Digest* everywhere: in my desk, in the car and in my pocket (so did President Kennedy).

Today, since learning how to erase and often prevent back spasm, I no longer need an assisting prop. However, if *you* have a dropped shoulder and a list to port (*or* starboard), you may want to use that wonderfully simple aid when you must sit for long hours. Use it *until* you can get the spasms under control, not *instead of* doing the Myotherapy you need. Once you have taught your back muscles better manners, you most probably won't need it.

Kyphosis, mentioned back with the Kraus-Weber minimum muscular fitness test, is another upper-back problem. The word *kyphosis* comes from the Greek word for humpbacked. It is an abnormally increased convexity of the *thoracic spine* as viewed from the side. By the time most people "view the condition from the side" with a question as to its normality, the condition is usually well advanced, and you don't have to be very old to develop it. We often see young children in the clinic that have been diagnosed as having *kyphosis*, and we are usually the last hope before operation.

Since bones neither advance nor retreat on their own, what would you say is pulling the spine into "an abnormal convexity"? It is primarily chest muscles that are doing a number on the back, with the arm muscles aiding and abetting. Discovering any aberration in early childhood is immensely helpful, for it is in childhood that most of these things begin. Adulthood is when they cause pain and a visit to the doctor. By then, the slender, pliable sapling, which could have been redirected, has become a gnarled oak with a whim of iron. The mother who ushers her twenty-year-old son into the doctor's office, complaining, "I kept telling him to stand up, but he wouldn't listen. Now look at him!" is on a par with the platoon leader who reports to his superior, "I kept telling them they had to take the ridge, but they wouldn't listen. Now they're all prisoners." That there was no *way* to obey those two orders without some form of outside help seems to be past understanding.

Outside help for *kyphosis* comes in the form of trigger-point work and stretch exercises. There is no possibility of *forcing* a spasmed muscle into compliance with your wishes. The frequency of use of traction and/or braces seems to have no bearing at all on the quality of results. You can't really *trick* muscles into relaxation with tranquilizers (even when called muscle relaxants). The thousands upon thousands of Valium addicts in this country attest to that. To entice a muscle to relax and *consent* to retraining, one must first find the cause of the spasm, the angry trigger points. When they are found, they must be neutralized with pressure so that the muscle *can* let go and can *really* be relaxed, not zonked silly while no attention whatever is paid to cause. As most people who have tried both traction and medication know, the spasm may ease a bit, but it is always there, ready to pounce again. That's what chronic pain is all about.

Before you start your work to relieve the muscles causing *kyphosis*, take the kyphosis test on page 137 and add one more, the table test for round back.

Have the subject lie supine on a table with arms at the sides. *Both* shoulders and arms should lie flat, touching the table from shoulder top down to the fingertips. If you feel that the shoulders are lifted even a little, press down on one or the other, and at the same time watch the wrist. It will rise appreciably. That means the muscles in both chest and arms are tight, typical in round back and a good check for improvement after trigger-point work, stretch and an exercise program.

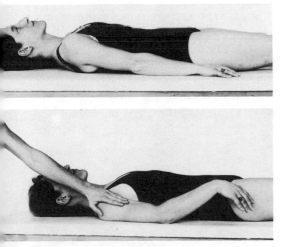

In *Quick Fix* you learned that a few key trigger points could relieve pain and stiffness and even weakness *for a time*. In *Permanent Fix* you are trying to make that relief permanent. Augment whatever you did before with a thorough search of the arms, the *axilla* and the chest. Leave no spot untouched. Hold the pressure

only when pain indicates or you will take forever and exhaust both yourself and the subject. Keep in mind that *quick* is not your aim now; *thorough* is. You don't have to do it all at once and will do the best job if you do one area one day and another area the next, with some rest time in between. There *is* a certain amount of discomfort involved, and discomfort is an energy drain. That's why people in constant pain are tired all the time and why many lack interest in doing anything more than they absolutely have to. Since they do less, they lose strength and *can* do less and less. The outcome is both predictable and bleak. If after doing all you can with permanent fix you *still* have some discomfort in the chest area, don't be disturbed. Just below it are the *abdominals*, which most people connect only with the pain of an upset stomach, cramps, appendicitis, gallbladder distress or some other awful-awful, almost never with trigger points; and yet look at the size of them! Note the large area they cover and remember what they do. Without them you would fall over backward. Some of you who haven't given much thought to them put too much fat behind them and stretch them. Some use them most effectively while having babies and then forget all about them, allowing them literally to go to pot. There are dozens of trigger points in the *abdominals*, and since they are situated so centrally, they can affect adversely a great many structures, one of those being the chest.

When you have completed your chest work you will need the proper exercises: the snap-and-stretch and the backstroke, on pages 69 and 70, in *Quick Fix*, and the shoulder rotations, on page 76. Add to these the handshake and the arm pump, on page 176.

The above are your stretch exercises, but you have an additional concern: The spasmed muscles have been pulling on their antagonists in the upper back for a long time, possibly since before birth. They are probably both weak and over-

FIG. 35: WEIGHT BAG

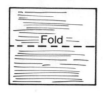

Fold

Stitch two sides,
turn inside out

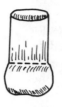

Half of shot
and stitch*

Rest of shot
and stitch top*

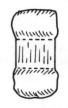

Turn upside
down, stitch*

*Use pins to hold shot while stitching

stretched. This is where weight training comes in.

First, let me explain, you won't get bulging muscles from weight work unless that is your aim, and even then it requires certain hormones, which women don't have in sufficient quantities. Using light weights and depending on repetitions for muscle strengthening will net long, smooth, very attractive muscle on either sex.

I have always preferred weight bags to dumbbells or barbells. They are far more versatile and easier to store or transport. They can go in a *small* corner of the closet or in the trunk of your car, and when I go on tour I take two in my pack. If weight bags are dropped they make no dents in either toes or floors. And they can be used by the whole family. To make weight bags, use either sand or lead shot. The latter is more expensive (hardware store), but requires less and is easier to handle and store. In order to differentiate the weights of the bags, use coverings of various colors. We use yellow for one-pounders, red for two-pounders and royal blue for five-pounders. To make up a set, we have two of each weight. For stronger than average people (or would-be stronger than average), we have additional five-pound bags. The covering material should be cut into rectangles: 7 × 12 inches for the one-pound weights, 10 × 12 inches for the twos, and 10 × 13 inches for the

fives. Denim or sailcloth coverings look attractive and wear well.

With a light weight in each hand, do both the snap-and-stretch exercise and the backstroke. You will need a fairly slow rhythm when you use weights, as you want to bring the resistance to bear all along the muscles involved.

Snap-and-Stretch, Bent Over

Stand with feet apart and do the same snap-and-stretch as you did standing, but with the torso at right angles to the floor. Do four for a start and then alternate with four standing upright. Do three sets. This will strengthen the upper back and arms while stretching the chest muscles.

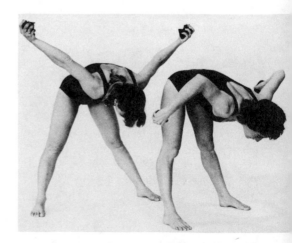

Weighted Prone Arm Lift

Lie prone on table or floor, holding a light weight bag in each hand. With arms outstretched, lift first one arm and then the other *slowly* as you did back in the correctives after the K-W test. Lower the arm as slowly as you raise it. Alternate for eight at the start, and then rest before doing a second and then a third set. As you improve, carry heavier weights.

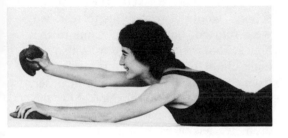

The Dead Lift

This is another strengthener for the upper back. Use a thirty-six-inch dowel that is one inch thick (hardware store) with two light weights hung one over each end. Stand with legs apart and knees

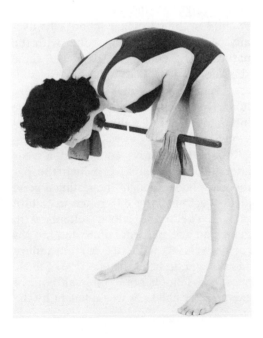

straight, bend from the hips and pick up your "bar." Let your arms hang straight as you lift the weights an inch or so above the floor; then, without changing the angle of your torso, which should be close to a right angle to the floor, raise the bar to your chest and lower to full arm-stretch eight times. Straighten up to rest, and then repeat the set three times. As you improve in strength, add both repetitions and weight.

Scoliosis

You have already met *scoliosis* a time or two in this book. The word means a curvature of the spine and is far more common than most people suspect. The word comes from the Greek word *skolios*, for twisted, and means an appreciable lateral deviation in the normally straight, vertical spine. As with headaches, there are many words used to describe the condition and the cause. Just reading about them will tell you what *doesn't* cause yours.

Cicatricial scoliosis, which means it comes as a result of a scar, should make you aware that there is more to scars than mere disfigurement. They and their accompanying trigger points can pull your body out of alignment. Not long ago a little boy was brought to the clinic. He was bent way over because of burn scars resulting from an explosion of firecrackers in his pants pocket. It took one session of Myotherapy to release him so he could stand and walk normally. The prognosis had been six months *if* he was given physiotherapy. *Scars should never be ignored.*

Empyematic scoliosis is connected with empyema, which is an accumulation of pus in the chest cavity. There's a good chance that the scar connected with drainage, *and the accompanying trigger points*, could have been at work there too.

Habit scoliosis is said to be caused by improper posture, but what causes "improper posture"? You already know at least one answer: trigger points.

Inflammatory scoliosis, said to be due to vertebral disease.

Ischiatic scoliosis is due to hip disease.

Myopathic scoliosis is due to paralysis of the muscles supporting the trunk.

Ocular, or *ophthalmic, scoliosis* is attributed to tilting the head due to astigmatism or muscle imbalance. Moral: watch your children for "tilts" of any kind and then ask yourself, "What muscle is pulling that head, that foot, that neck or that back that way?" Follow the questions with a trigger-point hunt; start that regime when the children are very little, so that it is the expected thing and brooks no resistance. After the hunt come the exercise and the awareness of what must *not* happen.

Osteopathic scoliosis is blamed on disease of the vertebrae.

Paralytic scoliosis is said to be due to paralysis of the muscles.

Rachitic scoliosis is due to rickets, but there isn't too much of that around these days, at least in the affluent parts of America.

Sciatic scoliosis is a list of the lumbar part of the spine away from the side affected by sciatica. And what do you know of the causes of sciatica? You already know that most of it can be relieved by chasing down trigger points in the gluteal and groin muscles.

Static scoliosis is due to a difference in leg lengths.

Idiopathic scoliosis is the one we see most often. *Idio* (Greek) is a combining form denoting relationship to self or one's own as something separate and distinct. That could be a good description for most chronic pain. *Pathos* is the Greek word for disease. *Idiopathy* is a morbid state of *spontaneous* origin. Spontaneous is medicalese for occurring without external influence. To us, however, *spontaneous*

usually seems to mean the surfacing of something that has been going on for a long time and usually has had a very definite external influence although the sufferer has forgotten if he or she ever knew. One such influence is an awkward posture in the womb; there are others that are equally unnoticed.

When we were giving the Kraus-Weber minimum muscular fitness test, we did *all* of the public schools in a large New England city. When we asked if the parochial schools would also allow us to test, we were refused, but when we came to the high school we discovered it was also the high school for the youngsters coming up from the parochial schools. So in order to get at least some information about the physical levels of parochial-school children, we asked each student what elementary and junior high he or she had attended. *Most* of the youngsters (and there were an inordinate number) who had scoliosis had come from the parochial schools. The major difference between the public and parochial schools (other than use of a gym, which the parochial schools lacked but which we did not feel could make much difference given the poor quality of public-school physical education) was in classroom rotation. A child in the parochial school was usually confined to one classroom with the natural light coming in over the same shoulder all year. The public-school children changed classrooms at least every hour. In this instance we felt that the influence was not only external but obvious.

In another study, conducted a year later in another area, in which the parochial schools thought the testing a good idea, we found the difference in failure rates between the public schools with gyms and a 58 percent failure and the parochial schools with a 60 percent failure and no gym, to be negligible. One of those parochial schools put in one half hour of exercise per child per week, taught by the school mothers in the cafeteria, and brought their failure rate down to the European level, 8 percent.

So if your child has a scoliosis and you can rule out scars (which you should go over for trigger points anyway), empyema (same), vertebral disease, hip disease, paralysis and rickets, what's left? Postural habits, uneven legs, sciatica and idiopathic scoliosis (which in essence means that nobody knows why). What those boil down to is a needed cleanup of trigger points that might be pulling on the spine, and you can find those by observing the curves. Then should come the retraining exercises, and if the legs are still uneven (which they might no longer be if the spasm has been relaxed) a lift on one shoe might help. However, if the difference is not extreme, the lift may cause more pain. I had to give mine up a week after I got it, and that was forty-seven years ago. In between then and now I have been a concert dancer, a skier, a sixth-degree mountain climber and an exercise teacher, all with one slightly short leg.

A full-blown scoliosis might look like this. Note how the back makes up for the primary curve by providing two secondary curves. What you want to do is prevent the first one.

Usually scoliosis becomes apparent at the onset of puberty; at least it becomes apparent to eyes accustomed to looking for such things. It *usually* sets and goes no further around the age of seventeen (no guarantee, just usually). As with a great many other things which you didn't know about before you read about them here, scoliosis should be watched for. Only in the past few years have the schools made an effort to pick up the child with the problem. The next problem is, what to do about it? Exercise is usually suggested, but which exercises? And can you get the youngster to do them? What is offered is usually without much value, boring and limited. Next step, brace; and the next, operation. This route is not for you if you can avoid it. Check with the scoliosis test, on page 136.

Don't wait until your child is eleven or twelve to check the back. Do it from the time he or she is two or three days old. It is far more important to note the curve of the spine than a child's height or first tooth.

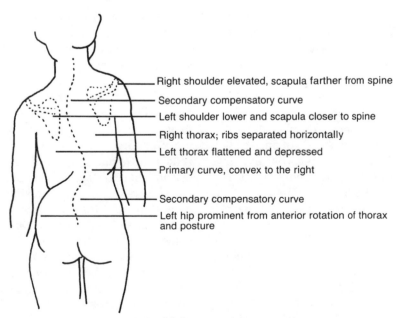

Right shoulder elevated, scapula farther from spine
Secondary compensatory curve
Left shoulder lower and scapula closer to spine
Right thorax; ribs separated horizontally
Left thorax flattened and depressed
Primary curve, convex to the right
Secondary compensatory curve
Left hip prominent from anterior rotation of thorax and posture

FIG. 36: SCOLIOSIS

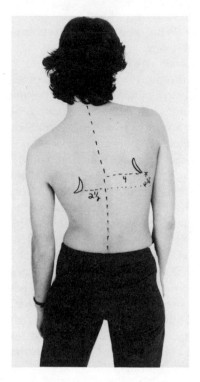

To check a back for scoliosis, you want to know four things: the distance of each scapula from the spine and the difference between the two measurements. Then you want the difference in level. Have the subject stand facing away unencumbered by shirt or bra. With a felt marking pen mark each of the vertebrae. Then mark the lower tip of each scapula. Measure from the tip of each to the spine. If the left is only two inches away from the spine and the right is three inches away, you have a discrepancy of one inch in your horizontal measurements. To get the fourth measurement, draw as straight a line as possible from the tip of one scapula to the other; then, using your eye or a level, determine the difference between the higher and the lower points.

There are many other tests, but these will give you the facts. One scapula is *x* inches from the spine while the other is *y* inches away. If that measurement changes for the better (more even distribution of space), improvement is taking place. One scapula is higher than the other by *x* inches. If that margin shrinks,

improvement is taking place. Now, how do you come by the improvement?

The first act is to hunt the entire back for trigger points. Follow that hunt with one in the chest, *axilla*, arms, neck and groin. How do you know where the boss trigger points lie? You don't. That's why you have to be so thorough. Follow the trigger-point work with the angry-cat and old-horse and the thread-needle exercises, on page 143, then the intercostal stretch, on page 155, but with a difference. The subject lies only on the side toward which the primary curve leans, and the folded pillow or rolled towel *straightens the spine* for the exercise. For the time being, have the subject stick to *bi*-lateral exercises—exercises that use both sides equally, such as swimming, rowing, gymnastics, riding, running, walking, biking, dancing and skiing. Until the back is under control, eschew such one-arm sports as tennis and bowling.

Where oldsters or merely olders are concerned, you *may* not be able to alter the measurements to an appreciable degree, but you can get rid of the pain. Painlessness is a sure sign of progress, but note also better range of motion and lessened fatigue. Clothes will usually fit better, and the adjacent structures— shoulders, neck and pelvis—will feel less strain. A young, painless body moves loosely. An older body, armored and trapped by spasm, moves *old*. Before you talk about cosmetic surgery for an aging face, think of a painless, youthfully graceful torso. Very often the face will reflect those pluses *without* surgery. It is certain that the surgery would do only half a job if the face presides over a creaky, painful torso.

And lastly, what of "arthritis of the spine"? Osteoarthritis comes to most of us with time. It shows up on the X rays we have taken when we suffer either a fall or "idiopathic" pain. When we are given the diagnosis, we are first horrified and then uneasily resigned as we wait to see exactly what "arthritis of the spine" means. Actually it means exactly that, some arthritis showing in the bones of the spine, and that's all it has to mean if you get rid of the trigger points causing the muscle spasm in the back muscles. Only 50 percent of those who actually have arthritis ever find out they have it. If it doesn't bother you, why bother about it? If your back with osteo and/or trigger points bothers you, fix it and go on about your business. You fix it by chasing down the trigger points and doing your exercises and never counting birthdays. I was thirty-five when I was given that unwelcome news, but I was too busy to pay much attention. Which is exactly what you should be. And incidentally, don't diagnose every ache and pain as arthritis, either. Dr. Desmond Tivy says that many people suffer from the arthritis that isn't, and those pains are 100 percent up Myotherapy's alley. And even if you see it on your X rays, remember that muscles are also involved and that heat, cold, pills, whirlpool, electrical stimulation, ultrasound, diathermy, massage, splints and braces are palliative. They don't go after the *cause* of your pain. *You* go after it with trigger-point hunting.

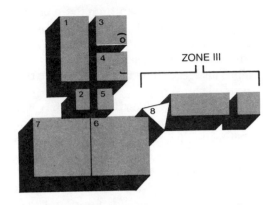

ZONE III, SEGMENT 8: THE AXILLA

The *axilla*, or armpit, has a great deal to do with pain, although because of Madison Avenue our major concern with it has been in connection with deodorants.

The *axilla* is loaded with lymph nodes, sweat glands, nerves, fat and muscles. The latter cross in every direction. They tie the arm to the chest, and no move is made by those muscles without signaling that move to the *axilla*. It plays a very important part in the rehabilitation of patients suffering from headaches, mastectomies, amputations and any shoulder, arm, elbow, wrist or hand pain. Those

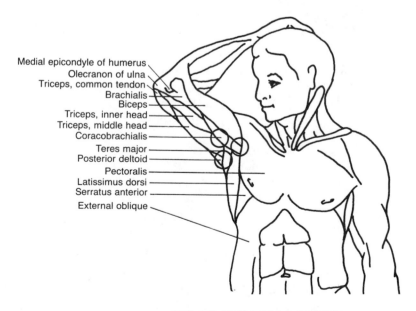

Medial epicondyle of humerus
Olecranon of ulna
Triceps, common tendon
Brachialis
Biceps
Triceps, inner head
Triceps, middle head
Coracobrachialis
Teres major
Posterior deltoid
Pectoralis
Latissimus dorsi
Serratus anterior
External oblique

FIG. 37: THE AXILLA POINTS

are fairly obvious, but then there are the upper back, the chest and both the *intercostals* and the *latissimus dorsi*. The lowly *axilla* is actually Rome, to which all roads lead, and it needs a lot more than Extra Dry Arrid.

When you work on the *axilla*, have the subject lying supine with the hand resting behind the head. If there is a lot of stiffness or pain in either the shoulder or the chest, you may have to support the arm with a pillow. Be sure the subject is comfortable before you start your hunt. You don't want to put any strain on a cold muscle, and until you have found some trigger points in that area and defused them, allowing for increased circulation and the warmth it affords, you are dealing with cold muscles.

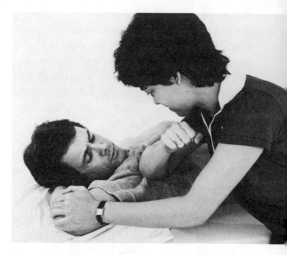

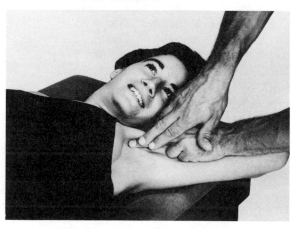

Place a damp washcloth over the *axilla* in order to prevent slipping. There can be trigger points anywhere, but the three large circles on Figure 37 will show you the major sites. Place your elbow first in the circle nearest the chest. Use your compass technique. Go gently and carefully; the *axilla* is not only sensitive, but there are emotional overtones connected with it. It is rarely exposed and is usually not only covered, but tightly protected by the arm. Also, the subject knows instinctively that there are some truly nasty spots there.

It should be noted that the *axilla* is the underside of the shoulder and the edge of the chest and upper back, especially

the *trapezius* muscle. Any injuries sustained by those structures will involve the *axilla*.

While you are about it with the subject in the ideal position, go after the underside of the *trapezius*. Place the fingers of one hand against the underside of the *trapezius* just below the two large circles that are one above the other in the *axilla* triangle. Cover the one hand with the other to increase your strength. You will be able to trap some of the meanest and most effective trigger points under your fingers. You may want to place a pillow under the near side of the upper back to make the subject more comfortable. Check again with Figure 5, page 71, and note the size of the *trapezius*. Understand that spasms in one part can cause trouble in any and every other part as well as in neighboring areas. It is important to do a thorough job wherever you find sensitive spots.

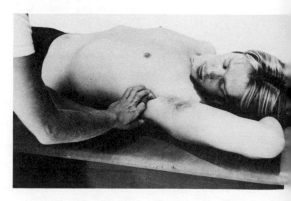

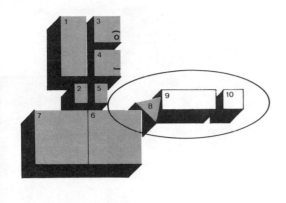

ZONE III, SEGMENTS 9 AND 10: THE ARM AND HAND

The arm doesn't seem to be terribly important to life and everyday living until one or the other can't work for you because of weakness or pain. If pain is involved in the arm, sleep will be interrupted, as the wise body tries to change positions every little while to prevent stiffness and is met with either a stabbing pain or an ache that increases in intensity the longer you lie on it. If the arm has pain, you can expect more of the same but in the neck, head, ear, upper back and chest. The reverse is, of course, true. Neck pain can lead to arm ache, and trigger points in the chest put typing, playing the piano or even sewing out of bounds. The mechanic may well lose his job.

Not long ago I was allowed to address the members of a famous orchestra, and several of them came to the lecture with their arms in slings. Being less politic than interested, I blurted out, "What are *those* things for?" Well, what the slings were *for* was to rest the arms when they were not actually playing in concerts or rehearsing, which make up most of a musician's life. What they were actually *doing* was something quite different. When a musician plays, motion in the arms and hands is limited to *exactly* that needed to draw from the instrument the most beautiful tones possible. The better

the musician the more limited will be the motion. It takes everything else in the musician's daily life to keep the entire muscle body in good tone. When a coffee cup is lifted, that is different from the way those muscles are used when playing. When he hoists his baby son overhead or she wrings out a dish towel or paddles a canoe, the muscles are used differently and more muscles come into play. Think now, what happens to muscles that hang in a sling all day because one of those muscles has a knot in it? The muscles atrophy and become weak, of course. What happens to them when they are used only in one way *and* there is a knot in one of them? The spasm spreads, the arm becomes weaker and more painful. What then happens to the musician's career as a musician? It's over. The same goes for the athlete who has to depend on rest and a splint. The more you rest and splint, the weaker the muscles become. Carry that a step older, to the elderly who give in to the doctor's siren song "Bed rest is the answer." Bed rest

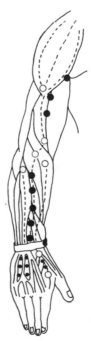

FIG. 38: ARM AND HAND, POSTERIOR VIEW

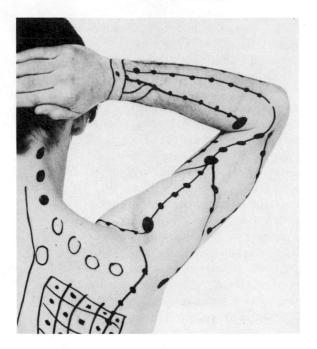

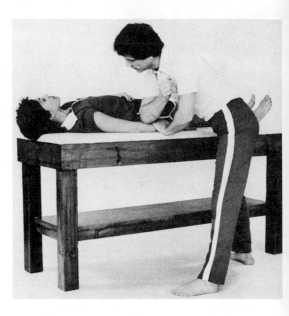

is just one step this side of the grave and should be resorted to only when there is no other way to go.

Zone III takes in the *axilla*, the arm and the hand; there is really no way to separate one from the others where Myotherapy is concerned. In *Quick Fix* you found a couple of key spots that would ease the arm and shoulder pain *for a time*, something you could take care of on the job or before a date. Now you need to go after *all* the troublemaking trigger points, and having a table to work on will make a tremendous difference. Now you can give all your attention to detail. Repeat what you did for the arm in *Quick Fix*, but this time as you descend toward the wrist note just how many muscles cross and how the edges of the many muscles come under your pressure, especially under the black dots. Pay attention to what the subject says as you press down on the dotted muscles. Follow the lines that start at the circles and apply pressure at one-inch intervals from fingertips to shoulders. Remember, the white circles are merely the worst trigger points *as a rule*, and your friend may not

be typical at all. His or her key trigger points may not even be marked on the maps. It's up to *you* to find and mark them on his or her individual scan. Put your name on it; you found it!

Always listen to what the subject says, and if you hear "Oh! That made my neck hurt," stop your work on the arm and go searching where the neck pain was felt. The trouble may be in the neck and felt only secondarily in the arm. When you go back to the troublesome spot in the arm, it may be much less sensitive or gone altogether. When you do Myotherapy, you are a kind of musician; you play on a human body. As the musician listens to the tone he creates, you listen to the results you are getting through the words of the subject. Do anything you can to get a response. You may have to ask the question "What did that do?" or "Did that refer anywhere?" In time you will get the cooperation you need; while "OOOOOOOAAHHHHH!" is response, it is not awfully helpful. Handling *that* requires: "That must have been a good one; what did it feel like, just a local pain or did it refer somewhere else? Where?"

If you have a tendency toward neck or arm pain yourself, keep a bodo handy and use it *before* you go to bed, *before* you sit down to write a chapter, *before* you go to rehearsal or drive to the mountains. You may avoid the pain altogether. If you have what is called "arthritis of the hand" use it *before* you exercise and be sure to exercise often throughout the day. Check with the exercises starting on page 217 and choose the exercises you *like* the most and that take in your trouble areas, and *do them often.*

The back of the arm is a veritable nest of awfuls. Most of those trigger points that cause numbness and tingling in the fingers can be found here. A lot of pain attributed to carpal tunnel syndrome in the wrist and hand really comes from here; it should be no surprise to you to learn that roughly half of the trigger points causing tennis elbow make their homes in the back of the upper arm.

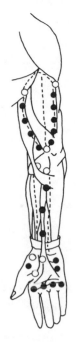

FIG. 39: ARM AND HAND, ANTERIOR VIEW

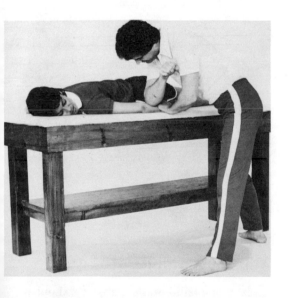

Have your subject lying prone with the arm stretched flat, palm up. Put a folded towel under the wrist to cushion unprotected wrist and hand bones. Have the subject turn her face toward you to relax the neck. You already know that most arm pain is labeled "arthritic" (whether it is or not, and either way it doesn't matter). Most shoulder pain is called "bursitis," which it almost always isn't. Most

elbow pain is called "tennis elbow," and most wrist pain now is called "carpal tunnel syndrome." Those names don't really tell you anything except *where* the pain is, but there is one pain that has escaped a name. It's the one that runs from the elbow to the *axilla* and feels like an electric shock. If you are not careful, someone will X-ray your neck and find signs of arthritis, and then if you aren't careful someone will want to fuse your cervical vertebrae because an electric-shock feeling must be connected with a sick disk in the neck due to your arthritis.

Think back over the years. Do you remember conking your funny bone on the car door, the shelf or the ledge? If you do remember that shocking feeling it wasn't funny at all. Most probably *there*, right at the elbow, you will find the trigger point that makes a full reach impossible without pain. Don't think, "nerve in the neck"; think, "trigger point in the back of the arm, which is *squeezing* the tail of a nerve leading to the elbow, because the muscle it serves is wide awake and caus-

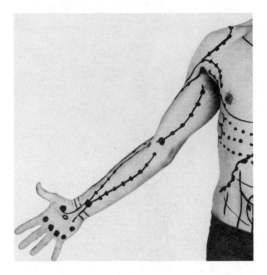

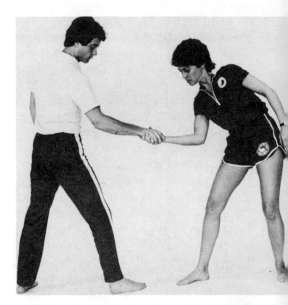

ing that muscle to go into spasm.'' Then go to work to get rid of the point or points, *all of them*, and start your exercises that will retrain the muscles.

Do the intercostal stretch, on page 155, and all the pulley exercises, page 157, plus the following exercises for resistance.

Handshake Arm Resistance

Stand opposite the subject and take the hand you have just worked over, and without putting on any pressure rotate your hand first inward and then outward several times so she will know what to expect. Set up a slow rhythm and when the movement is going well start to give a *little* resistance. This is when you play the whole thing by ear. You need to give just enough resistance to make the muscles of your subject work, but not so much that there is strain. Err on the side of too little rather than too much. It is the same procedure as that used for neck stiffness. The antagonists of the contracting muscles *have been patterned to give up tension*, and they usually do, especially after trigger-point work. This allows for further stretch. Do about a minute of this exercise, being careful not to tire the arm.

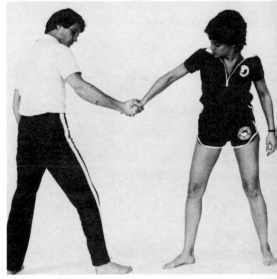

Arm Pump with Resistance

Place one hand on the subject's shoulder to prevent substitution (raising up) and take the hand of the arm you have just freed of trigger points and raise it slowly, stopping at that level where pain is felt. Then have the subject press the arm down to the vertical against a *little* resistance on your part. Each time you raise the arm, try to see if it will go a *little* higher before the pain interferes. When it does (if it does), stay at that level for

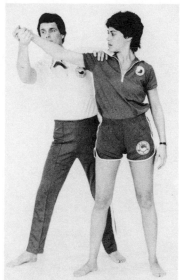

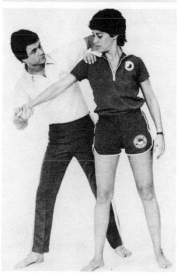

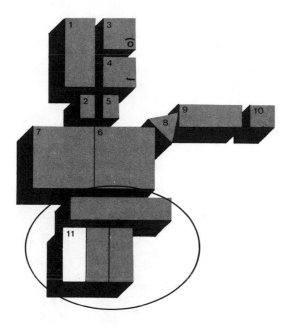

ZONE IV, SEGMENT 11: THE LOWER BACK

While the *uterus* is the most sinned against part of the body, at least half the population is safe from the often unnecessary operation hysterectomy, but almost *nobody* is safe from low-back pain. If back pain comes to you, you too will be in danger of an unnecessary operation in which there will be a search for the cause of that pain. In back pain there is no discrimination as to sex.

The lower back is the most expensive structure we have, because it causes more lost pay, lost jobs, lost opportunities, more exhaustion, more despair and faster aging than any other area of the body, including achy heads.

The first time you refer to Charlie as "good ol' Charlie," as opposed to "that young fella Charlie" is the day he comes to work all bent over. The first serious sign of slippage is when the foreman says, "Get Charlie to help you with those crates. No, wait a minute, Charlie's got a bum back, get Jim!" Raise that up to the executive level, and you've got the same story with a tie on it. "Haven't seen you at the gym lately, Charlie." A goodly

a few raises. Do about ten and be sure not to exceed the strength of the arm by offering too much resistance. After doing the two exercises, ask the subject to raise the arm without assistance. It usually goes up without difficulty or pain *or* substitution. That's what you are after, that and the pleased look on the subject's face, which is what Myotherapy is about: getting rid of pain.

The lifts with resistance can be (should be) done a number of times during the day without help from you. The subject's other arm can provide both the lift and the resistance. (See page 80.)

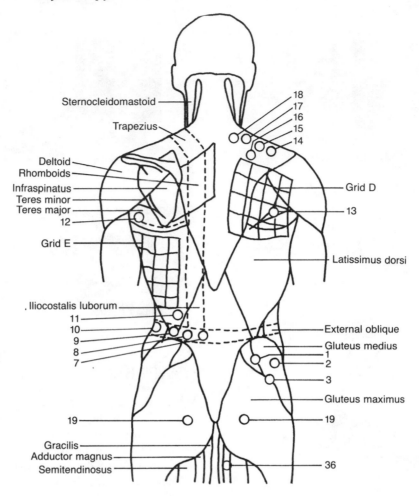

Sternocleidomastoid

Trapezius

18
17
16
15
14

Deltoid
Rhomboids
Infraspinatus
Teres minor
Teres major
12

Grid E

Grid D

13

Latissimus dorsi

. Iliocostalis luborum
11
10
9
8
7

External oblique
Gluteus medius
1
2

3

Gluteus maximus

19   19

Gracilis
Adductor magnus
Semitendinosus

36

FIG. 40: THE BACK

number of companies provide on-the-premises gyms as a precaution against losing a valuable employee to a heart attack. While nobody says Charlie *has* to show up for a workout, his promotion may depend on just that.

Now move the bad back into the home. It really doesn't matter who has the back pain; still, some folks are more indispensable than others, and if the housekeeping and childbearing and -rearing depend on the woman of the house, a "sacroiliac," "degenerating disk," "arthritis of the spine," a "pinched nerve," "spondylosis," "spondylolisthesis," "spondylarthritis," "myalgia," "myasthenia," "myogelosis," or just plain low-back pain, can lay her up for weeks. It can also

turn her into "Poor Mrs. Smith, she must be a lot older than her husband." Now, there's no sin in being older than your husband. Sometimes that's the best way to be. You just shouldn't *look* it. If there's one way to age fast, it's to suffer with a bad back. There's no way to hide it even if you still can get out of bed, out of your chair and out of the car. Every move screams pain even when you don't. The only good thing about back pain is that it is the easiest of all chronic pain to fix.

All through the book, you have been learning how interdependent the various parts of our bodies are. You also know that the closer the various parts are to one another, the more suspect they are

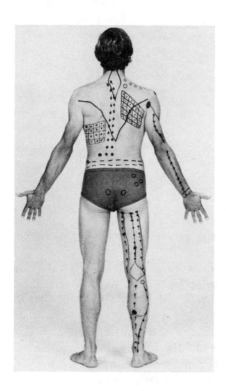

when it comes to sharing the blame for pain. Take a good look at Figure 40 and observe how much overlapping the back muscles do and also the size of those muscles, and think for a minute about their job descriptions. You can't stand up without them, or pick up your child or even a kitten. They are at work all day and often half the night. You can't walk to the refrigerator or lean over to reach the pie at the back. As a matter of fact nothing much goes on without the back taking part.

What is usually done for back pain? Muscle relaxants, analgesics, X rays, myelograms, heat, cold, rest. Some folks even take Doan's Pills! That is just one wall of the torso that is nothing if not neighborly. The opposite side of the back is the abdominal wall, which has a goodly amount to contribute when it comes to back pain, and what is usually done for that? Laxatives, antacids, tranquilizers and diets. Some folks who watch TV rely on Pepto-Bismol!

Those are just two sides of the torso; there are also the two lateral aspects: the

sides of the pelvis padded, over by the *gluteals*, the *tensor fasciae latae* and the *iliotibial band*. Pain in those areas is usually called "hip pain," even though the cause of the trouble may be elsewhere. The roof, or top of the area, is called the "*diaphragm*," which can refer pain upward or downward. Good examples are chest pain, heartburn, abdominal cramping and even a distinct feeling of anxiety.

The floor of the pelvis is a whole other story. Supporting, as it does, many organs, each of which can refer pain, pressure and a sense of foreboding, it is also the housing for our sex organs, the means of our sexual pleasure *and* the results of that pleasure, the next generation. Keep in mind that back pain can affect any of these structures, and that trouble in any one of them can be the cause of your backache. After your doctor has ruled out pathology connected with the organs and has said that no, you don't have a fractured back and no tumor is growing there, then, before you think spine, think muscles and do something about them.

We are all victims of superstition, ignorance and either little education concerning our bodies or none at all. When we are given body education in school, it is usually poorly organized and badly taught when it is not downright nonsense. I knew that when I wrote my first book on pain, *Pain Erasure the Bonnie Prudden Way*, but now it is four years later and there have been thousands of letters bearing out the two suspicions I have harbored a long time: the first, that what we were taught in school had little bearing on anything, and the second, that people are really very bright and, given the truth, they know very well what to do with it. Ignorance always was costly, but now hospital bills, laboratory bills, doctors' bills and medicine bills, which are the practical considerations in the prevention of disease and dysfunction, are out of sight. The cost of pain and the results of pain cannot be estimated financially. The cost in suffering is also incalculable, and as of now you are not going to contribute any to the growing mass. It *is* growing, too, because of the sedentary way in which many people live and the insane way in which others try to get into condition (see the section on *Sports*).

Learn as much as you can about the back and you will be able to help about 80 percent of your family and friends. That's a good percentage of folks owing you goodwill for more than just getting rid of their back pain: You will free them from analgesics, tranquilizers and corsets. You will free them to exercise and improve their lives. You will free them to make love without pain or the fear of pain; and that may be best of all.

The pelvic bones look like a Rorschach inkblot and, depending on the kind of mind you have, you can turn it into a portrait of Mickey Mouse or a sex symbol. Actually it's both, and a lot in between.

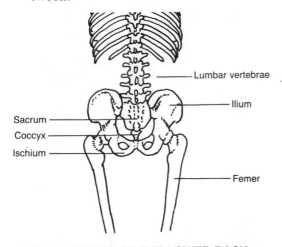

FIG. 41: BONES OF THE LOWER BACK

Pelvis comes from the Greek *pyelos*, which means trough. The lower (caudal) portion of the trunk is bounded posteriorly by the *sacrum* and the *coccyx* (tailbone), and anteriorly and latterly by the two hipbones, the *ilia*.

The *sacrum* is that triangular bone just below the *lumbar vertebrae*. It is formed usually by five fused vertebrae, the *sa-*

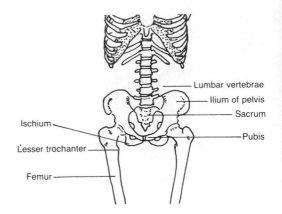

FIG. 42: FRONT OF PELVIS (GROIN)

cral, which are wedged dorsally between the two hipbones. The word "sacroiliac" doesn't tell you much about your back pain. It's just a spot on your body map denoting the articulation between the *sacrum* and the *ilium* and the associated ligaments and where the pain is *felt*. Not a word about what is causing the pain or what to do about it. When your friend says, "Oh, my sacroiliac," the proper response is "Hmmmmm."

Coccyx comes from the Greek word *kokkyx*, for cuckoo. The bird has a bill that resembles the tailbone in a human being. The *coccyx* is formed by the union of three to five (usually four) rudimentary vertebrae.

The upper boundary of the pelvic cavity is known as the *inlet*, *brim* or *superior strait*. The lower, "true" pelvis is limited below by the *inferior strait*, or *outlet*. It is bounded by the *coccyx*, the *symphysis pubis* and the *ischium* on either side.

So much for the box called the pelvis; now look where it is: right in the middle of everything. Notice that there are three roads leading toward or away from the pelvis. They are the spinal column and the two *femurs*, the bones of the upper legs. The muscles strapped over, across, along and around any of those structures can contribute to low-back or abdominal pain. Spasmed muscles in the pelvic area can cause pain down the legs or up the back even as far as the head. Two particularly vivid and distressing examples of this referral of trouble are impotence and frigidity. Hardly anyone would tie either condition to a fall on the *coccyx*, say at age twelve, or to a chair being pulled out from under the sufferer by a classmate in the eighth grade, but there it is: damage to the pelvic muscles, which, like a lot of damage, waits to make itself known until there is emotional stress. For a great number of people stress accompanies intercourse, and the muscles respond by going into lesser or greater spasm. Almost invariably the sufferer is told the trouble is in the head, and it's hard to tell what the psychiatrist will ask him or her. What is almost certain

is that no one will ask, "Did you ever fall on your *coccyx* or get kicked in the groin, jog on the road or take an 'aerobic' dance class?" More on this later, and yes, there *is* an answer, once you have asked the question.

The back of the pelvic box is upholstered with an impressive array of muscles. It is easily dismissed with words like "rear end," "seat," "butt" or "buttocks." That's too easy and, it is similar to dismissing Michelangelo's *David* as "a statue." It is, of course, but there is more to it.

Under the *gluteus maximus* and the *gluteus medius* is the *piriformis*, which attaches to the *ilium*, the second, third

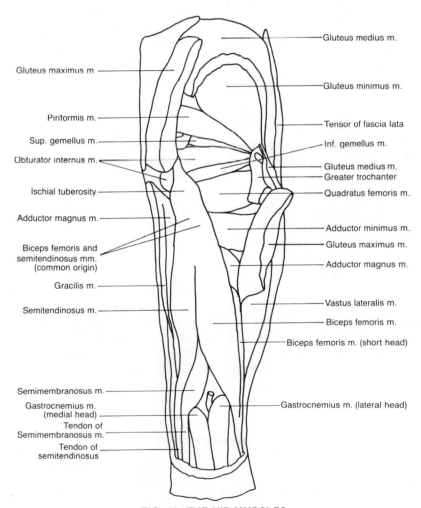

FIG. 43: THE HIP MUSCLES

and fourth sacral vertebrae, and the *femur*. Spasm in the *piriformis* can cause that infamous "sacroiliac pain."

The *superior gemellus* and *inferior gemellus* muscles run from the *ischium* to the *femur*; spasm there has a way of making the sufferer feel as if the bottom is dropping out and everything inside with it.

The *adductor magnus* has the same quality, since it attaches to the *ischium*, the *pubis* and the *femur*. If you have menstrual cramps, the *adductors* may respond appropriately to give you aching legs as an added problem.

The *semimembranosus*, which runs from *ischium* to *tibia*, can do the same thing. If you were running on the pavement or taking "aerobic" dance, muscle spasms in the legs may refer pain to the pelvis and provide the menstrual cramps that ruin the day.

The *obdurator internus* takes in the hipbone, the *ischium*, the *pubis* and the *femur*.

The *quadratus femoris* is special. It is often referred to in athletic circles as "the quads." It is the name applied collectively to four muscles and often dismissed collectively as having nothing to do with back pain. But it does. The *rectus femoris*, from which it takes its name, attaches to the *ilium*, the rim of the *acetabulum* (hip joint), the *patella* and the *tibia*. The *vastus intermedialis* attaches to the *femur* and the *patella*. The *vastus lateralis* attaches to the hip joint, the *femur* and the *patella,* and the *vastus medialis* attaches to the *femur* and the *patella*. All four attach to the common tendon that surrounds the *patella* (kneecap) and the *tibia* (the larger of the two lower-leg bones). After the uterus, the knee is the structure next in line for unnecessary operations, and this time the male sex is more in danger—through sports. Why? You have just read the names of four very good reasons if you couple those names with the word spasm. You have just been given an antidote

against most knee operations. It is called information. Use it. You will learn how when you come to the information on knees, page 235.

Lordosis

While the upper and mid back are hosts to *kyphosis* (round back) and *scoliosis* (curvature), the lower back has two postural anomalies of its own, *lordosis* (swayback) and the less-well-known flat back. *Lordosis* is caused by an anterior concavity in the curvature of the lumbar spine; the compensating curve will be found in the cervical spine, in the neck (see page 137). We see this most often on little girls; part of the cause is the attitude of adults toward little girls which fosters a self-image of cuteness and helplessness.

Body language is now known to be as effective in setting stages (and lives) as any spoken order. Little girls are *taught* to be helpless and to expect tender, loving care. It is called "The Daddy's little girl syndrome" in *The Cinderella Complex*, by Colette Dowling (Summit Books), which you should read if you are female, both for yourself and for your daughter. If you have a daughter who is being raised as "cute," you'd better hurry.

It is *not* a natural stance for a little girl. Tomboys don't stand that way. Poking the tummy out and turning one foot in (a la Hummel) is exactly the same message as that given by the puppy in the presence of a large adult dog when he rolls over and urinates. He and the little girl are saying, "I'm little. See? *I* can't hurt you. Please be nice to me." Just for the fun (or the horror) of it, look around at your adult women friends who stand that way. You'll be lucky if they don't simper, too.

If the damage is not already wrought by parental attitude, a sure way to damage an unprepared six-year-old is a ballet class. Since something like 85 percent of our six-year-olds in America would qualify as unprepared where muscles are concerned, that puts a lot of little girls in jeopardy. See the *Sports* section to learn how to prepare your small dancer for both dance classes and the sports she *must* embrace one day.

Another activity that contributes to swayback is gymnastics taught to the same age group by instructors who know very little about the human body, especially the very young human body. The rate of chronic injury from gymnastics in *the under-nine crowd* is now epidemic.

The test for *lordosis* is the psoas test, the third in the Kraus-Weber minimum muscular fitness test, on page 133. Repeat that test with some additional information. Have the subject lie on a hard surface. There may be a greater or lesser arch at the waist, but the important second for observation comes just as you give the command "Raise both legs about eight inches above the table." Before you do that, place your hand under the arch and against the spine. The swaybacked person usually has to *increase* the arch to provide help to the *psoas* in order to raise the legs, and the spine will leave your hand. There is also a slight (or not so slight) hitching movement of the pelvis instead of a smooth lift of the legs. If this person is in an exercise class taught by an incompetent teacher who asks the class to raise and lower both legs at the same time as an exercise, she will soon have low-back and groin pain. If this condition is discovered, spend some time every day on the correctives (page 135).

The muscles playing an important role in *lordosis* (and therefore in danger of harboring trigger points) are the abdominals, the *psoai* and the neck muscles.

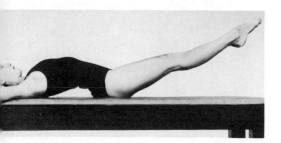

You have already learned about the neck although you probably never suspected that neck pain can come from a swayback. Those trigger points are secondary to the real culprits coming up.

Flat Back

The flat back is less discernible than the swayback. The lumbar curve is less than normal; you can see its presence by the way clothes hang on the back at the waist. There is no indentation at the belt line, and both pants and skirts hang flat, as if painted on cardboard. While there is too much give at the waist in *lordosis*, there is not enough in flat back.

Have the subject get onto hands and knees and hump the back up as in the exercise angry cat, page 143. Next tell her to drop her back into a sag like an old horse (same exercise). It may drop a little but usually very little past the horizontal.

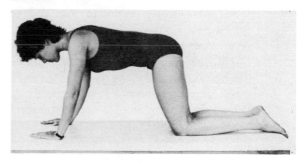

To get rid of back pain and to improve posture, have your subject lying prone on the table. Lean across the back and begin with circles 1, 2 and 3 as you did in *Quick Fix*. Use your compass every time. Hold any trigger points discovered for seven seconds.

Next, move on to the circles on either side of the *coccyx*, 19. If your subject suffers from the type of pain associated with *hemorrhoids*, you may be able to relieve it. Varicose veins in the legs respond to Myotherapy when the pressure caused by muscles in spasm is released. Perhaps hemorrhoids respond similarly.

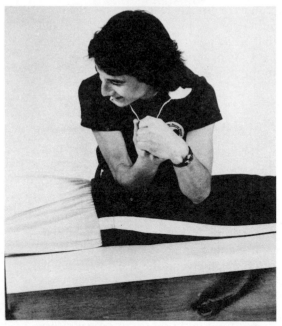

It is worth a try; we have had good luck with circles 19, plus the rest of the *gluteal* work and also the groin. You will find it a little farther along.

Follow the trigger-point work with the side-lying stretch exercise you did in *Quick Fix*. To that, add the limbering series, page 185.

The subject lies on one side and draws the bent knee to the chest, then stretches it full length to a point a few inches above the resting leg and then lowers it to relax. Do four *slowly*. Don't forget to do both the exercises and trigger pointing to *both* sides.

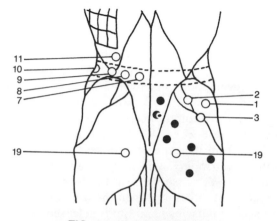

FIG. 44: THE LOWER BACK

If you really can't find someone to help you when you need it, the bodo can be a good friend. Attach it to or hold it against a wall. Some people find that the tape that holds carpet to flooring will also hold a bodo to a polished surface. It has glue on both sides.

Back into the bodo slowly, hunting for the right place. It can be used for trigger points in the side of the hip, circles 4, 5 and 6, as well as the *gluteals*, circles 1, 2 and 3. Circle 11, in the belt line, will respond to bodo pressure as well. That should take care of the lower back *if* those are the trigger points causing the misery.

In *Quick Fix* you worked over circles 9 and 11, in the waist area. Do that work again and add circle 8. In other words, go right across the belt line at one-inch intervals and give extra attention to circle 11.

There is a second way to get at circle 11, which is a key trigger point, especially where there has been whiplash or if the subject is involved in a sport requiring

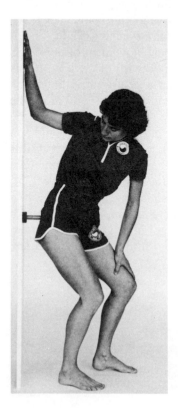

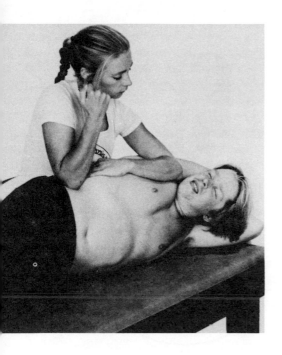

Lie supine with knees bent, bring your right knee as close to your forehead as you can, but don't strain. You have time; it will come. Next, lie back down and extend the leg straight out and down to a point six to eight inches above the bed, and then bring it back to the starting, knee-bent position. Alternate four to a side and then roll over onto your left side, knees slightly bent and relaxed.

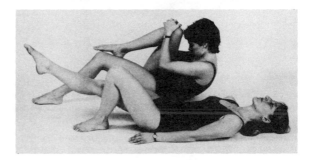

Draw the top knee as close to the chest as possible, extend the leg straight down about six to eight inches above the resting leg, and then bring it to relax on that leg. Rest for at least three seconds. Repeat four times.

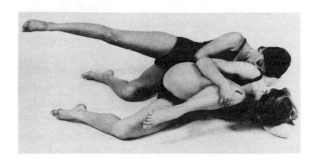

upper-body rotation as in tennis or golf. Have the subject lie on his side. By stretching the upper leg as long as possible and reaching overhead with the arm on the same side, you will make the space between the hipbone and the rib cage wider. The point of entry for your elbow in this position is straight down, directly into the side. Press straight down and then pull toward you. Hold for seven seconds and then use the stretching done for the *intercostals*, on page 155. Hold a weight bag in the stretching hand and allow the hand to fall over the edge of the table above the head to stretch all the muscles of the side. Inhale as you bring the arm to the overhead position and exhale as you bring the arm down to your side. Do ten.

The Limbering Series

The best exercises I know for the lower back are a set of five. Do them *before* you get out of bed in the morning if you have the slightest tendency to back pain or stiffness.

Roll to the prone position and relax your *gluteals* by turning your heels outward. That is the *rest* position. Roll the heels in to touch and tighten first the gluteals (buttocks). Pinch them together as tight as you can. Holding the contraction, add the abdominals. Pull them in as far as you can possibly manage. Finally add the *sphincters*. A *sphincter* is a ringlike band of muscle that constricts a passage or closes a natural orifice. The ones you want are in the floor of the pelvis, and if

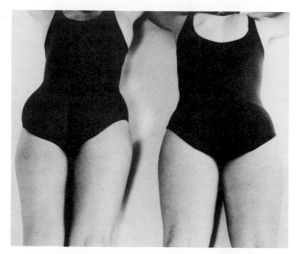

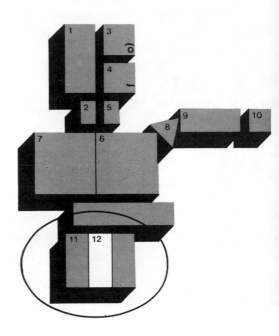

you had to get to the bathroom right away or disgrace yourself, the muscles you would tighten are the *sphincters*. The constant tightening and relaxing of those muscles will do several good things for you. Improve your sex life, keep the floor of the pelvis well exercised, and prevent leaking if you elect to jump rope or bounce around on your mini-trampoline (see page 283). After childbirth, these exercises are a must. Relax. Hold the *rest* for four seconds, then tighten for four. As you improve, rest for only two. Do four. Roll to your right side and repeat the side-lying exercise.

Roll onto your back and bend your knees with feet about a foot apart. Keeping your seat and shoulders on the bed, arch your back as much as possible and then flatten it *hard*. Try to round it at the waist by tilting the pelvis forward. Do four. Two complete rollovers is better than one if you are hurting, but one is a must for backachers. If your back is kicking up, get someone to check your trigger points and then do the series every two hours for two days.

ZONE IV, SEGMENT 12: THE SIDE OF THE PELVIS

The sides of the pelvis are extremely important where back pain is concerned. The *gluteus medius* lies under circles 4, 5 and 6, and it is the *gluteus medius* that keeps you standing there all day at the blackboard, counter, stock ticker or back of the theater (Fig. 45).

Maintain the same side-lying position you put your subject in for circle 11, at the waist, and start with circle 5, which is on the seam of the pants midway between the waistband of the underwear

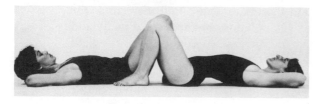

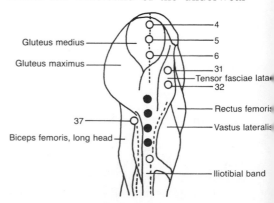

FIG. 45: THE SIDE OF THE PELVIS

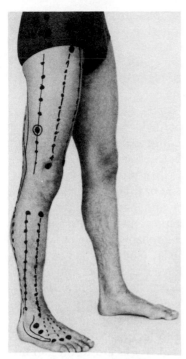

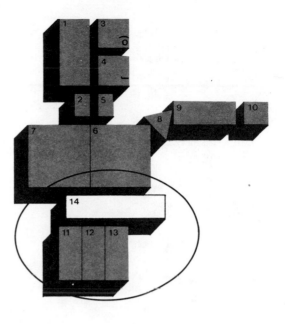

and the leg hem. Circle 5 is usually very sensitive. Hold your elbow in place with the other hand so it will not slip off the bony pelvis. Follow up with circles 4 and 6.

Standing at the subject's back, reach over the midline of the leg to press on circles 31 and 32, the *tensor fasciae latae*, *very* sensitive spots in any athlete or dancer. Anyone who has had to stand for long periods will also respond with alacrity if not enthusiasm.

As long as you have the subject in the right position, cover the black dots down the *iliotibial band*. Very few people escape with no trigger points in that area; they affect the knee as well as the back.

To stretch the side of the pelvis, have the subject remain in the side-lying position and drop the top leg over the edge of the table. This is often enough to stretch the muscles; but, to increase the stretch, place one hand on the near hip while leaning over to place the other hand on the hanging thigh just above the knee. Stretch in *easy* bounces about four times and then rest a second or two. Repeat three times.

ZONE IV, SEGMENT 14: THE ABDOMINALS

The abdominals cover the front of the pelvic box; most people think of them as being flat (good) or bulging (bad) or perhaps rounded (sexy). Of late some people think of them as being strong or weak, and a lot of people refer to them (wrongly) as "the stomach."

The abdominals take in the front of the body from the bottom of the *thorax* (chest) to the bottom of the *pelvis*. The abdominal cavity is separated from the thoracic by the *diaphragm*. What's inside? The *viscera*, which are enclosed by the abdominal muscles, the vertebral column and the *ilia* (pelvic bones).

The treasures in the abdominal cavity include the *adrenal glands*, so important where stress is concerned, and the *appendix*. This structure was once considered superfluous, and snipped almost as a matter of course. Time has shown us the folly of this, but a goodly number of several generations sport half a chevron on their bellies, a sort of Purple Heart. Then there is the *colon*, yards of it, and the *duodenum*, the *fallopian tubes*, *gonads*, *ovaries*, *uterus* and *prostate*, de-

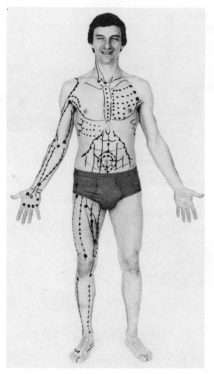

that President Johnson, who didn't fit at least four of the five Fs, did have a troublesome gallbladder.

When there is pain behind the abdominal wall, it is blamed on a host of conditions: spastic colon, menstrual cramps, appendicitis, colitis, gallbladder or a bug. When the doctor says, "No, you don't have any infections, inflammations, perforations, obstructions, infarctions, or ruptures . . ." then probably Myotherapy will help. In the past year we have added spastic colon and nervous stomach to menstrual cramps and "pseudo gallbladder," which is probably a form of nervous stomach. And if, God forbid, you do fit the fat F, go on a diet and get into a good exercise class or use the *Self Center* section and change things. Forty is a very nice age to be, as is any age in which you are fulfilled and happy. You know very well what to do if you are fertile, so do it. And lastly, that crack about being female: about half the world is, and if longevity is any criterion, I think the females have it.

pending on your sex. It also contains the *jejunum*, *kidneys*, *liver*, *pancreas*, *rectum*, *spleen* and *stomach*. In addition, we have a *gallbladder*, but there is sex discrimination with that one. The Five Fs for Gallbladder Diagnosis, learned by all too many medical students, are "Fat, Fertile, Flatulent, Forty and Female." I can tell you, I was mighty pleased to learn

Sometimes there *is* something wrong inside, but sometimes isn't always, and when health experts look at you as if to say, "You don't have anything the matter with you, it's all in your head, or maybe you like it on compensation," don't panic

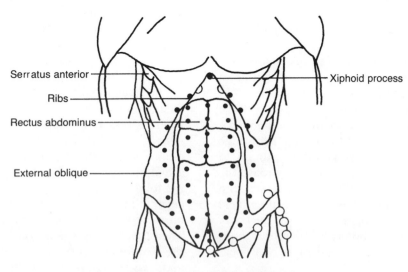

FIG. 46: THE ABDOMINALS

Serratus anterior

Xiphoid process

Ribs

Rectus abdominus

External oblique

and don't shoot anyone either. The first will aggravate the pain and the second is rather final all around. Try Myotherapy rather than the psychiatrist, for starters anyway.

Back in *Quick Fix*, you used the wraparound technique for menstrual cramps on the borders of the rib cage and hipbones. Do those same points all along the rib cage and pay special attention to the *xiphoid process*, at the spot most people recognize as the *solar plexus*. If that spot is unusually sensitive, know that it is on just about everyone else. That's why you give it special attention. See Figure 46 and follow each line of black dots from rib cage to groin. As you *gently* sink fingers into the softness looking for trigger points, have a felt-tipped pen ready.

work onto the scan you have made for your friend by tracing the muscle chart. If the pain should return, you have a good map that will, at least, cut the time in half.

Trigger points in the abdominals may cause pain that is attributed to adhesions. "Adhesions" often occur at the site of an operation. What else shows up at the site of an old wound? Scar tissue. What do you find in a lot of scar tissue? Trigger points. What do you do then? You find the sensitive spot and press for the required seven seconds. If the cause of the pain is trigger points in scar tissue, it should respond. If it responds, it was trigger points, not "adhesions."

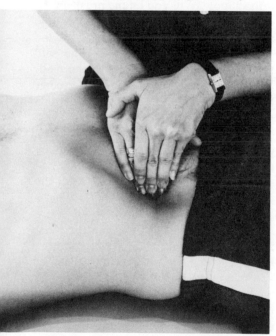

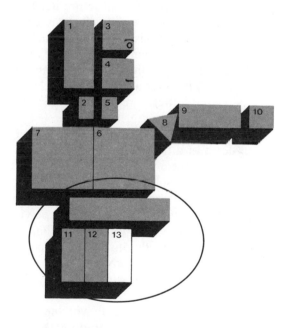

Leave a dot of ink at each point where you pressed but did *not* find a trigger point. Put an *X* at each point where you did cause pain. You may find that the abdominal trigger points correspond with some you found in the back and some will refer pain to other parts of the body. Circle those and go at once to the referred point and see what you can find there. After you have finished, copy your art-

ZONE IV, SEGMENT 13: THE GROIN

If you complain inelegantly of a bellyache, who is going to ask you if you have checked out your groin lately? Nobody. If your menstrual cramps lock you out of the office two days a month, will there be a single finger pointed at the probable (not merely possible) cause,

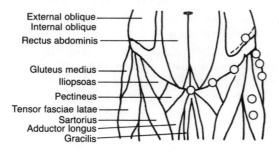

External oblique
Internal oblique
Rectus abdominis

Gluteus medius
Iliopsoas
Pectineus
Tensor fasciae latae
Sartorius
Adductor longus
Gracilis

FIG. 47: THE GROIN

your groin? Not likely. If you have a "bad back," an "aching back," or a "sacro-iliac," is the doctor even going to *think* groin? Doubtful. Yet the groin plays a star part in every one of those complaints and in a great many more miseries that are far removed from the structure itself.

The groin, like the abdominals, is a part of the front that also affects the back. It lies below the abdominal curve and is the anchor to which the abdominals are attached. That fact alone tells you that in its vicinity there are possible lairs for trigger points.

The massive leg muscles pass over, under and attach to parts of the groin, and while the abdominals pull *up* against it, the leg muscles pull *down*. Nor is that the end of the tension. There are muscles in the back and in the floor of the pelvis, each with its own groin connection. As a matter of fact the inside of the pelvis looks like a series of complicated spider webs, and the groin supports every filament.

What has the groin to do with hip pain? Everything! What has it to do with back pain? Plenty! When you find trigger points in the groin, many of them will refer down the inside of the thigh, which means the reverse can occur. The *psoas* muscle, which attaches to the *lesser trochanter* in the groin, also attaches to the *lumbar vertebrae* and passes behind the kidneys. A spasm in that area can make itself felt anywhere along the line. If it's

in the kidney area, you might be tempted to take pills for it or worse.

A lady once came to a book-signing where I was autographing and occasionally working on an elbow or knee and said, "I wish it worked for kidneys." She had just been told she had a kidney problem and was due for a cystoscope the next morning. I asked where the pain was and sure enough she covered her kidneys with both hands. "Right here." I asked if that was the *worst* spot and she replied that no, the worst was in her groin, which she'd had ever since last week's "aerobic" dance class. Ugh! You can't imagine how that hits me every time. "Aerobic" dance, done as it is without proper warm-up or direction, accounts for many of the injuries sustained by females trying to get into shape. "Will you let me press on the spot that hurts in your groin and a couple in the backs of your legs?" Those are the "aerobic" dance injury sites. She said sure, and I did it right there in the mall. When she stood up I asked her where her pain had moved to. She stood there a second or so and then she leaned over. Then she stretched backward and lifted one knee. "It's gone. Even my kidney pain is gone." I asked if the doctor had asked her about what she did to get the pain, but no, he hadn't. That's what's happening today. People everywhere are trying to get healthy by doing the most unhealthful things, and the doctors haven't caught on to a new disease, sportsitis. The kidney pain didn't come back and that lady didn't go back for the rest of her "aerobic" dance classes either. How did you get *your* pain? A sure way to develop this kind of pain is to run on the road, dance on tile over cement or do straight-leg sit-ups, which P.E. teachers, coaches and DIs have been addicted to for generations.

The last side of the pelvic box to interest us is called the floor of the pelvis. It is *essential* that you know more about it than you do, simply as a matter of self-

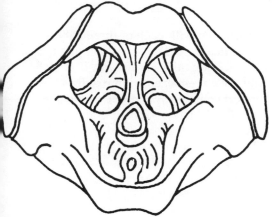

Male pelvis (from above)

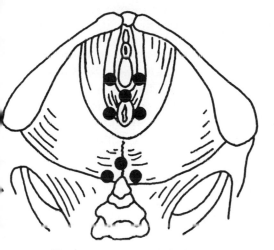

Female pelvis (from below)

FIG. 48: PELVIC FLOOR

familiar with the words *vagina, rectum, anus* and *prostate* (although it is often called prostrate!). There is some tissue between the *anus* and the *genitals*, and while we all know it's there, most don't know its name, the *perineal fascia*. Anyone who has had an *episiotomy* knows it well, too well. When faced with the many six-syllable words denoting muscles and the attachments of muscles, just remember the *sternocleidomastoid* and what that word taught you.

One injures the pelvic floor in many ways, the most universal being a fall that hurts the *coccyx*. Then there are people who have either pronounced tailbones or not much in the way of gluteal muscles and fat to cushion and protect a normal one. Doing many sit-ups on a hard floor can injure that area just as severely, although very few people know what they are doing to themselves or their students at the time. Any woman who has been forced into the *lithotomy position* for childbirth can wonder about injury to the *coccyx* and its muscles. The *lithotomy position* is flat on your back with legs strapped apart and up into metal stirrups It is the position that has necessitated many *episiotomies*, which are routine in the United States but nowhere else in the world. This mostly unnecessary surgery causes spasm and pain, and who needs that!

Rape is a contributor to injuries in the floor of the pelvis, as is sexual child abuse. Inept lovemaking isn't much of an improvement when little or no preparation is given to relax the muscles and provide lubrication. Boys' bikes have contributed to a number of pelvic floor injuries, as have English saddles and pronounced backbones on horses being ridden bareback.

The rough use of a cold *speculum* in a pelvic examination can injure the pelvic structure, as can careless use of instruments in the rectum. Any operation in the abdominal area can produce pain at a

protection. It is involved in every move and even when you sit. It is the floor of the pelvis that determines how good your lovemaking will be and, one day, whether or not you will need diapers for incontinence.

The muscles we will now study have long and hard-to-remember names unless you take the trouble to dismember them. Then it is easy. *Coccyx* is part of most of the muscle names and *pubis* is part of most of the rest. That's the back and the front of you. Pretty nearly everyone is later date, as can any work done on the pelvic floor. Trigger points in that area *can* cause impotence and frigidity, which of course will be blamed on just about everything else, including your mother.

The pelvic box is closed at its nether end by the *coccygeus* muscle, the *levator ani* and the *perineal fascia*. The *coccygeus* attaches to the *ischium* and the *sacrum* at the *coccyx*, which it supports and raises.

Levator ani is the name applied to important components of the pelvic diaphragm; they include the *pubococcygeus, levator prostatae, pubovaginalis, puborectalis* and *iliococcygeal* muscles. Levators are designed to elevate the organ or structure into which they are inserted. These muscles *all* play an important part in lovemaking, and all you thought you needed was another person!

The *pubococcygeus* originates in front of the *obturator canal* and extends to the *anococcygeal ligament* and the side of the *coccyx*. Keep remembering that any injury to the *coccyx* can come back to haunt you sooner or later, and later isn't much better than sooner. Spasm in the muscles under the scalp will be called a headache; in the gluteals it is called a backache; but what do you call a spasm in the pelvic floor? Sometimes it's called over-the-hill, and a little later on, incontinence.

The *pubovaginalis* is the name applied to a part of the anterior section of the *pubococcygeus*; it inserts into both the *vagina* and the *urethra*. It is involved with the *control of urine*. The *levator prostatae* is also a name applied to part of the *pubococcygeus*; it is inserted into the *prostate* and the tendinous center of the *perineum. It too is involved with the control of urine.* Would anyone ever think that a fall or a blow sustained fifty years earlier might account for the fact that Old Uncle Charlie dribbles down his pants leg in public? And did anyone blame the same problem or those called "female troubles" on the "routine" *episiotomies*

you sustained with each of three babies? For that matter, did anyone think that the babies had anything to do with it at all? If you cough, sneeze or jump across the floor in exercise class and wet your pants, you probably have trigger points in the pelvic floor.

The *iliococcygeus* is the posterior portion of the *levator ani*; it originates as far forward as the *obturator canal* and inserts on the side of the *coccyx* and the *anococcygeal* body. Again, if varicose veins in the legs improve after spasms in the leg muscles have been eased, what happens to hemorrhoids if spasm in the pelvic floor is released? For that matter, did you know that hemorrhoids are varicose veins?

Before you start your pelvic floor search, do quick fix for the groin (page 92). And *after* you have stretched, do the following. Have your subject lie supine with hips supported by a pillow. The knees should be bent and held apart by the subject's hands. Use your fingers to find the central tendinous point of the perineum, between the anus and the genitals, male or female. Press straight in *gently*. There may have been trigger points there for years, gone unrecognized, unsought and certainly unfound. Use the compass technique and then

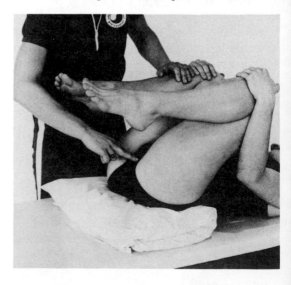

move on to the four outlying trigger points.

Next, have the subject take the knee-chest position by kneeling and bringing the shoulders as close to the table as possible and resting the head by turning it to one side. The arms are brought back along the sides of the legs. Use the third finger to slide in under the tip of the tailbone. There is usually a very sensitive trigger point there. Also, nobody likes having a tailbone disturbed, and there will be some tension. Perhaps this isn't exactly in your training either, so take your time; both of you will get used to it. A well pelvic floor is worth whatever it takes. Use the compass technique east and west and you will probably pick up trigger points along the sides of the *coccyx*. Finish by pressing down on the outside or top of the tailbone and follow with the side-lying stretch you did for the lower back (page 89). There are excellent "sexercises" in my paperback *How to Be Slender and Fit After Thirty* and *Exer-Sex*. See the *Sources* section, at the end of the book.

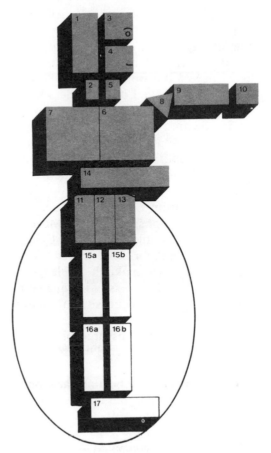

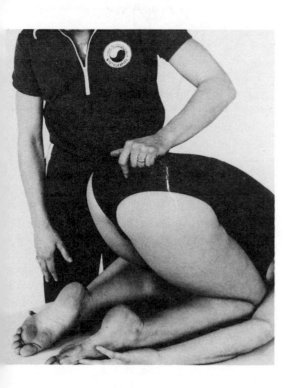

ZONE V, SEGMENTS 15, 16, 17: THE LEGS AND FEET

"The legs go first," say the old athletes. And do you know why? It is certainly not due to age per se, although "old legs" do indeed go first on athletes. They fail their owners because they have been overused and undercared for since the athletic career began, often in Little League. Little Leaguers are taught to pitch and bat and run bases. They are exhorted to win, but to be good sports while they are doing it. They are told to be good sports when they lose, too, and they are taught to be on time, have clean uniforms and to *play through* the "minor" pains that Little Leaguers are heir to. Those "minor pains" are usually called "Little League elbow," "growing pains," "muscle cramps'' and ''shin splints.'' If they strain something, they are taped. If they sprain something, they are X-rayed and then taped. But at no time are they taught to take care of the wonderful bodies they are starting to ruin. Little Leaguers know where their *biceps* are—they are always flexing them to see if they are growing— but they wouldn't know a *tibialis* from a *frontalis*, not even that one supports their socks and the other their caps.

Move up from Little League and see what high school sports teach. More of the same and as little of the same. College is no better, and for those, called ''meat on the hoof,'' who make the big leagues, it's worse. To the stress of playing competitively, add the necessity to make a living and to that add today's economy, in which the best jobs are going glimmering with the same wind that blows the pennants.

Legs start taking a beating early on in America, and that goes for everyone's legs. Athletes' legs, while important, are only important to a few. That's how many athletes we have, compared to the general population. The average leg, on the average boy or girl, suffers from the start from a *lack* of exercise. Beginning in baby carriages, playpens and strollers, the will to move is systematically starved. The muscles don't atrophy from nonuse; it's worse than that: they never develop in the first place! It is fairly easy to put older people into good shape even when they have let their bodies deteriorate over the years. They *walked* everywhere as children. It is all but impossible to put today's teens and twenties into top shape, because, when their bodies were forming, they never walked at all. That is also why we spent *two billion dollars* last year on ''sports medicine.'' That money wasn't spent just by athletes, but by the average John and Jane who want to be fit. *Wanting* fitness isn't enough. You have to know how to rehabilitate the young person who doesn't know he or she is half crippled to begin with.

The legs are important in their own right, but they also contribute to the well-being of many body structures. Since they are right beneath the pelvis, any injury they sustain can refer messages into the floor of the pelvis, making sex less than a joy, and on up into the back, which turns everything off. They can refer pain to the abdomen, the chest, and the upper back, and they aren't blameless in some headaches, either. The first thought when you are faced with an aching back should be the *gluteals*, followed immediately by the legs, even if they are completely free of warning pain.

What sort of leg pain do we see most often? Cramps in the backs of the legs and ''shin splints,'' which are really just leg cramps too but in the fronts of the legs. We see knee pain that is called ''trick knee,'' Osgood-Schlatter disease and *chondromalacia*, which is called

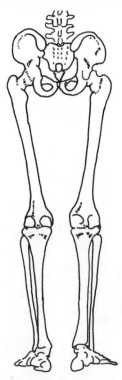

FIG. 49: BONES OF LEGS, POSTERIOR VIEW

"growing pains" in the young. The same thing is simplified to arthritis in the old. All these names in spite of the fact that, like headaches, most knee pain is muscular and of the same cause: muscle spasm.

We see varicose veins, which pop out sooner in the legs of the pregnant but sooner or later in the legs of almost everyone else. The aches are treated with heat, cold and tape, the varicosities with elastic stockings, which exacerbate the condition. The spasmed legs are having trouble enough getting nutrition down to the feet without being squeezed even further.

We see swollen ankles without a history of sprains, and we see (or rather hear about) fatigue, feelings of pins and needles, numbness and poor balance. We are told of "sciatica," "heel spurs," and "sore bones." If we have the patience to watch the crowds in air terminals, we can observe every kind of terrible walk there is. We will wait all day, however, to see a good, healthy, strong, energetic gait. If someone has the misfortune to trip, he or she usually goes down. The development

of proprioception has been one of the lacks in American physical education.

Have the subject lie prone on the table with legs a little apart and feet hanging over the edge to prevent straining the muscles in the fronts of the legs. If the leg is at all painful, slip a pillow under its length.

Standing to the outside of the leg you are about to work on, reach over to put your elbow into the spot marked circle 36. Press down and toward you at an oblique angle. Use a strong compass, especially north and south. Then go down the line at one-inch intervals to the *popliteal* (back of the knee) as you did in *Quick Fix*.

Instead of doing the back of the leg piecemeal this time, do the entire line as shown by the black dots. Take it all the way to the ankle. Keep in mind that no matter what you find in the rest of the leg, circle 47 and the edges of the *gastrocnemius* and *soleus* will be extremely sensitive. As you approach the ankle, switch from your elbow to either your knuckle or a bodo.

You should note that when you are working on one of the subject's legs, the

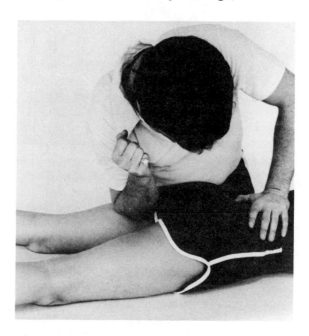

FIG. 50: LEG. POSTERIOR VIEW

other is free to kick back against your head. With or without a shoe, this can be a jolting experience. Certified Bonnie Prudden Myotherapists have been knocked cold with such a blow, much to everyone's dismay. Avoid that by having someone protect you by laying a hand on the free leg. Either that or keep your eyes open. When you do the outside of the leg, you lean over the free leg and your own body will protect you against any reflex jerk.

Now we come to the middle of the back of the leg. This line is the Ma Bell for the legs, because under it runs the *sciatic nerve*, the nerve that is blamed for far more discomfort than it deserves, since it is more sinned against than sinning. Look carefully at Figure 51 and also read what various medical dictionaries say about sciatica. Here's how one dictionary puts it:

> **Sciatica** . . . a syndrome characterized by pain radiating from the back into the buttock and into the lower extremity along its posterior or lateral aspect, and mostly caused by prolapse of the intervertebral disk; the term is also used to refer to pain anywhere along the course of the sciatic nerve.

Since the *sciatic nerve* is the widest nerve in the body and one of the longest, that gives a great deal of leeway, and if it really is "mostly caused by prolapse of the intervertebral disk," there must be a great many "prolapsed disks" around. Another dictionary goes on:

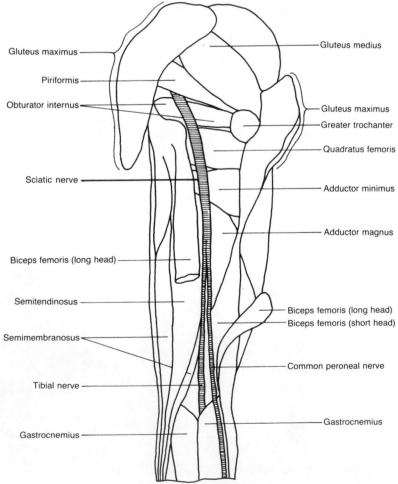

FIG. 51: THE SCIATIC NERVE

Because of its length the nerve is exposed to many different kinds of injury and inflammation of the nerve or injury to it. This causes pain that travels down from the back or thigh along its course in the leg and into the foot and toes. Certain muscles of the leg may be partly or completely paralyzed.

This particular dictionary does not claim that *sciatica* is commonly caused by a prolapsed vertebra, although it does list herniated disk along with back injury, arthritis of the spine, pressure by certain types of exertion, toxic substances such as lead or alcohol and pain referred on connected nerve pathways to the *sciatic nerve* from a disorder in another part of the body. That pain would be called "idiopathic," which, as we have already seen, means "nobody knows why."

With all that information and Figure 51, what have we got for you to work with? The plate shows that the nerve is in great danger from spasms in the *gluteal* muscles; since it enters the pelvis passing under the *piriformis* (no slouch when it comes to spasm), it is surprising that there isn't more *sciatica*. Aside from disk disease, we are offered back injury as a cause. That's legitimate enough and rather cheerful news, since *most* pain due to back injury can be erased with Myotherapy, and that includes taking care of the scars due to operations. *Arthritis of the spine* shouldn't be a stumbling block either, since arthritis seems to be secondary to muscle spasm when it comes to *causing* pain. When they say *toxic substances* you should remember that drugs are toxic substances and go over yours again in the P.D.R. (Physician's Desk Reference) in the library. When the dictionary speaks of "idiopathic causes," that means the tests have been negative and your guess is as good as the next one's. Try a complete trigger-point hunt. You may well be agreeably surprised.

First check out 1, 2 and 3 in the seat and then start your run down the center of the back of the leg right over the *sciatic nerve* as it begins its descent into the leg at circle 38. If the subject does have *sciatica* or any other painful condition of the leg, put a pillow under its entire length. Have him or her tell you any time a trigger point refers to another area, and then interrupt your search and check out that spot at once. Be sure to note those spots on your tracing map. You may want to check both later for a sending or receiving station.

Try to get in between the muscles as you use your compass technique in an east-west direction. You should think of it as a hunt for a trigger point *hiding* under one edge or the other, because it probably is. As you work your compass at one-inch intervals, there may be response from the groin, the inner surface of the thigh and even the knee. Should the subject ever complain of knee pain in the future, you will know that wearing an elastic knee bandage, rubbing it with ice or drawing off fluid are unlikely to be the answers. Check your map for trigger-point information and go right to those referring spots.

About one third of the way down the thigh, the *sciatic nerve* splits into the *tibial nerve* and the *common peroneal*. The latter runs down the outside of the lower leg. That area will be extremely sensitive in athletes and dancers and may well contribute to the plethora of low-back pain in those who indulge in either activity. When you approach the *Achilles tendon*, use your knuckle, or even better, the shaft of the bodo laid across the tendon. It will give you more control. You may find that the *Achilles tendon* is shortened and extremely sensitive. This is often found in women who wear high-heeled shoes exclusively and in athletes who either stretch *before* warm-up or omit stretch altogether.

Start your work for the outside of the back of the leg at circle 37 and proceed down the entire line at one-inch intervals. You will find this outside line to be less sensitive than the other two.

Stretching the back of the leg requires

two separate stretches. Check back with the calf stretch, in *Quick Fix*, on page 102. That is the stretch in which you bent the knee while pressing down on the ball of the foot. First, press the toes straight down toward the knee and, after doing three press/release stretches, turn the foot inward and repeat. This stretches the outer side of the lower leg. Follow that with three presses with the toes turned outward. This will stretch the muscles in the inner side.

A "normal" leg should bend far enough to allow the heel to touch the buttock. If you measure the distance from heel to buttock *before* you do the front of the thigh and again afterward, you can get a good indication of the progress you are making in releasing spasm in the *quadriceps*. If, when you do the calf stretch and approach the buttock with the heel, the seat rises with tension, it is a clear message to go for muscles in the groin and front of the thigh.

Whenever the subject lies down either supine or prone, check out the directions to which either the toes or heels point. If they are uneven, one muscle (at least) has spasm, felt or *not yet* felt. If, when the subject is prone, one heel leans out farther than the other, do the trigger points all along the *outside* of the leg right up to and including 1, 2, 3, 4, 5 and 6, the *gluteals*. If the subject is supine and one foot rests quite comfortably at a better turnout angle than the other, do the *inside* of the less relaxed side first, then the outside of the relaxed. Each time, the leg with spasm will tell you where it is, with pain.

If your subject has observable *pigeon toes*, the trouble lies in the muscles on the inner aspects of the legs, in the *groin* and in the *gluteals*. If the subject is a baby (see *Pain Erasure the Bonnie Prudden Way, Sources* section), teach the parents how to find the trigger points and how to stretch the little legs by turning the whole leg outward *many times a day*. The trigger-point hunt should be confined to a few minutes every other day, with only

enough presses to elicit a wail starting from smiles. That number is usually three, but it is enough. Have the parents keep track of where they press each day so that they don't overdo in one area and neglect others. If your subject walks like a duck, with feet turned out (remember, that walk often accompanies swayback and often flat feet, so if you see one look for the other), do the outsides of the legs up to and including the hips. The turn for those people is *in*.

Before stretching the backs of the upper legs, take the trigger points out of the muscles in the fronts of the legs and both the inner and outer aspects.

The leg is a beautiful column. Even when it has too much padding, one can look at Figure 52 and say, "*My* leg looks like that *somewhere*." It's almost enough reason to take off some unneeded and usually unwanted pounds.

In the front of the leg, as in the back, you have three lines running from ankle to groin. Probably the best place to start is at circle 35, on the *rectus femoris*, in the center of the leg just above the *patella*.

Press into the muscle as usual and then, keeping the pressure on, cross over in the compass technique as far as the skin will allow and then pull back under the edge of the *rectus femoris*. That will allow you to include the *vastus intermedialis* and the inside edge of the *vastus medialis* (inside) and the edge of the *vastus lateralis* (outside), depending on where you have positioned yourself. Cross back with the pressure still steady and do the opposite side. Proceed with this east-west compass action at one-inch intervals all the way to the groin. Notice that where the muscle is fullest, you may have to stretch the skin considerably in order to encompass both edges. Usually the most sensitive area will be about halfway up, where the inward reach of your compass will catch the first large black dot on the *sartorius* (Fig. 53). Each of the other two *sartorius* dots will probably be sensitive as well. If

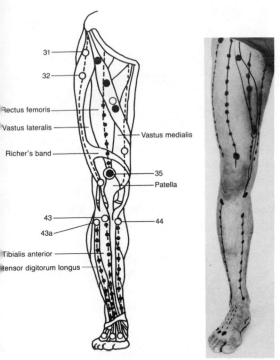

31

32

Rectus femoris

Vastus lateralis

Vastus medialis

Richer's band

35

Patella

43

44

43a

Tibialis anterior

Extensor digitorum longus

FIG. 52: THE LEG, ANTERIOR VIEW

you are a yoga neophyte you should be given the warning needed by every *American* who would partake of that ancient wisdom and activity. *Warm up before stretch; you are hurting yourself.*

Stand to the outside of the leg you have just worked on and have the subject turn slightly away from you. This will give you a good angle for circles 31 and 32, on the *tensor fasciae latae*. Your compass technique inward toward the median line of the body will not be very sensitive, as a

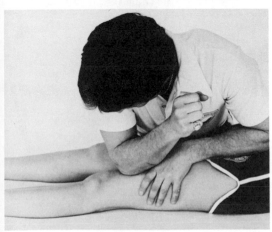

general rule. However, when you pull toward the back, it may be startling in its response. The pain will probably refer to the outside of the leg, to the *iliotibial band*, and you may feel it in *both* the groin and the knee. It may also refer to the *gluteals*, in the seat. Starting at circle 31, follow the line down the leg to the knee at one-inch intervals.

The innermost line begins just to the inside of the *patella* and proceeds up to the groin. If the knee is a "trick knee," "arthritic," or has ever been operated on, even with an arthroscope, all three lines will be extremely sensitive. Arthroscopy is an operation, and although it may do less overall damage than an operation that lays the knee wide open, it does cause tissue injury and it does leave scar tissue behind it . . . *inside*, where it can't be seen.

The front of the lower leg houses many trigger points, not only because the muscles are numerous, but also because it is they that manage the small movements that maintain constant balance. To observe them at work, kick off your shoes and stand on one foot with the knee slightly bent. The sinews in the top of the instep and at the ankle will keep up a continuous flutter. The *extensor digitorum longus*, circle 43A, which attaches to the four outer toes, will be under the first line you tackle. If the subject has a "classic Greek foot" ("long second toe") or "Morton's toe," you will discover a hornet's nest of trigger points starting on the instep and going right up that outer line. Use the compass at one-inch intervals up to the knee.

When you have completed the outer line, locate the *tibia*, the long shinbone. To its outside lies the *tibialis anterior*. Start at circle 43 and go down the leg at one-inch intervals. This particular muscle is responsible for making even feet that are flat work well. It *must* be kept clear of spasm. It also plays a major role in balance, and this applies as well to the skater as to the elderly person whose brittle bones should be protected from falls.

The third line starts at circle 44 and covers the edges of the *gastrocnemius* and *soleus*, in the back of the leg. You have already had experience with those in *Quick Fix* and just a little while ago in this chapter. The golden rule should apply with that line. Try to imagine *yourself* under your subject's elbow.

There are only the inside and the outside of the leg left to do, but these two lines are the most important of all and often the most sensitive. The inside of the lower leg has been covered, but not that of the upper leg.

Have the subject lie on her side and pull the top leg up and out of your way. Begin at the lowest of the large black dots, near the knee. Your initial pressure will be on the *sartorius*, but as you bring your compass technique to bear and press away from you, you will take in the *vastus medialis*, one of the key muscles in knee injury or disease such as arthritis. *Take it easy* or you may lose your subject's confidence. Watch the response carefully and stop your pressure when it is too much or you are told it is. The second black dot will almost always be worse, and the third not much better. When you have come to the fourth dot, you have reached a crossroads. Since you started facing the subject's back, your best leverage will be with the line that includes circle 42, toward the front of the leg. Follow that line at one-inch intervals doing an east-west compass. As you press toward the medial line, you will be covering the *gracilis*, and when you press away, you will take in the *adductor longus*. No matter which way you go, it will be painful. When you have worked right up into the groin, go around the table and, starting at the crossroads, go up the line next to circle 41, which traverses the *adductor magnus*. Your compass will take in the side of the *gracilis* and, in back, the edge of the *semitendinosus*. Yes, they *all* affect the knee.

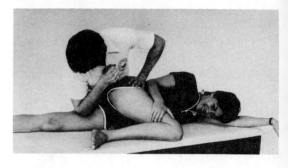

For the outside of the leg, have your subject lie on one side with a pillow between the knees. Do the upper leg first, starting at the knee on the black dot between circles 48 and 43. One of the *most* sensitive spots will be about one third of the way up the leg, at the fourth dot on the huge *vastus lateralis*.

You will remember that earlier we were talking about the muscles of the lower back and mentioned the *quadriceps femoris*, or "quads" (*vastus medialis*, *vastus intermedius*, *vastus lateralis* and *rectus femoris*). I call them the O'Quads,

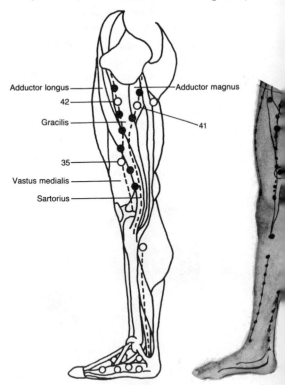

FIG. 53: LEG, MEDIAL VIEW

because they are like a family of fighting Irish. They not only take on all comers, but fight even more effectively (or destructively) among themselves. If either the *vastus medialis* or the *vastus lateralis* is in severe spasm, it will pull the knee in its own direction against the best strength of the other. I have a knee that houses just such a belligerent pair, and often as I'm walking along there will be a snapping sound and the knee feels as though it might lock. It never does, though, because I recognize the warning. Since it always pulls to the outside, I know it's my *vastus lateralis* that is flexing itself into a fist. I have a choice: stop and fix it with pressure to the *vastus lateralis*, or ignore it until one day when I really need that knee it will lock on me for real. When you, the athlete, the dancer, the semipro, weekend athlete or just plain average get-through-each-day-as-it-comes person, hear and feel that snap . . . get rid of your trigger points, because it's Saturday night in Dublin for the O'Quads.

A knee that harbors chronic spasm in any one of the four *quadriceps* muscles is always in danger, and sometimes the slightest insult is enough to ignite the touchy O'Quads. Also keep in mind that the attachments for them are the *common tendon of the patella*, in the front of the leg, and half a dozen anchors in the lower back. A bum knee can cause back pain, and back pain can refer to the knee. Is it any wonder that ice and taping and resting a knee falls short of finding the cause of the trouble and often in giving any relief from pain?

For the outside of the lower leg, just continue your compass at one-inch intervals to the ankle between the two dotted lines, circles 43 and 48. You will be covering the *peroneus brevis* and the *peroneus longus*, often the culprits when tendinitis is the diagnosis.

To stretch the lower leg, use the calf-muscle stretch with the foot pointed in all three directions (page 102), and then, lying supine with legs outstretched, point the toes downward (pronation) and then, keeping the pronated position, point the toes first inward and then outward. Do this exercise at least five times.

For the upper-leg stretch do the flexibility bounce with hands behind the back and the *head up* (page 99). To get at the inner and outer aspects of the upper leg, do the straight-leg hip wag: Stand with feet apart, leaning forward from the hips. Keep the legs straight and the shoulders still and wag your seat from side to side. Start with eight and work up to thirty-two. Take your time; an increase of eight a week is fine.

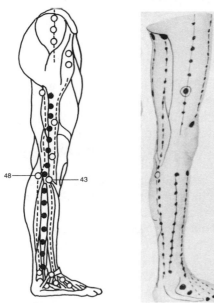

FIG. 54: LEG, LATERAL VIEW

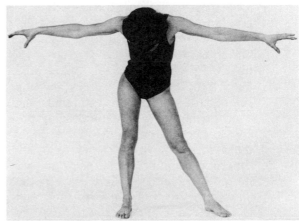

To stretch the front of the thigh, have the subject lie prone and try to bring the heel of first one foot to touch the buttocks by pressing down in short, *gentle*, rhythmic bounces, then the other, and finally both. If you use music, you will get results faster, and that goes for any stretch exercise. Measure results from time to time. If you have done well *and then all of a sudden there is a relapse* and a tightening of either the *rectus femoris*, in front of the leg (tested by the heel-to-buttocks press), or the *biceps femoris*, in the back of the leg (checked with the BHF test in the Kraus-Weber minimum muscular fitness test, page 134), ask your subject what's wrong with his/her life. Something is almost always causing stress when muscles suddenly shorten, especially those muscles.

The Feet

When you did the quick fix for the feet, you did almost all there was to do except the only prop we offer, "The $1.50 Fix for the Long Second Toe." Long second toe is often referred to as "Morton's toe," named after the Dr. Morton who first understood its enormous influence on the rest of the body as well as the feet. Dr. Janet Travell calls it "the classic Greek foot," because she noticed that the people who posed for all the ancient Greek statuary must have had such feet. The Greeks were more fortunate than we are, however, because they wore sandals, which allowed the toes to spread wide and thus provide the balance those who have the problem need. We, on the other hand, box our feet into shoes and consider pain, hammertoes, bunions and even aching legs the natural aging process. Aging isn't that destructive. Many older people have their own teeth and they don't bumble in the half-light permitted by cataracts. There are aids that allow them to hear whatever they *want* to hear (which appears not to be every-

thing). There is no need or excuse for most postural faults, and there is no reason to accept ugly, bumpy, twisted feet.

Do *you* have a long second toe? "No," you say, "mine are all even." Take a different kind of look. With one hand, bend all your toes downward and, with a felt-tipped pen, circle the first joints of the first two toes. If the joint of the second toe is farther forward in your foot than that of the big toe, you have a long second toe, no matter how far the *tips* reach. The placement of the joint is what counts.

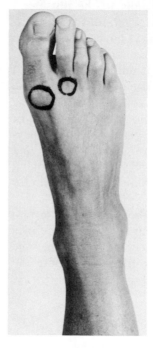

A "good" foot lands on its heel and as the weight is shifted forward onto the front of the foot it lands on the ball of the foot just behind the big toe and on the outside edge of the foot. This provides a solid tripod, a well-balanced base for the column of the leg, above. The foot sporting the long second toe is different. From its landing gear, the heel, the foot drops forward onto the joint of the long second toe, which is in the middle of the *metatarsal arch*. On the feet of people who have this condition and must wear shoes, especially tight shoes such as those worn by women, there is usually a large callus

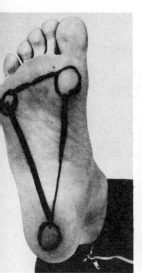 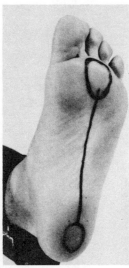 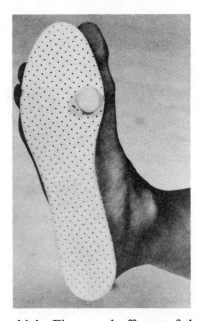

at the point where the front of the foot strikes and another on the outside of the big toe where it constantly grabs for balance, and a *hammertoe*, or bent second toe. And the start of a bunion.

If you walk behind a woman who is handicapped in this way and is wearing high heels, the heels will teeter laterally with every step, which is as nothing compared to what is going on in the feet and legs. Since these feet are not tripods, but knife edges, the ankles are being stressed, the knees are being stressed and so are the hips, as is every muscle that holds these structures together and provides locomotion.

The worst trigger points will be on the insteps just back of the toes, especially the second toes and the soles of the feet. The lower legs will have garnered a goodly supply in each: the *tibialis anterior*, *extensor digitorum longus* and the *flexor digitorum longus*. No muscle in the lower leg will escape; it is merely a matter of time and degree.

What is "The $1.50 Fix"? The prop itself is a pair of Dr. Scholl's innersoles. To these you will affix a couple of pads. Ask the druggist for a sheet of adhesive foam. It is about one eighth of an inch

thick. First, peel off part of the backing and then cut out a circle about the size of a quarter and stick it to the *bottom* of the sole. It should be stuck right on top of the circle over the ball of the foot behind the big toe. Look at the picture showing the tripod action of a "good" foot. Then cut a second circle about the size of a nickle and stick it onto the first. Put the inner soles, pads down, in your shoes. This should be just enough to lift your weight from the long toe joint and move it onto the ball and outer edge of your foot, providing the stable tripod base.

If you wear sandals, you can stick the circle pads to the balls of your feet and get the double benefit, both the lift and the freedom to spread your toes. If you must wear high heels, then make use of your own home to go shoeless and stockingless as well. Do *not* walk around on wooden or tile floor in socks or stockings. They are like footed tights and cause many falls, some of them serious. As for footed tights on wooden floors of gyms or dance or exercise studios, if your instructor permits them she should immediately invest in more insurance.

Sports in America

In the fifties, when I was in Europe giving about three thousand school-aged children the Kraus-Weber minimum muscular fitness test (page 131), the people wanted to know what I was looking for. I explained that we had given the same test to thousands of American children and had found them seriously lacking in both strength and flexibility. We were testing the European children so we could make some comparisons. When I told them that, while Americans failed at the rate of 58 percent, only 8 percent of Europe's children had less than the minimum needed for healthy daily living, they were astounded. I kept hearing "But Americans are so sporty! How is such failure possible?"

Most of the Europeans we talked to were meeting their first real American: me. But they were sure they knew all about us. To begin with, we had just won a war, and then too they had seen our Olympic athletes, our rodeo riders, our tennis and golf players on the European equivalent of Pathé News. They were well acquainted with our prowess as polo players and mountain climbers, so of course Americans must be "sporty." They had a lot of information about us, but their conclusions were inverted. Those top athletes were definitely Americans, but not all Americans were ath-

letes. Most definitely not; nor are we today.

Now, in the eighties, we are as confused about sport in America as the Europeans were thirty years ago. Now *we* think we are "sporty." There is one clear reason for this muddled thinking, and in two words it's *Madison Avenue*. We read articles in our newspapers and magazines about the fitness boom. Our children will ride nothing but ten-speed bikes and wear no shoes without three lateral stripes. Most of the products advertised on TV are framed with healthy people in silk shorts, tank tops and running shoes. Polls announce to the world that 50 percent of Americans exercise daily. This is backed up by the sight of several joggers bobbing along the highway, a couple of mad marathon melees and the weekly membership special at the "spa." We are told we are becoming the fittest nation, although no one says fitter than whom. We are told that everyone is dieting. If so why are we so fat? We are told there is more interest in sports, but no one specifies that the interest is in watching, rather than in participating. We are told . . . we are told . . . and by whom? Actually the polls ask the wrong questions of the wrong people. The athletic shoes and sports clothes are mostly for appearance, and Madison Avenue is getting the workout. This is not to say that America is not listening and trying. It is doing both, but what are the facts in this matter? There is a wonderful old story that explains us as a nation.

Long ago two thieves, abhorring work but well informed on human nature, descended on a peaceful little country, determined to fleece the populace. Dressed as tailors they set up shop in the center of the marketplace. They spent their days pretending to cut and sew, often standing back to admire each other's work while commenting on style, color and workmanship; they would also enlist the opinions of bystanders. At first they were considered mad and given a wide berth, until a rich and curious merchant asked them what they were about. He was told that they were making the wonderful clothes he was looking at from material that only the pure in heart could see. The scoffers had hearts so black that to them the material was invisible. The merchant, who was not given to purity in any aspect, was suddenly filled with fear. Struggling with guilt and anxiety, he immediately not only "saw" the material but ordered himself measured for a coat. Stalking off, he left a confused and also guilt-ridden group of people. Afraid of being considered less than honest, they too began to "see" the gorgeous bolts. The two thieves did a roaring business for a week. Then word reached the king, who commanded them to appear at the palace.

The very next day, the self-appointed "tailors" presented themselves at court. They were accompanied by many well-paid "assistants," who carried in bolt after bolt of the now famous "material." The king was really a good and humble man, but, like many others, he felt he was neither good nor humble enough, and he was quickly made aware that he was not. His doctor exclaimed over the materials, as did his Master of the Sword. The prime minister was especially vociferous in its praise, and suddenly his wife, the queen,

stated that she *must* have a gown in that heavenly blue. So shaken was the king's confidence in himself that he too ordered a suit of clothes, in crimson, and commanded a parade in which all might display their finery *and the purity of their hearts*. The tailors went to work with a will and a cart filled with gold.

The day of the great parade dawned bright and still and the royal road was lined with peasants come to observe the wonders. The bugles sounded and the richly caparisoned horses of the nobles pranced in the invigorating chill.

As the great assemblage approached, a silence fell on the people. Not a word was spoken and the watchers stood as if turned to stone. Suddenly, as the king passed close to a small family group, a little boy whose clear eyes and innocent face gave ample evidence of a still-pure heart, piped up, "But, Papa, the king is *naked!*"

We, the American people, are that king. We have accepted as truth so much nonsense put about by venders of "material" that only the "smart," the "educated," the "fit," the "Beautiful," the "with-it" can see, that our nakedness is startling to other nations. "Pure in heart" they are not . . . but, for the most part, when they are taken in, it is not by dishonest makers of dream cloth.

We are not a nation of athletes or even would-be athletes. In fact, a great number of us really want to be matadors, *but* we don't want to fight the bull. Some of us do what other people do because we think they know more than we do. Most of us fall victims to chicanery because we not only lack the facts, but the good sense to apply such facts as we do know, to ourselves. Instead, we follow "tailors" who not only make up "facts" to suit themselves, but with time and repetition come to believe what they are saying . . . and then act on it. Take a look at what our "tailors" have wrought in these United States.

1. We have one of the highest infant-

mortality rates in the civilized world, and it isn't just because of hospitals and the American Way of Birth. It is also due to poor nutrition and a lack of physical exercise in the maternal population. There is the key to fitness in a nation, *the maternal population.*

2. Preschool children in the United States watch an *average* of forty hours of TV a week. Doesn't "the maternal population" know that inactivity in small children has the same effect as would imprisoning a young animal? Doesn't "the maternal population" know how to bring activity to little children? Certainly not. Where would they find that out? There was no physical fitness in either their homes or their schools when *they* were growing up. They never suspected there were dangers in sedentary living, not even that there was a better way to live.

3. As a result of the above, *most* American children enter school failing the minimum muscular fitness test, which *most* European children pass easily. Our children are either weak or inflexible or both. If a child fails two or more parts of the test, it is usually an indication of unrelieved stress. *No* European child failed two, but 32 percent of the Americans failed two or *more.*

4. We "sporty" Americans have almost no physical education worthy of the name. *Almost* stands for the very few schools that are the exceptions, *not* the rule. Private schools, however, are often excepted. While the majority of our children enter schools, both public and private, as physical failures, graduates of our better private schools are far fitter than those graduating from any public school. Why? Because their P.E. programs are better. Why? Parental interest. Why that interest by parents? Because they are paying the bills directly and they expect their money's worth.

5. On graduation day, the already unfit young people face the real world. They become deeply involved in making a living, making a marriage, making a baby, making their mark and in making mistakes. Taught in school to believe the "experts," they go right on following the very same people who have been so *in*expert that they have made us physically the weakest nation in the world, starving nations *not* excepted.

MISTAKES MADE BY THE EXPERTS

Circa 1930 it became accepted in educational circles that John Dewey's ideas on creativity and latitude were important if education was to progress. At that time the physical educators understood that to mean a letup on discipline and demands for excellence. All children love to play, so "play" would be provided instead of all those "sweaty calisthenics," gymnastics, rope climbing, and so on. Since there can be no excellence without effort, we now get a good look at what that incredible decision has cost us, as a nation as well as individually.

The children who entered school with the best bodies and the greatest fund of healthy energy made the demanding first teams. The others became Tail-End Charlies. The team members built better bodies, honed their skills, enjoyed their positions and won. The lesser-endowed were repeatedly shown up, defeated and ultimately bored. They grew to hate gym and they lost. They lost the chance to better themselves during the best years for physical development. They developed neither skill nor interest. They became what we have as a vast majority, the Sedentary Americans—a nation of Tail-End Charlies worshiping a handful of stars.

At about the same time as Dewey, another "expert" interpreted Freud for Americans. Children who are unhappy develop into unhappy adults was translated to mean "Children must never be allowed to be unhappy." They must "develop creatively at their own speed."

No demands must be made lest we stunt their "creativity." Education entered the "progressive" stage. Today we can see the results of that misinterpretation everywhere.

In order to upgrade education, we emptied our few-room schools and built regional schools, which were "centrally located." The idea was to provide more educational specialists, but there was a serious catch. To move the children to the centrally located schools, busing was required, and thus began "The Great Migration." Off your feet and onto your seat, child of mine. We'll ruin your body to improve your mind. They accomplished the first but not the second. We are only beginning now to wonder if we might not have spent our tax dollars more advantageously had we built walkways to less prestigious schools to which children could walk and where smaller groups would learn basics safely.

The war changed things too. It ushered in television, and American children learned to put their feet up before learning to walk, run, jump or skip. While there were "experts" in hordes teaching how to brush teeth, take college boards, drive a car and stop perspiration odor, *not one said put a lock on the TV set and get the kids out of doors*. So America sat down.

In the thirties, doctors who were taught nothing about exercise in medical schools were telling men over thirty-five to "sit down, for God's sake; do you want to have a heart attack?"

Women were told by physical educators that if they jumped they would scramble their reproductive organs. That surfaced again from the same "experts" a year ago in connection with jogging.

Girls were told to "rest" during their menstrual periods, and they soon learned that a menstrual period guaranteed freedom from gym, which they considered, in one word, yuk! The effect of that was to develop a nation of girls who "menstruated" nine months a year, September through May.

The "experts" in physical education considered girls so fragile that they were denied the more exciting and faster rules of boys' basketball. Marathon running was considered impossible for them, and they were told they could not do "boys' push-ups" because they were "built funny." Although girls of the previous generations had done chin-ups on the bar in the cloak room doorway, those of the thirties were convinced that they were too weak to attempt them.

An "expert" from Texas sold the public schools on the "fact" that duck walking caused meniscus injuries in football players and that deep squats for weight lifters did the same thing. Therefore no one should do deep knee bends. Knee bends were forthwith banned in public schools, but expensive private schools ignored him.

In the seventies another physical education "expert" stated that "static stretch" should replace the tried and true "ballistic stretch." In "ballistic stretch" increased flexibility is attained by *gentle* bouncing, usually to music or a count. In "static stretch" the stretch is pushed to its extreme and held between twenty and sixty seconds. To see firsthand how inexpert this advice is, go to a dance school where "ballistic stretch" is used and then visit a P.E. class where "static stretch" is used, and compare the flexibility of the two groups.

Prior to 1954, when we presented the findings of our study on the lack of minimum physical fitness in American schoolchildren, there was virtually no interest in fitness at all. Even when President Eisenhower said he was shocked by the report and that he would appoint a presidential committee to look into the matter, we were not allowed to use the word *physical*. The committee preferred "Youth Fitness." This left the door open for every kind of nonsense, mental fitness, emotional fitness, social fitness and maybe, yes, a little physical fitness. No matter the name, nothing changed except the attitude of the YMCAs. They began to think "Family Fitness."

When President Kennedy came in, he (or some of his advisers) realized that the President's Council on Youth Fitness and its Citizens' Advisory Council was a do-nothing group, so out it went and the name was changed to the President's Council on *Physical* Fitness. He also decreed that there should be fifteen minutes of exercise daily for schoolchildren. Nothing happened.

The manual for the Division of Girls' and Women's Sport did come out with a remarkable statement. Those "experts" said, "Exercise will not harm girls and women." Late, weak and one step up from the negative, but at least a step.

In the early sixties we started the first Baby-Swim-and-Gym classes at a YMCA in Detroit. The idea spread all over the country, although the "experts" fought it tooth and nail. Babies would drown, they would develop ear infections and meningitis, they would urinate in the pool. They might even "soil" in it! Baby-Swim-and-Gym is still flourishing, because people with common sense began to question the "experts."

Where there's a market, sure enough there will be "tailors," and the vendors began to smell money. The first "health clubs," later called "spas" as well, began to appear. Wall-to-wall carpet, wall-to-wall chrome, saunas (then very chic) and adult wading pools. Designed to increase memberships while at the same time discouraging members from overusing the facilities, they spread like measles across America. The attrition rate is 75 percent. The first rash went out of business, but the second attack was launched by market-wise men. They hired Madison Avenue and added Jacuzzis.

Slenderella gave them a bit of a run for a while, because all you had to do there was lie on a table and you were told it would jiggle your fat away.

Then came Adidas, to change the feet

of America. Like previous styles (saddle shoes and loafers), running shoes were "in," and along with them came a tidal wave of other fads.

Coupled with the fad "aerobic," the fad Adidas ushered in running as the be-all and end-all of fitness. Dr. Paul Dudley White had brought Eisenhower back to the country with exercise, and the YMCAs were promoting "run for your life" programs for postcardiacs. The "stress test" rose out of Texas, where the "no knee bends" edict came from. It became a real money-maker and the smell of dollars grew stronger. The two thriving "tailors," who had been nickel-and-diming it up to then, really went to town. Y's were for middle America, but the big money was with the corporations, who were ripe for picking. It wasn't that they weren't pure in heart, it was that hearts were quitting, and there's nothing better than fear of death to sell a product. The stress test might not make you safe, but it could tell you you were, and that was enough for the corporations. The big boys headed for the test and the track, all paid for by the company.

The billions flowed in, and soon there were hordes of "tailors." Vitamin salesmen who knew as little about their products as the salesmen for the pharmaceutical houses know about theirs, worked overtime. Health-food stores, formerly patronized by dancers, the followers of Gloria Swanson and little old ladies in tennies, began to prosper. Rachel Carson made history with her book *Silent Spring*, and Americans began asking questions about pollution. Bill Longgood brought out his book *The Poisons in Your Food*, and I went on the "Today" show. It was the first time people had fun exercises brought into their living rooms. I had written my first book on physical fitness, *Is Your Child Really Fit?* and was doing one for adults, *Bonnie Prudden's Fitness Book.* It was a compilation of all the many exercises I had done for *Sports Illustrated*. These opened two doors: one was for a spate of fitness books and the other the start of the endless exercise columns in women's magazines.

Madison Avenue shifted into high gear, and physical education, that Sleeping Beauty of stirring America, slept on, leaving each generation that passed through the schools as innocent as babes and as vulnerable.

Madison Avenue told them they were fat. They felt terrible about it.

Madison Avenue said, "Thin is in." So they dieted.

Madison Avenue said, "Fit is it." And they said, "Right on!"

Madison Avenue said, "Aerobic." And they went aerobic.

Madison Avenue said, "Run." They ran.

Madison Avenue said, "Buy." They bought, oh, how they bought. Bikes, slant boards, rowing machines, treadmills, rubber suits and memberships in health clubs and spas.

Madison Avenue said, "Lift weights." They lifted.

Madison Avenue said, "Dance." And ready or not, good dance or not, they "danced" through pain, muscle spasm, shin splints, heel spurs, aching knees, low-back trouble and migraines.

What's the matter with me? Isn't that what I wanted, fitness for everyone? Yes, I wanted fitness for everyone, but no, not physical destruction for too many; and *one* is too many. Let's see what has happened because of our energetic "tailors" and sleeping "experts." Begin with the children.

Ballet we have always had with us, and when little girls had to walk to school they built enough strength to withstand the very abnormal posture of ballet's fifth position, the one used to develop "turn-out." Today's sub-nymphettes are too weak to tolerate safely the least abnormal pressure, and they develop swayback (lordosis, see page 137) by the thousands. They also get a good start on painful feet and knees.

Little guys, many also candidates for rehabilitation, join Little League and similar clubs that took over from the perpetual pickup games that went on in every neighborhood before the advent of television. Those little boys don't stand up to abnormal stresses very well either. Repeated pitches can be called an abnormal stress on both elbow and shoulder. Check the professionals for injuries. What they suffer as adults started in the leagues for "littles."

The football leagues are at least as dangerous for *today's* little boys. Even when nothing as extreme as a fracture occurs, the lesser strains and sprains prepare weak knees, backs, necks and shoulders for what is yet to come: contact with a charging truck on the high school field.

One of the worst developments is the new interest in gymnastics. Gymnastics took off in America with the advent of two rocketing stars, Olga Korbut and Nadia Comaneci. Those were two little girls chosen for their superior potential from thousands upon thousands of Soviet and satellite children. Once selected, they were subjected to intensive training by the greatest gymnastics coaches in the world. The natural ambition of those two youngsters was fed by the hope for riches and fame in countries where the average citizen is less than nothing. Try to imagine what went into their training and that of their teammates, also selected for superiority *at a very young age*. And compare what you feel with what you may feel about what happens here.

A host of little girls in this country saw those marvelous kids on TV. Mothers gasped with admiration as they balanced, twisted, turned and flew through the air. So did fathers and older brothers and sisters. They saw the tiny slender bodies, so feminine and yet so strong. They compared those bodies with their own, pudgy ones. The saucy, beribboned heads bobbed with pleasure as they racked up 10.0 after 10.0. Applause denied American girls except for skaters and swimmers (one year there was an Olympic Gold Medal skier, Andrea Mead Lawrence). The whole world loved Olga Korbut and Nadia Comaneci, and so gymnastics, a sport of consummate difficulty, came to America, the land where there is absolutely no natural preparation whatsoever. In 1960 we could not find eight hundred competitors in the United States and Canada to try out for the Olympics in gymnastics. The Communist world had over a half million, and the number grew every year. The *best* were selected for further training. In this country, all that is needed is the price of the class, and thousands have found the price. Remember, between 85 percent and 100 percent of the children entering school flunk the minimum test, but they are going out for *gymnastics*!

To become a competing gymnast with any hope for the big time (and every little girl dreams of the big time), you must be a gymnast by age ten. Gymnasts today are over the hill between fifteen and seventeen. Russian girls start their training as soon as they can walk, because that's the only way to get where they are going. Exercise is a part of nursery schools. There are keen eyes watching little children in every school. If one shows promise, she goes at once to a special school. In America, few elementary schools have any physical education at all, and nobody watches for superiority or would know it if they saw it. Nor would there be a place to send such a child. By the time the Russian would-be gymnast is six, she is already a long way along the road to perfection. She already has the basics: a good body, strength, flexibility and coordination. The American child has hardly started, and few have even the minimum needed for daily living, let alone gymnastics. And that is only the beginning.

The Russians work many hours a day, not just on the gymnastics themselves but on the contributing arts: dance and music.

Most of the time, we include dance as part of gymnastics, rather than as a separate art, and music is usually ignored altogether, at least by the gymnastic coach, who, reflecting the typical American P.E. college education, is no musician. *Some* of our coaches have had firsthand experience with gymnastics competition. Most come right out of physical education schools and should not be called coaches at all, but what does the American mother know? Remember, today's mother belongs to the maternal population that was totally ignored where physical education was concerned. She may lack knowledge, but all too often she, like some Little League parents, has an overabundance of ambition.

As in much of our education, we are short on basics, and basics in gymnastics makes the difference between a good and safe performance, and a poor, dangerous one. And everybody is in such a hurry. *Years* should be spent *preparing* the body for what are termed "stunts" or "tricks." *We* want results *now*. So, with inferior bodies trying to ape stunts designed by competing athletes of Olympic caliber and executed by superior bodies after many years of basic training, weight training, dance training and total discipline, we reap dismal rewards. Failure to win is only one of them. While it is easy to understand injuries resulting from contact sports, what we are now seeing is an epidemic of chronic injuries to feet, knees, ankles and backs *of little girls, nine and ten years old*. With conventional treatment, ice, rest, taping and orthotics, most injuries to joints become chronic. The problem is due to repetitious strain on muscles already housing trigger points, which can increase the slight spasm to the point where severe damage is done to the muscle by the muscle itself.

American boys and girls are victims. They are victims of a way of life that no other nation on earth "enjoys." Ease is deadly in war, and competition *is* war. These children are also the made-for-plucking victims of the "tailors" and the "experts." The one sells them the excitement of sports on TV, and the other uses that excitement to get them into schools, and camps, leagues and clubs that are forced to produce instant "stars" or go out of business. The real winners are the sports-medicine doctors and someday the rheumatologists.

The weight-training world has its "tailors" and "experts" too. Weight training is invaluable when it comes to building strength. Done correctly it develops strong, healthy, *flexible* muscles. Back in the forties the "experts" were against "pumping iron." Dr. Peter Karpovich, of the famed physical education college Springfield, in Massachusetts, wrote *books* on what it did to ruin flexibility in muscles. One day he walked into the weight room and saw a student standing with straight legs pressing his palms to the floor. Something was wrong. "You can't *do* that. You lift weights. Nobody who lifts weights is flexible." No student at Springfield ever willingly contradicted the great Karpovich, but this one already had. He lifted weights and was flexible. "How did you do it?" He had done it by finishing each lift with a stretch exercise for the working muscles. At the end of the session he had put in a concentrated half hour of stretch exercises while the muscles were both hot and in need of stretch to counter the shortening that occurs with contraction. Since "experts" are constantly contradicting themselves, Dr. Karpovich felt no qualms concerning his about-face. He immediately started writing *in favor* of weight lifting. But who was the real expert in this instance? It was the young, intuitive student who did what he *felt* right. He'd been doing it since he was fourteen and had never read any of the "experts."

Barbells have been on the market since before the days of the ninety-seven-pound weakling, but at first only small-time "tailors" were dabbling with them. The only thing they could think of to spruce up the black, greasy, sweaty, under-the-stairs-at-the-"Y" image was red, white and blue paint and chrome sleeves. Small dumbbells were painted pink for weird women who wanted to build-a-better-bust.

In the sixties, however, the distinct clink of gold pieces could be discerned in the iron department. A *machine* was developed, an *expensive* machine. Now the weight people started to talk American. It was chrome. It had pulleys, levers and padding. It was impressive. It was not for the steamy body builders, who were suspect at best. No, these moneymakers were for the college crowd, the pros and the rehab centers. And as Madison Avenue pulled out all the stops, it joined the treadmills, stress-test paraphernalia, stationary bikes, and rowing machines in the corporate gyms, which were burgeoning as big companies beefed up their images.

The grandpa "tailor" didn't really get going until the seventies, when franchised "spas" and "health clubs" had designed the format for get-rich-quick-and-the-devil-take-the-hindmost schemes. These schemes invariably bilked the physically ignorant public, often ruined the eager franchisers, but were a gold mine for the "tailors." Weight centers for the Flabby American are now as common as movie theaters once were.

A good case in point are the thousands of weight-training centers. One company alone claims 2,400 shops with 175,000 members. Weight training done well and under expert supervision makes an excellent adjunct to a fitness program *if* the rest of the program includes calisthenics, stretch and endurance training. Alone, it is like a half-built house on a wintry day— inadequate. In addition, since the supervision is usually anything but expert, arms, legs, chests, abdominals and *backs* are laying up a stack of trigger points that will provide quite a different image from the one so sought after, and soon. *One* of the dangers lies in the fact that the "experts" running the centers are usually inexpert indeed. In addition, all it takes is one nut, determined to bust his gut, and he sets the pace for half the room. Americans are nothing if not competitive, and we seem to be born with "If he can do it I can do it" tattooed on our hearts.

The greatest weight man of all, Arnold Schwarzenegger says, "When you compete, you always injure yourself. You have to decide if it's worth it." I would give that man the title *expert* without quotation marks. He really is. He is also the first expert I've ever heard admit that, yes, sport does injure. That's quite different from thinking, "I might be injured." All athletes and all dancers injure themselves, all the time. The trick lies in correcting the damage and preventing it from multiplying itself into seriously disabling problems at the time *and ten years down the road.*

There is no need to mention "spas" and "health clubs" again other than to remind you to read the small print on the contract somewhere away from the premises, without the "help" of the salesperson. Remember, too, that a "Lifetime Membership" only means the lifetime of that club. Many such clubs have a reputation for folding their tents like the Arabs and silently stealing away between Saturday night and Monday morning. One thing more: see if there is a cancellation clause in the contract; if there isn't and you are forced to move away or give up going due to an injury you may well have sustained there, you are still stuck with the payments.

"Aerobic dance" is the next major fad on the list. Aerobic dance is just part of the aerobic craze. The word simply means "*able to live, grow, or take place only where free oxygen is present.*" In other words, everything you do is aerobic to a degree. "Aerobic dance" just means dance, but the fad sells it. In the fifties, "chlorophyll" sold green toothpaste. In the sixties, "hormones" sold everything. In the seventies, America went "aero-

bic." The eighties will see the rise (and probably fall) of the word "natural."

Aerobic dance as it is conducted in most classes today could hardly be called *dance.* Not by a dancer, it wouldn't. Jumping up and down, snapping fingers, clapping hands and shouting is certainly action, but dance it is not. However, it filled the vacuum in the lives of girls and women left by the failure of physical education. Madison Avenue has decreed "exercise." So what's around? What's handy? What's *in*? Aerobic dance.

If a real dance teacher calls what she teaches aerobic dance in order to get clients, it is understandable, but the clients at least should know the difference between the hop, skip and jump routine and other forms of exercise in the category labeled "dance." There *are* distinguishing features.

Starting at the bottom, check the footwear of the teacher and her clients. If the group wears sneakers, you are in the wrong place. There might be *one* little old body with feet so wracked with hammertoe, bunions, corns and calluses that for the good of her own self-image she chooses to hide them, or someone with feet so eaten away with athlete's foot that she would be a danger to the others, but if the *teacher* wears them that should send you elsewhere. Sneakers or gym shoes are protective coverings designed to save feet from injury during a wild game. They are essential in *spike sports*, which depend on quick starts and stops and in which action is unpredictable. *Dance* depends on none of those things. The dancer (except for the ballerina on point and the tap dancer, whose shoes are percussion instruments) needs ten toes for balance, and the ten toes of everyone need exercise. The sneaker turns the foot into a hoof.

Next, there is a garment made up of an elastic pantie and two elastic stockings. This is a part of the aerobic dance uniform. Elastic stockings are splints, props and unhealthy. *They compress vessels* and prevent good circulation. Far from helping in cases of varicose veins, they force the heart to work harder, pushing blood down to the feet and back up to the heart *against resistance*. If you have aching legs, don't think "varicose veins," even if you can see them. The veins are present, but the *ache* probably comes from your trigger points, which are causing spasm from overwork. Spasm can make the veins stand out. Drop your arm to your side and grasp your forearm tightly. Hold that squeeze for five seconds and watch the veins in your wrist and hand swell. Why would you do that to your legs?

So much for the clothing. Next, watch the program *before* you sign up. How much and what kind of exercise is provided in the warm-up session? If the warm-up is composed of stretches, the teacher is ignorant of the first rule of safe exercise: *Never stretch a cold muscle*. The warm-up should be vigorous, lots of waist twisting, arm swinging, knee lifting, shoulder and hip rotating, *but not a single jump*. It should last from five to ten minutes in a standing position and, if the class is really good, proceed to kneeling, sitting and lying exercise. Such work is rare in "aerobics," as it is not considered "vigorous enough." If the class is required to blast into off-the-floor action without preparation, take your business elsewhere or you will soon be taking it to a doctor.

It's hard to believe that not long ago we could not mention the word exercise around women. Now if you don't exercise you are definitely not one of the girls. Unless you can *talk* the lingo—pulse rates, stress factors, peaking, isometric, isotonic (whether you use it or not)—you just don't belong.

A *good* exercise class actually does what an aerobic dance class *says* it does. It improves the quality of both heart and lungs, but it does that without damaging the legs and back. In addition, a good exercise class improves the strength of the whole body *and its flexibility*. Women go to aerobic dance and jazzercise because it's fun, and they use music. A good exercise class uses music too but with many tempos and moods, which not only develop differing levels of coordination but feed the emotional needs. Not every hour is noon nor every day full of sunlight. There *is* music other than rock.

If your dance class or exercise class leaves you feeling exhausted and/or in pain, or if you can hardly get around for the next day or two, you have been injured *and your instructor did it*. The words dance and exercise are not to blame; the instructor is. In spite of the emphasis on aerobics, it is *not* necessary, nor is it healthy, to lie gasping in a corner after a particularly vigorous workout. It could well mean that you are outclassed and should start with something less violent. What's good for the movie star is not necessarily good for the moviegoer.

If you are bored by your exercise program, be it at a spa or at the local Y, you are going to drop out sooner or later. If the adult ed. class is taught by a schmoo who is gearing the program to the least fit (often herself), leave. She should not be encouraged. On the other hand, if your instructor got his training in the Navy and runs the class by the count, which not only bores you but hurts (he does small arm circles, double leg lifts and begins the class with jumping jacks), get out. Both army and navy exercise instructors have been developing G.I. and middie bad backs for years.

Nobody could have guessed that Hula-Hoops, skateboards and Frisbees would become national fads, nor would most people in the fifties and sixties have considered that running could involve sixty million American feet in the seventies. About the time that we made the report on American unfitness to the President, you could walk into a YMCA anywhere in the country and, except for a few overage regulars, nothing much happened before school got out. Then, until evening, it was a boys' club. In the evening the bigger "boys" came over. Women could use the pool on Thursdays. Little children and dogs were not allowed in the building. Many of the gyms had upstairs tracks, but few used them. On the corporate level there wasn't much action either, except at the golf club. A visit to the New York Athletic Club gym didn't provide much in entertainment or even an inferior workout. A few men would lift a few weights, run around the track for a couple of laps, toss the basketballs and head for the showers, without having worked up a sweat. At the famous health center in Aspen, Colorado, the picture was the same. Everything lacked challenge and excitement. Then along came running.

Running is an excellent exercise, and cross-country running, with its changing terrain, twists and turns, and even different resistances as grass replaces hard earth, which replaces rocky surfaces, sand and sometimes soft mud, is best of all. Of all the advice the "experts" provided, and a lot of it was very bad indeed, the one thing they could have mentioned had they had any smarts at all, was to stay off the road, that ungiving surface that no flesh, bone and blood can long withstand without injury. Not *one* ever said stick to the cinder track, the golf course, the bridle path or the beach. Not even the soft side of the road was ever suggested. Then, when they told runners to land on their heels, that cinched it. Even a child understands why a cart without springs is harder to ride in than a car. There is *no* cushioning spring.

When runners began to injure themselves, the art of orthotics, a very remunerative line for "tailors," came to the fore. Soon you weren't really a runner unless you had been fitted for orthotics, and at the White House Conference on Sports Injuries in 1980 one of the chief proponents of orthotics was asked what they could do for the runner. The answer

was, he can run twice as far before he begins to feel pain. When the question "What happens then?" was put, he answered, "I tell him to take up biking."

We would never run a valuable horse on cement; never. It's bad for his legs. If running is your thing, get off the road.

Then there was the question of what to do *before* running. The right answer would be "Warm up," but the "expert" said, "Stretch." So all over the country one could observe runners sticking feet up onto fences to "stretch" cold, tense muscles. Every stretch damaged a few fibers; not the whole muscle (that would come later), but a few fibers hurt on every run will soon be enough to end a running career.

Told to "run through pain" or to "run it out," the poor physically ignorant but game American grits his teeth and tells his weeping body to shut up and get on with it. He then proceeds to spread and multiply the damage, or he buys another pair of shoes in the vain search for relief. If he is on a team he will be sent to the whirlpool bath and then taped. Soon enough the pain will transfer from his legs to his back, and that usually settles it as far as running goes. It also settles it for tennis as well.

Action is essential to the human body, and sports like running, climbing, tennis, other racket sports, riding, swimming, biking, all ball games, tumbling, gymnastics and dance are all attractive, exciting and productive when the right body is matched to the right sport; and when the proper preparation has been observed and the right coach employed. There is no one sport that will answer all the needs. Running works the legs, lungs and heart but does little for the upper body. Same with biking. The male gymnast very often builds a strong upper body but may neglect the legs. The swimmer uses arms, legs, chest and shoulders but does little for the abdomen. The dancer, like the runner, builds legs but rarely arms. Most sports develop strength but interfere with flexibility, and flexibility is one half of coordination.

Sports are like language. If you speak two languages, a third and fourth are easier to acquire. The more catholic your interest *and participation* in sports, the easier it becomes to add other skills and the more complete will be the body development. Dance improves flexibility, weight training improves strength, swimming works for endurance and rhythm, rock climbing increases courage, the ability to plan ahead and allotment of energy. The more you can do the more you will be able to do. Basic to that of course is the *pre*training of the body. The earlier any skill is begun the more it becomes a *part* of the body. The reflexes require no overlay of direction. The action becomes subconscious, leaving the brain free to observe, plan and use the exigencies that come to hand.

So much for what is going on among the average Americans striving for a higher level of personal fitness *without* the information that should have been provided during the eight years in elementary school, four years of high school and, for many, four years of college. But what about the elite, the ones who *were* given some training and guidance? Those were the varsity football players, varsity baseball and basketball teams, the cheer leaders, those in gymnastics clubs, and a few swimmers. And what about the pro, the player who went on to make a career out of athletics? He (and it's mostly he, even today) gets the best that's available. And what's available?

R-I-C-E
R . . . Rest
I . . . Ice
C . . . Compression (taping)
E . . . Elevation

There hasn't been an advance in the care of athletic injuries for decades, other than cortisone, which is a mixed blessing since while we are counting the blessing we also have to count the side effects. True, they have lots more tests today, but the care is the same. They had ice when Mighty Casey struck out; only, today it comes in Dixie cups and is rubbed on the injury by the player instead of shredded and packed around it. This new way is a little like telling the distraught expectant father to go boil water for the coming birth. It keeps him busy and out of the way while the game goes on without him.

Today the top teams are pretty evenly matched. All of them get the same type of training from well-known coaches and trainers, and their training tables are supervised by reliable nutritionists and dieticians. They all have team doctors. The championship, however, is determined by which team sustains the fewest injuries to top players. *And so far, nothing has been done about prevention.* Nor have they found a way to cut sideline time. One act by American trainers practically guarantees injury on the field, since it *causes* micro-injury every time it is used: *stretch before warm-up.* The second incredible error made by these trainers and coaches is also born of ignorance. They have no idea what constitutes a good warm-up, what it is supposed to do or how to go about one.

Anytime you stretch a *cold* muscle, you tear muscle fibers, and this is especially true of athletes, who are already loaded with scar tissue from years of practice and competition. Every time an athlete goes into action, some muscle fibers are torn by virtue of the strain put upon them. When these *micro-injuries* heal, they leave behind *micro-scars*, where the edges of *micro-wounds* were drawn together. Scar tissue, whether it is very obvious in a line running from neck to navel, as in chest surgery, navel to pubis in order to extract a baby by C-section, or around and over the stump of an amputated arm, is different from uninjured tissue. It is thicker and less flexible and needs watching, because wherever it is it is apt to harbor trigger points, and trigger points cause *spasm*. Those hidden trigger points don't need a special invitation to light up the scene either. The Rose Bowl game might do it, but a slip on the shower floor, going up or down stairs, even getting out of bed can throw a muscle into spasm. If the emotional climate is right (competition) and the physical climate is right (trigger points in muscles from hard work at endless practice), an athlete can, as Randy Gardner did in the 1980 Olympics, lose the chance for a medal. It should be noted here that his skating partner, Tai Babilonia, went down with him as well. This happens to many teams, be they twos, fives, nines or elevens, when a key man or woman is injured . . . and all of them work just as hard for the championship as the injured player did. *A lot of injuries can be prevented.*

Coaches and trainers will tell you that stretch is essential, and they are right. They know that a tight hamstring doesn't permit as long a stride as a free one. They also know that the player with the tight hamstring has a good chance of pulling it, somewhere along the line. What I rarely hear from them, however, is that *flexibility and strength, in the proper timing and intensity, yield coordination.* One tight muscle can throw off the whole mechanism. *One trigger point in one muscle can do it.* Why was your aim bad? Why did you double-fault three times in a row? It wasn't your eye or your aim, it was a firing trigger point, probably on the scapula (under circle 13, on Fig. 9). The next time it happens, have someone check that trigger point and improve your score.

The muscles of athletes should be constantly worked for flexibility, because scarified muscles shorten over the years. If you began in Little League, "over the years" means college days. When muscles shorten, the joints lose full range of motion, which sets the body up for other injury. If your chest muscles are tight and your antagonist hits your shoulder, it doesn't give back like a young sapling, it separates.

WARM-UPS . . . WHAT ARE THEY?

The word *warm-up* means precisely that, exercises to warm up muscles. In the forties, athletes used to jump around a bit or run in place to "loosen" themselves up, but really warm up? Most of them never heard of it, and even today they don't know how. What they *call* warm-ups are part of their injury program. Basketball players come into the gym and run around bouncing balls, passing them back and forth and tossing them into the baskets. It's called a "lay-up drill"; in essence it is a mini-basketball game without the competition. *The movements are exact copies of what they will do when they play.* They do the lay-up drill with cold muscles. Hockey players mostly warm up by skating slowly around the rink, and with their level of expertise on the smooth ice, it does practically nothing, since it calls for virtually no effort. Football players often have a "light" contact drill, which amounts to bumping into each other without intent to maim. Actually they are ramming cold muscles with cold muscles, and if a muscle is tense and in even a slight spasm it can set the player up for catastrophe. Tennis players begin with rallies, and golf players, nothing at all. The rest of us uninformed American would-be athletes or weekend athletes are told to emulate our betters and do what professional athletes do! And we do—even though we would only have to put two and two together when we read the lists of casualties on the sports pages to see DANGER. With those records, we should do virtually nothing the professionals do to get in shape either for the long haul or in the warm-ups before the game.

For starters, those activities done before competition aren't really "warm-ups." Warm-ups are a series of exercises to *warm* muscles—*all* the muscles. They are supposed to warm the muscles *before* any spike action or even coordinated action takes place.* *Warmed* muscles are required for jumping jacks or running in place or around the block, and *hot* muscles are required for anything other than a light stretch done *ballistically* in easy, short bounces.

A good warm-up is done standing in one place so the cold muscle does not have to lift the body off the ground, especially in an explosive effort like a drop into the basket or reaching for a errant backhand in a rally.

A good warm-up includes the whole body, not just the legs as in slowly skating around the rink.

A good warm-up involves rhythm, because muscles respond to both natural and imposed rhythm with a minimum of direction from the brain. And if they have been trained with good warm-ups for months, the muscles move easily within a safe parameter, never overreaching. A *light* stretch is built into a good warm-up, but only after the muscles are warm and loose.

A good warm-up is designed to speed up the heart action (without straining cold muscles) and increase circulation. That's one of the reasons for waiting a while after meals before you play anything. If the blood needed for digestion is drawn off for the muscles used for action, one area is going to be shortchanged, and if it's your stomach you may have to forfeit because of stomach cramps. If it's the extremities, you won't play as well as you can.

Warm-ups *should* be done to music, and it *should* be the right music. In the forties and fifties, we used Leroy Anderson's music, such as "Sleigh Ride" and "Fiddle Faddle." Over the years we went through Burt Bacharach, Herb Alpert, Ray Charles, Percy Faith and dozens of others whose music fitted the times and the tastes of America. Of late it has been the music of Abba, the Village People, Diana Ross and the Bee Gees. We let the "Top Ten" guide us *if* it makes the muscles *want* to move. *If* the music is right, Americans will do *anything* (even warm up) to it.

When doing warm-ups back at the gym, when the young athletes are first exposed to *your* methods of training and you have decided to give this a whirl, have them work in as little clothing as possible so *you* can see what's wrong with the muscles of each one. You will see that there *is* something wrong later, out on the field or court, but only by observing inferior performance. The player has a better chance of perfecting his game if he or she does not have tightness or substitution working against him or her. The best position for the class is in a circle around the leader, who can then be seen by everyone and can see everyone. A good aid is an assistant who circles the circle correcting wrong movements. Choose an assistant who knows a wrong from a right movement.

The Swim

With feet apart, lean forward from the hips and do a straight crawl stroke to the front for eight counts, then right, then left and back to forward again. That makes a set. Do two sets.

What to Watch Out For

If the upper body bobs with the beat. It should be level and still. All but the arms and shoulders are held still. Shoulders should reach with the rhythm. If the back is rounded instead of flat. This usually means the hamstrings, back muscles and groin are tight.

If either knee bends *at all*. The same

---

*Spike action involves sudden starts, stops and bursts of effort. This translates to most American games.

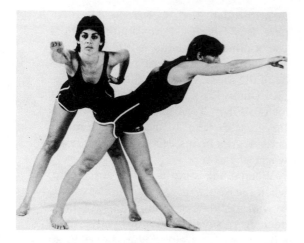

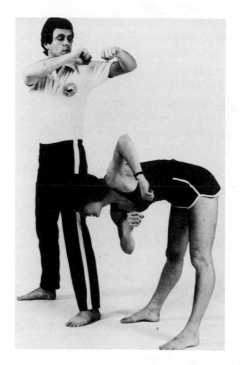

hamstring or back tightness may be the cause or perhaps the individual has little ability to see and translate what was seen to the muscles.

If the strokes are shortened and do not reach full stretch easily. Means either tight shoulder girdle or laziness. In the first, play will be limited by poor tools, and in the latter, play will be limited due to attitude. Either way, not a winner. Both can be improved.

All sports require waist flexibility, and yet all sports militate against it. The *internal* and *external oblique* muscles, the *latissimus dorsi* (in the back) and even the *rectus abdominus* (in the front) come under terrific pressure in forced twisting motions found in most sports other than swimming, but if these muscles are not flexible, it is difficult to isolate the upper from the lower body, which limits competency. All those muscles are snug harbors for many trigger points just waiting for the right climate or a call from a neighboring structure in spasm trouble, such as the leg.

Waist Twists

Again with feet apart for stabilization, keep the legs straight and raise bent elbows to shoulder height. Turn the upper body to the left as far as possible, initi-

ating the movement with the left elbow *pulling back*. Then do the same to the right. Alternate with a brisk rhythm for eight. Then drop the upper body forward until it is at right angles to the floor. Continue the twists with the back as flat as possible and the head still. Do eight. Two groups of eight make up a set. Do four sets.

What to Watch Out For

There may be little flexibility in the shoulder girdle. This tightness involves the *pectorals*, the *axilla*, the *trapezius* and the upper-arm muscles. In most weight lifters there will be considerable limitation in arm movement and trigger points in the trapezius, especially under circle 13.

You have now used the arms for one exercise and the torso for a second. You have spent roughly fifteen to twenty seconds on each. One of the keys to a good exercise class is constant change of area while not stopping action. This permits the absorption of lactic acid, a fatigue product. Anytime the leader spends longer than twenty seconds on any single exercise or area, he or she does not know the main point: give the muscles a chance to rid themselves of waste. Now change to the legs.

Hip rotation is essential for any sport requiring quick changes of direction; when flexibility is lacking in this area, trigger points mount in the groin and *gluteals*, and that spells back pain even for the ordinary citizen, and the athlete is no ordinary citizen, not even the weekend athlete.

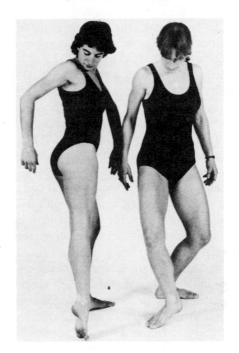

Hip Twists (Rotations)

Stand on one foot and, stretching the other leg *forward*, twist the foot in as far as possible touching the floor with the toe. Next turn the foot outward as far as possible, again touching with the toe. If a player detects any tightness or pain in the groin with this exercise, a good bit of your wondering and worrying about his performance now has an answer. There are trigger points in the thigh, usually the *adductors*, but take no chances, check the *gluteals* as well. If you don't find the cause of the stiffness or pain, do the entire leg as in *Permanent Fix*. Do four twists to a side to make up a set. Do two sets.

Hip twists to the side are helpful as well. Just make the toes touch the floor. Four to the right and four to the left. Do two sets.

Hip twists in the air, you will have to wait a while for. When dealing with most athletes, unless they have had dance, you are going to have to work with a very limited movement vocabulary and will have to proceed slowly unless you want either discouragement, substitution or revolution.

Doing hip twists in the air with the foot about six inches above the floor removes a point of reference. Raise the foot and, *keeping it in one place*, try to work the hips as before, forward and to the side.

Overhead Reach (Lateral Stretch)

With feet wide apart and knees straight, place one hand at the side of the knee, which will bring the upper body over to one side. Place the other arm over the ear for a starting position. To the beat, stretch that hand overhead and as far to the side as possible, then back to cover the ear. Do eight to a side for a set. Do two sets and proceed to the next position.

Place one hand at the side of the knee but farther to the back. Repeat the same action, bringing the other hand to the ear,

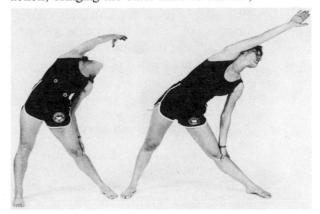

and this time when the stretch is made, reach back on the oblique. Do eight to a side for a set. Do two sets.

This is what we call a *light* stretch. The muscles are not required to *feel* stretch, but they are stretching gently all the same and will be gaining flexibility at about the same rate that the sports lessen it. Then, even if you did nothing else to stretch this area, you would not lose ground.

Ideally the young athlete should come to the sport with maximum strength *and flexibility*, but given the American way of life and limited physical education, this is rarely the case. The coach wanting a winning team and the trainer desiring one free of injuries should watch each player for tightness in the muscles, for that is the area at the greatest risk and the one most likely to fail in a pinch.

In "olden days," when calisthenics were a part of every gym class, the following exercise was called a "charge" forward or to the left and then right. It develops the *quadriceps* muscles, which control the knees. If you have a player with a "trick knee," take the trigger points out of the *vastus lateralis* and the *vastus medialis* before he or she does this exercise. Any player wearing the telltale elastic knee bandage has probably suffered for quite a while with a knee injury or instinctively feels all is not well with the knee and is trying to protect it. An elastic knee bandage may lend support to the psyche, but it won't do a thing if either of those muscles obeys the behest of a trigger point and collapses entirely or goes into massive spasm. It would be far safer and the results far better if the muscle were cleared of danger.

Charges and Groin Stretch

Standing with feet together, drive forward with one leg into the "charge," or half-knee-bend position. Return that foot to the stand position and alternate legs forward for eight, using two beats for each charge. Next, do the same to the sides. Next, spread legs wide and drop into the knee-bend position on one leg. Return to the standing spread-leg position and drop to the other side. Alternate for eight.

Next, keep the same spread-leg position and drop into the knee bend on one side. Stay low as though there were a low roof overhead and carry the body to the other side. Start with only four and work up to eight. Use four beats for each crossing.

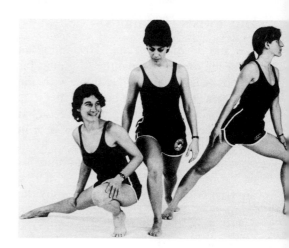

What to Watch Out For

The forward-charging foot may have an extreme turnout with pronation of the ankle.

The side-charging knee may lean inward. The knee should cover the foot. The crossover in the deep knee bend may not be kept level and the torso rise at midpoint, indicating groin inflexibility.

Muscles that have been put under stress profit from what is called a "break." The leg, hip and groin muscles have just been stressed, so the "break" should cover those. Any dance-floor frequenter has done it hundreds of times; most athletes will look as though both legs are lefts.

Alternate Leg Twist (Break)

Stand with *most* of the weight on one foot and the toes pointing outward. As you put *all* of the weight on that foot, twist the hip so that the toes point *inward*, and at the same time plant the other foot down firmly with the toes pointing *out*. Repeat that with the other foot. Take all your weight on it as the hip twists the toes *in* and the first foot comes down with toes *out*. You are back at the starting position. Once the rhythm is going, keep it going for four sets of eight. It's a great loosening feeling and one of the dance movements permitted American boys, who are not, as a rule, taught to dance. One of the reasons it is easier to put older people into shape than it is to do the same for young ones is that they all danced at one time, even the men. I'm not sure exactly when this was lost, but today, unless you do disco, which is done opposite a partner or alone, you cannot find anyone to dance *with* under the age of fifty.

At the end of that series you will have used up three minutes of your warm-up time and the muscles will begin to feel *warm*. It is now safe to add a little *ballistic stretch* to the back and hamstring

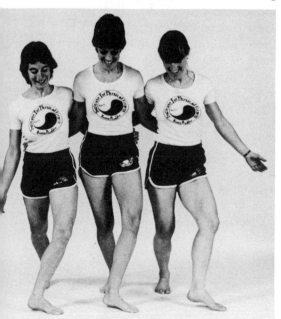

muscles, the muscles that play such a part in sports injuries and backaches for everyone. There is no excuse for tight hamstrings unless there has been severe injury or an operation, and even then the right exercise would probably provide the stretch if trigger points were attended to.

Flexibility Bounce

Stand with feet apart and *knees straight*. With hands behind the back and *head up*, bounce the upper body downward in eight *short, easy* bounces. There is no need to strain at all; just go as far as the muscles will go *easily*. This exercise can be done all day long even without warm-up. Just don't *push*. It is most helpful in offsetting sitting.

Next, allow the upper body to drop down with head and arms hanging loosely. Do eight more easy bounces. Repeat the head-up and head-down set to the right and then to the left and once again in front. That will require forty-five seconds. Repeat that entire flexibility series again, which in all will use up a minute and one half more of your warm-up time. If you are doing warm-ups twice daily, morning and any other time, once through the series would be enough. If you are using them in preparation for sport, dance or demanding exercise, go through them twice. That usually

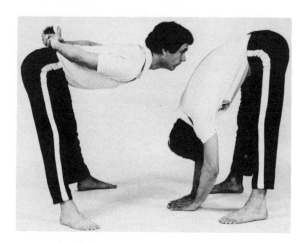

amounts to the time required for two pop tunes.

Having just given two examples of ballistic stretch, I think we should look a little closer at that controversial subject static vs. ballistic stretch. Since we are not, as a nation, educated physically, we have to use common sense and observation when it comes to "new" modalities of any kind. Not only are we endangered by people who make the results fit the premise, but by others who misread the results of studies, by some who misinterpret the results of studies and even by some who misreport the results of studies. Medical literature is fraught with examples of every one of these, which, picked up by succeeding generations, have affected those generations adversely. Dr. Travell gave me the following one recently, showing how dangerous it can be to depend on "experts" and how you should make up your own mind in whatever *you* accept.

During World War I, a German scientist wanted to know the average lengths of the various bones of the human body, and he used the thousands of cadavers brought back from the front for burial for his measuring. He noted ankle to knee length and then knee to hip, hip to shoulder, wrist to elbow, elbow to shoulder and so on, then published his results. Innocuous so far and typical of millions of studies that seem to be of no consequence other than to satisfy one man's curiosity. The study was published in German, and somewhere along the way, either in publication or translation, the measurements from ankle to knee and knee to hip became inverted. The measurement for the lower leg was listed as longer than that for the upper leg. "So what?" you ask. "What has that to do with me or ballistic or static stretch?" Try this for the answer to the measurement error: *The entire furniture industry has used those mixed-up measurements to make chairs for over*

sixty years. That's why the heels of many people swing in the air when they should be flat on the floor. That's why the backs of many thighs are compressed, with resulting poor circulation, and that's why a lot of chairs are uncomfortable and so are a lot of people.

Somebody said, "This is the way it is," and the rest of the world, if they thought about it at all, which is unlikely, said, "OK, they must know, they are the experts." That is not necessarily so, and the controversy over deep knee bends is a case in point.

In the sixties, a man working with football players and weight lifters (male) whose knees had been damaged by those two risky sports, reported that the injuries of this very small group had been caused when in the deep-knee-bend position. The football players had first noticed their pain doing duck walks, and the weight lifters when in a deep squat supporting hundreds of pounds. Not your everyday activity, to be sure. The investigator came to the conclusion all by himself that it had to be deep knee bends that did it, so he published a paper that recommended all deep knee bends be abolished. And would you believe it, although most people dealing in joints and muscles know that they have to be put through full range of motion daily to remain healthy, nothing was done to stop that misinformation from spreading. All over America, children in the public schools were not *allowed* to do deep knee bends, but without batting an eye we sent those unprepared legs to Viet Nam. They were to carry our sons into a stooping, running, crawling war. One can wonder if some of them did not return as a result of their lack of training. You can't do in six weeks what you have left undone for eighteen years. Still today there is always someone in my audience who says, "But I thought you weren't *supposed* to do deep knee bends." *Supposed.* In the dictionary, "supposed" means "*presumed* to be true."

Now we have ballistic vs. static stretch. In *ballistic stretch* the muscles are stretched by *gentle* (*never* to discomfort), easy bounces, preferably to music that the muscles seem to "hear." In *static stretch* the limit of the stretch is reached at once and held from twenty to sixty seconds. The proponents of *static stretch* say that *ballistic stretch* sets up tension in the muscles and damages them. The aficionados of *ballistic stretch* seem to feel the same way about *static stretch* when they consider it at all. I say that *any* extreme stretch can damage a *cold muscle*, including the stretch you do in bed before getting out of it in the morning. That fact can be borne out by thousands of back-pain sufferers who did just that and went into such spasm they couldn't get out for a week.

Since, in the end, you are going to do one or the other, if you will remember to warm up first, your chances of getting results *safely* are good. However, if you want to see which gets the better results, as we said earlier, watch a dancer, trained with *ballistic stretch*, and then the average athlete, trained with *static stretch*. Don't take my word for it or anyone else's word for it. Check it out for yourself. This is America, land of the ivory lean-to and outhouse, where you can get a doctorate by doing a paper on the arc of the badminton bird. What we are almost totally lacking in is the power to observe and good plain common sense. Again, whatever our milieu, *we* are responsible for ourselves, and our muscles are a very large and important part of each one of us.

When, then, should you stretch for extremes? The answer is, When the sweat is pouring off of you, when you have worked up to that point in an exercise class or when you have finished your run, your weight workout or your sport. In short, while you are loose as a goose.

A good exercise class should *not* begin

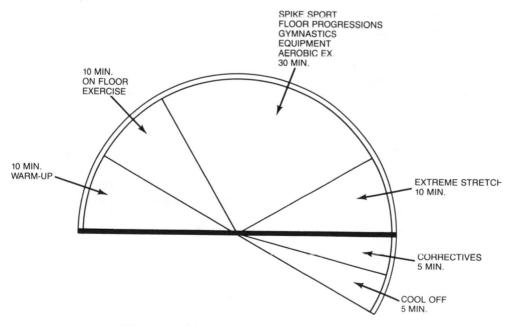

FIG. 55: TIME OUTLINE FOR EXERCISE CLASS

SPIKE SPORT
FLOOR PROGRESSIONS
GYMNASTICS
EQUIPMENT
AEROBIC EX.
30 MIN.

10 MIN.
ON FLOOR
EXERCISE

10 MIN.
WARM-UP

EXTREME STRETCH
10 MIN.

CORRECTIVES
5 MIN.

COOL OFF
5 MIN.

and end with aerobics. It should begin with a ten-minute warm-up, and that warm-up should be like prayers: don't miss them or the world will come to an end. Follow that with ten minutes of concentrated calisthenics sitting, kneeling and lying, both prone and supine. Leave a half hour for floor progressions, a spike sport, gymnastics, exercise equipment and *some* aerobic work other than that attained by floor progressions or dance, whatever your class is built around. *After* the class has really put out (and volley ball with twenty to a side cannot be called putting out), do your extreme stretches. Follow the stretches with correctives (nobody's perfect), then cool down for five minutes. Expensive horses are walked, and it's good enough for humans, too, but your class may duck out, so do your first warm-ups again, but slowly and easily, at about half time.

The above class would require seventy minutes. If you must shorten it by ten minutes, have those needing correctives come in early and leave the cool-off up to the class to do on their own. If *you* do one, even if it's just walk around the room, most will follow.

If you intend to incorporate exercise with practice for a sport, you merely extend the section allotted for spike sports or the like for as long as you please and do the stretch after that session is over. *If* some of the players have been sitting on the sidelines, they are *not* warmed up and would have to do more warm-ups until sweaty again.

If you intend to use the warm-ups before golf, tennis, skiing or the like, then you have a choice. You can do your warm-ups in front of God and everybody or you can do them in the locker room. My guess is that sooner or later people will do them as a matter of course before sports, because it's the thing to do. Who could imagine sedate matrons in bright shirts, shorts and helmets whipping by on ten-speeds, twenty years ago? Nobody, that's who.

STRETCH EXERCISE

There is as much misunderstanding as to what stretch exercises are, as there is about when and how to do them. There are all kinds of stretches, some for general use and some for very specific use (like the "hurdler's stretch"). There are easy stretches, such as the flexibility bounce, and some impossible stretches, like some of the yoga positions. Yoga exercises consist primarily of *static stretch*, *but* yoga came to us from India, a land where it is one hundred and twenty degrees in the shade. Everyone is *always* warm in India.

Then, too, the Indian personality is entirely different from the American personality. Indians are more contemplative, and we are more outgoing at our best, and at our worst, violent. The Indian body in India is *always* ready to stretch. The American body, *even* in India, is *rarely ready* to stretch, and since our heat must come from within, we must generate it with warm-ups. Since ability to contemplate is spotty at best and our body awareness virtually nil, we have to develop both. I find that music is one of the best aids; we use it both for warm-ups and for stretch—and for almost everything else, including presport training. For the following stretch exercises, use slow, slightly hypnotic music.

Spread-Leg Stretches: Ear to Knee

There are a number of ways to do spread-leg stretches. Start sitting with legs spread wide. Sit up straight and raise both arms overhead. Drop to one side as both hands reach for the foot (or at least in that direction), and try to bring the ear toward the knee. Bounce gently eight times when you have reached your farthest point of stretch. Return to the upright position, arms at rest, and then repeat to the other side. If there is difficulty and you have Fluori-Methane (the coolant spray, see page 232), use it to help you attain better flexibility. Alternate sides eight times.

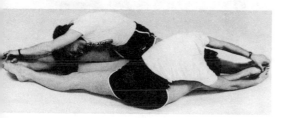

Spread-Leg Stretches: Chin to Toes

First let me assure you, the chin never gets there, it's merely used as a direction. Grasp one ankle with both hands and, *keeping your head up* as you do in the first half of the *flexibility bounces*, pull your chin toward your toes for eight bounces. Repeat to the other side. Alternate for four.

Spread-Leg Stretches: Chest to Floor

You may not be able to accomplish this beautiful end result, especially if you have come lately to stretching, have had poor or no coaching *at the start* of your sports history, or even if your present life is stressful. It is not important that your

chest reach the floor, only that next month it is nearer than it is today.

Spread your legs as wide as you can. If that's not very wide, check out the groin for tightness. Grasp as far down the legs as you can with both hands and pull your head toward the floor. Use eight bounces and then sit straight. Do four.

What to Watch Out For

In all these stretches, watch the knees; they must be straight.

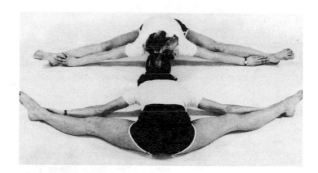

Back Arch with Pelvic Tilt

Lie prone with your head resting on your arms. Raise your pelvis as high as possible *while you keep your chest glued tight to the floor*. Lower, and repeat eight times. If you have difficulty with this exercise, check for trigger points in the pelvic area and fronts of the thighs. Check also for flat back (page 183), and if this condition exists, do the corrective, the old-horse part of the angry cat/old horse (page 143).

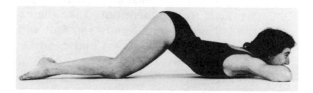

Pelvic Tilt Standing and Kneeling

Stand with feet slightly apart and knees slightly bent. Tilt the pelvis forward. Then, maintaining the same position for the rest of the body, thrust the pelvis back. Do sixteen.

Kneel with insteps flat on the floor. If yours won't go flat, put a rolled-up towel under your ankles until you can stretch the tight foot muscles. Tilt the pelvis forward, but don't come off your heels by more than a couple of inches. Then press back as you did standing. Do eight.

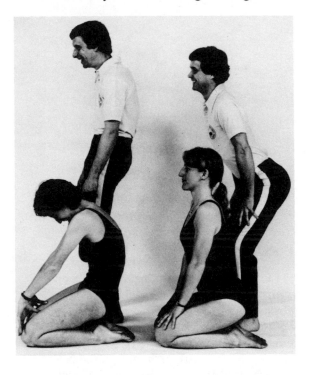

Crib Rock

To relax the muscles you have just worked, stretch them out. Take the extended position on hands and feet with the feet pointed forward and head up. Keeping arms straight, press back to bring the heels flat to the floor and your head dropped between your shoulders. Do eight.

What to Watch Out For

In back arch with pelvic tilt, check to see that the chest remains on the floor. In the pelvic tilts the *pelvis* moves, nothing else. In the crib rock make sure that the feet point forward.

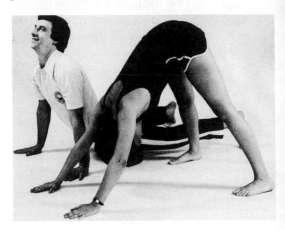

Hurdler's Stretch

Sit down and extend one leg forward. Bend the knee of the other leg and pull the foot back until the lower leg lies parallel to the thigh. Grasping the ankle of the outstretched leg, pull your head down toward your *unbent* knee in eight easy bounces.

Lean your body back to rest on the floor for a count of eight. *Feel* where the tightness is in the leg and the pelvis, and try to relax that spot. Repeat twice to each side.

What to Watch Out For

Many athletes are "crotch-bound." Those that are will have a difficult time getting the buttocks to lie flat on the floor. Check for trigger points in the front of the thigh and along the inside lines (adductors).

Working in pairs is fun and gets better results than working alone. You are going to want a partner later, to help you when you start using Fluori-Methane and for "seeking massage."

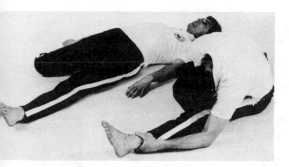

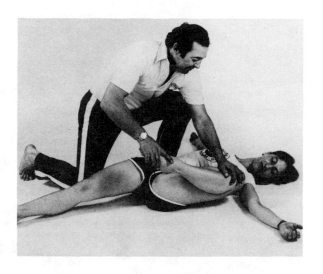

Lower Back and Hamstrings, Sitting

One partner sits with outstretched legs and grasps his ankles, but not to use for pulling. When you use your own body to do the pulling, you can direct only one action fully: pulling or letting go. Concentrate on letting go while your partner stands or kneels behind and presses down on your shoulders and upper back, in eight easy bounces. Straighten up to relax. Do four and then change positions with your partner and repeat the stretches.

Hamstring Stretch, Supine

One partner lies supine and the second kneels away from the leg to be stretched. Place one knee *lightly* on the supine partner's near thigh to prevent the knee from bending. Grasping the other leg at knee and ankle, press the leg back overhead in eight easy bounces. Relax and repeat four times. Do the same to the other leg and change off.

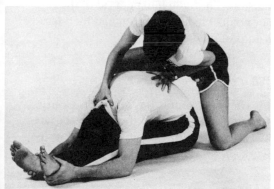

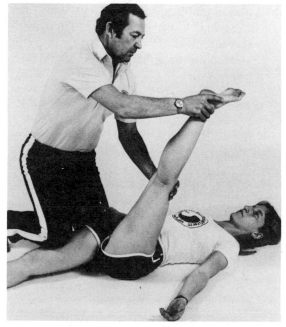

Groin Stretch

One partner lies supine, as relaxed as possible. The other presses the knee first straight up toward the chest for eight bounces. Then turn the knee outward and into the armpit to stretch the groin for eight bounces. Open the thigh as much as possible. Do each leg twice and then change off.

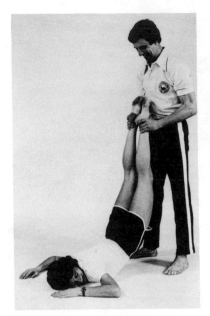
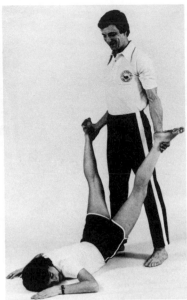
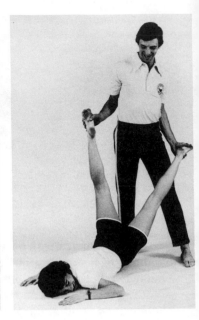

Abdominal Stretch

One partner lies prone and the other picks up both legs. In the instance in which the partner to be stretched is much larger than the other, put two stretchers to work, one on each leg. Raise both legs straight up while the chest remains still on the floor. Raise and lower slightly eight times. Keeping the stretch on the abdominals, spread the legs wide and raise and lower eight times. Then, with the legs wide, twist the lower body to stretch on the oblique. Do eight and then change off.

Crotch Stretch, Sitting

The first partner sits on the floor with the feet *held* drawn in as close to the crotch as possible. The second partner presses down on both knees for eight easy bounces and then returns the knees to a closed position to rest. Repeat four times and change off. Don't be surprised if your crotch seems to have no give at all. You weren't always that way and you *can* improve with time and work. Strength is a lot easier to come by than

flexibility, but the one is equal in importance to the other.

Light and easy stretches should be done often and lightheartedly. You cannot *force* a muscle to relax or give up its tension. First you must get rid of the trigger points binding it in iron and then *tease* it into obedience.

What to Watch Out For

Flexibility cannot be hurried. Consistency and many repetitions are the answer. Never force; it just plain doesn't work.

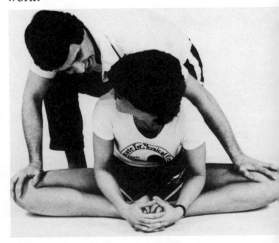

Last summer I did a lecture-demo in Texas for S.W.A.T.A., the Southwest Athletic Trainers Association, and I was talking about stretching and warm-ups as well as the prevention of and care of injuries. One man asked, "How am I going to get a whole bunch of guys to do that stuff?" I asked him if he was the boss. Well, some trainer who *is* the boss is going to do it. And he's going to stretch their muscles *after* they are hot, and he's going to check out his players for trigger points before the game. And that man's team is going to win.

Women are in exactly the same boat, only worse. Despite Title IX, the federal law that was supposed to end discrimination against girls in physical education, which never did get very high off the ground, girls and women in America have gotten a very bum shake when it comes to athletics. When I was telling folks, back in the sixties, that most of their kids were weak and inflexible, there was always some irate parent who would rise in anger to say, "*My* child isn't like that. We have *good* physical education at *our* school." I would reply that I was very glad for her, while wondering if her youngster was one of the elite who got everything, or if perhaps she ever visited the child's P.E. class and really knew. But there *are* some good schools with good P.E. teachers who have good training. There *have* to be *some* principals who back up the teachers and who really believe in the adage "A sound mind in a sound body." But they are few and far apart. Again, don't believe *me*. Borrow a stopwatch and go sit in your youngster's (or *some* youngster's) P.E. class with that stopwatch held on that kid when he or she moves productively, which is not jumping up and down and watching some other kid move.

Because girls are discriminated against all through school and many are still brainwashed at home ("Nice girls don't throw themselves about. Only tomboys run around like that"), they get off to a bad start if they start at all. Women *can* be as strong as men of like weight (and you'd never know it, because unless they *choose* to flex muscles like the girl weight trainers, it doesn't show). The uterus doesn't fall out during the game, and if you don't have cramps, menstruation interferes with no sport. Girls don't become masculinized with training, and girl jocks get married, have children and cook every bit as well as home ec. majors. I know that the prevention of injury with proper warm-up and stretch training done at the right time and with Myotherapy to free the muscles of spasm, will make them better athletes. Maybe a woman will be first to try it out. If she does, *her* team will win, everything else being equal.

Prevention of Injury: Seeking Massage

The human body can be a beautiful thing. It can also give every appearance of a sports injury just waiting for Friday night. You already know that you collect trigger points all of your life and that you probably have a goodly supply, except you're not sure just where they are. Get a friend and some oil. Oil one leg, climb up on the table, and lie face down. Have your friend make a fist and run her knuckles *slowly* down the center of the back of your leg on the line starting at circle 38, just under the buttock. If there

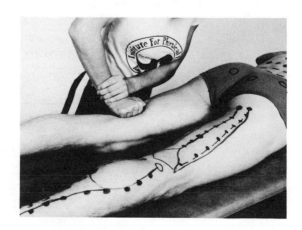

is no sensitivity under the moving fist, fine. If there is, tell her to hold it right there and put a seven-second pressure on the trigger point just found. There are usually one or two on that center line in the upper leg and up to six in the lower. Do the two other lines on the back of the leg and three lines in the front as well. Add to that the inside of the thigh and the outside. Average time per leg, about three minutes, less if the trigger points are few. You will have quieted the trigger points, which are potential booby traps should you step wrong, throw wrong, hit wrong or *be* hit wrong. When that happens, there's a searing pain that ends the game. How can you help win if you are sitting on the sidelines?

When you finish the legs, do the arms, chest and upper back. Don't bother to do seeking massage on the *gluteals*. Just figure there will be the usual trigger points in that area for any athlete. They almost all have them. After you have finished taking out the trigger points, do your warm-ups and a few light stretches such as the overhead reach, the flexibility bounce, the snap-and-stretch and the backstroke (pages 219, 221, 70 and 69). Do a few deep knee bends and then go out and win.

You think you don't have time for all that before a game? Well, there are players who have been spending *hours* trying to get kinks out with massage and strength in with tape. Time is relative to the reward, and your teammates won't thank you if you lose them the game or the medal *if you knew what to do but didn't take the time*. And twenty years later you'll wonder why your old injuries won't let you finish eighteen holes.

After the game do two things. Use as many of the stretch exercises as you can as well as you can even if it's not all that wonderful at the start. You will improve and so will your game. Follow that with another quick go at seeking massage to see if any old trigger points lit up or new ones were added during that dash to the net in the third set, the stumble at the fourth turn or when the guard landed on your foot just before half time. Sports are unpredictable, and they don't have to be contact sports. Football is equated with skiing and mountain climbing when it comes to risk, and the contacts in the last two are with nothing human at all.

Treatment of Sports Injuries

The conventional treatment of sports injuries, as reported earlier, depends on R-I-C-E. *R* is for *rest* and rest is nice unless you *have* to pitch, and many baseball pitchers may not get a day off for weeks at a time. It's lovely unless you have to run tomorrow, dance tomorrow, skate tomorrow or, heaven forbid! kick off tomorrow.

I, for *ice*, according to doctors, doesn't just ease pain (which is what the player believes it does), but shrinks the torn blood vessels and prevents the blood from leaking into the wound area, which then slows healing. For certified Bonnie Prudden Myotherapists ice is nice, but not really much of an answer to the problem of swelling, torn vessels and pain.

C is for *compression*, which means wrapping with an elastic bandage, or taping. It is supposed to limit swelling, but a lot of swelling goes on anyway, and if it gets bad enough the taping has to be cut off and replaced to encompass the progressive edema. Doctors say that uncontrolled swelling also retards healing, and it certainly does. Certified Bonnie Prudden Myotherapists would rather not wait several days for the swelling to go down, but take measures to get rid of it at once so healing can begin at once.

E, for *elevation* of the injured part to a point above the level of the heart, uses gravity to help drain excess fluid. There hasn't been a sensible argument against gravity since 1687, when Edmund Halley helped Sir Isaac Newton publish his *Philosophiae Naturalis Principia Mathe-*

matica, *but*, if the dirty bath water is leaking slowly from the tub due to a faulty or plugged drain, it does make sense to hurry the drain along by unplugging it, gravity notwithstanding. When all the ducts leading to and from the injured part are very nearly closed by muscle spasm, it's going to take forever, and the athlete hasn't got more than a couple of days, if that. For the seriously injured, there's plenty of time, at least this season, for he's out of it. But there's always next season. For the strained and sprained there's Saturday's game, Sunday's dance concert and next week's Olympic tryouts.

IMMEDIATE MOBILIZATION AND MYOTHERAPY

Immediate mobilization isn't new (almost nothing is). I saw it used first in Manchester, Vermont, when an obese gentleman crossed over the ski tips of a skiing companion who was a European-trained M.D. The doctor fell to one side, spraining his ankle, but he continued to ski all afternoon, which you know you can do if you've ever sprained anything. The constant use of the muscles keeps squeezing the fluids out of the injured area, and the pain doesn't set in until later, when you *rest*. That evening, with the help of a coolant spray, the doctor exercised his ankle every two hours, from the last run down by the ski patrol at 4 P.M. until nine the next morning, eight times in all. Lo and behold; there he was on the slope at nine with a perfectly good ankle. It was colorful all right, but it wasn't swollen and had full function. I never forgot it, and that example, put together with Myotherapy, has netted us enormous success with athletic injuries. Two certified Bonnie Prudden Myotherapists who are also trainers and working constantly with athletes report that 97 percent can be made pain free, while 94 percent can function within half an hour to an hour. Many can go back into

the game immediately. But 3 percent have reactivated old injuries and require two or three sessions, and 3 percent are usually stress fractures, which won't show up on X rays for a couple of weeks, when callus forms. One of these trainers, Darlene Jones, has coined the Myotherapy word for what a certified Bonnie Prudden Myotherapist does, M-I-C-E.

M, for Myotherapy to the damaged muscles, comes first. The second an ankle is sprained, every trigger point in the leg as high up as the hip is thrown into action by a master switch labeled DAMAGE CONTROL. What does that mass of multiple spasm do? It closes off most of the traffic in the leg, and that includes both the fluids that must be flushed *from* the injury site so healing can begin and blood bringing help *to* the injury. If you put a tight band around your wrist, it will be no time until your fingers swell. If your cast is too tight, your toes will swell and may turn purple. If a constricting band is around your neck, the same color will suffuse your face. Spasm, like those tight bands, constricts the muscle area through which the conduits pass. When the borders are closed and the fluids can't get through, the ankle, the foot and even the lower leg swell. As with the skier, if your injury is such that you choose to keep going, your muscle action alone will keep squeezing the fluids past the spasm barriers, but once you rest, you are done. Swelling increases immediately, as does the pressure on the injury. Pain prohibits all further movement. That's usually when it occurs to you to elevate your leg; you can't do anything else!

The certified Bonnie Prudden Myotherapist's aim is to get rid of the spasm, even that which started high up in the thigh, just below buttock and groin. *If the athlete is known to have a "trick back," start your hunt in the gluteals and groin.* Using the quick-fix technique, work rapidly down *to* the ankle, but not into it. Then begin at the toes and work up *to* the ankle. Then, and then only, do you *gently* tackle the ankle. By the time you arrive at that point, the swelling will be reduced considerably and the area much less sensitive. Same as with rheumatoid arthritis in the hand when you begin in the shoulder.

I can hear you screaming already, "WHAT IF THE ANKLE IS BUSTED?" You have a team doctor, don't you? Just who is it that says, "Get back in the game, Buddy, all you've got is a strain." Who says, "Sit over there, Johnny, and rub your ankle with this Dixie cup of ice. It'll feel better in a couple of minutes." Somebody takes charge. Somebody makes the decision as to whether the injury is "minor" or of the sidelining variety.

If a doctor is present, then by all means ask him; you would anyway. If he isn't, then by all means follow whatever your routine is: have the youngster sit out the game and go to the hospital for X rays or send him home to his mother, *but*, if you take the trigger points out of the entire leg, avoiding the ankle altogether, you will lessen the swelling and pain and, even with one go-round, hasten healing. You've seen enough sprains to know the usual course: swelling, pain, immobilization, taping, crutches and elevation. They can take days or weeks to repair themselves, and some (usually in older people) never do. If *your* kid is sprained, get the doctor's diagnosis, sprain, and go on to the next step, full range of motion first without resistance and, later, with resistance. The exercises can be done without any assistance other than the removal of trigger points from the entire leg, and that's what the average Joe and Jane and their children, dogs and cats (Myotherapy works for animals and birds too) need. The work will be quicker and less painful, as it was for the skiing doctor, if either ethyl chloride or Fluori-Methane is used. The trouble with them for the average person is that they are prescription items. EC and F-M are like Cain and Abel. Cain was older and did a bad thing. Abel came later and, though

he wasn't bad at all, he got done in. Ethyl chloride is explosive; it has been known to blow people up. It is so cold it can be used for minor operations, but it can also freeze the skin. It has such excellent anesthetic properties that it can be used as a general anesthetic, but has been known to kill users. Fluori-Methane, the younger product of the same company, in exactly the same bottle, isn't so cold that it insults muscles and freezes skin. You can't use it for operations, although it's great for bee stings and before injections. It isn't explosive, and the only thing that happens if you inhale it is a stomachache. Pretty dull! But it is fabulous when it comes to muscle spasm. Trainers can get it, as can doctors, dentists, and veterinarians. That tells you whom to ask for a prescription.

When something is injured, it flashes a message along the nerve pathways to the autonomic nervous system, yelling, "Hey, we've got trouble down here, send *spasm*!" Response is instantaneous and help is on its way. As soon as the spasm (meant to put the part out of action and safe from further damage) hits the injured area, *there is more pain*. That too flashes back to the brain, and the area plus several others not involved get a second order to spasm. In no time flat, a spasm-pain-spasm cycle is in effect, and that's when you can't straighten your back, lift your head off your shoulder or put any weight on the ankle. The longer the spasm-pain-spasm cycle stays in effect, the harder it is to retrain the muscles, and even for the spasm to "let go." One more reason for breaking the cycle as quickly as possible is that muscles have memory. They never forget what they learn, good or bad. You know from experience that if you go down the wrong street once, it's no big deal. You find the right one and take it every time. *But* if you stay on the wrong street for hours, days, weeks and sometimes years, it's very hard not to take the wrong turn ever after. The "wrong turn" for a muscle is into spasm.

Fluori-Methane is rather like a four-hundred-dollar TENS unit (transcutaneous electrical nerve stimulator). The needle-like spray travels along those nerve pathways, and its message gets to the nervous system ahead of the pain messages. Instead of hearing "Hey! We've got trouble down here. Send more spasm," it hears, "It's cold down here, Charlie, how about closing the window?" If the autonomic system responds at all, it's with a desultory "Do it yourself. I'm Damage Control, not a janitor."

Since you already know what to do in the case of a stiff neck, let's use the familiar for your introduction to Fluori-Methane. *After* you have taken out the trigger points from the *splenius capitis* (at the back of the head), the *trapezius* (on either side of the back of the neck), the other end of the *splenius capitis* (at circle 18, on the upper back) and the *sternocleidomastoid* (on each side) and are ready for the resistance exercises, get your bottle of Fluori-Methane ready. Do the resistance as you have already learned (page 55), but when you have finished and asked, "Where is the pain now?" and the subject says, "Right here," pointing to one spot or another, put that muscle on a gentle stretch and spray along the line of the muscle in stripes about half an inch apart. The resisting knot *usually* gives in. If it doesn't, you have missed an important trigger point somewhere. Try again.

Back to the leg. After you have done Myotherapy on the whole leg of the injured player or of your visiting aunt who just hobbled in after falling over your Great Dane, do the range-of-motion exercises for the ankle (page 114). Start with *plantar flexion (pronation)*, pointing the toes downward like those of a ballet dancer. The first move will be tentative, but you will improve. The second move is *dorsiflexion (supination)*, or pulling the toes upward toward the knee to stretch the back of the ankle. The third is *inward rotation*, turning the foot inward, which

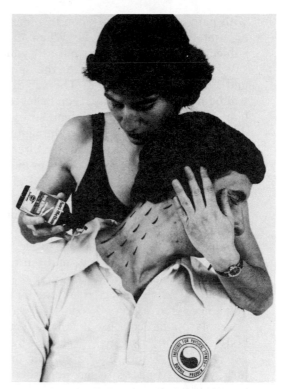

is apt to be more painful, since most strains occur when the foot rolls over to the outside. Finish with *outward rotation*, turning the foot outward. Do those exercises two or three times, and then move on to resistance exercises for the ankle. If you have Fluori-Methane, use it here.

While the simple contraction of the muscle in the range-of-motion exercises and the Myotherapy will have helped to bring the swelling down already, watch what happens when you apply resistance, which you could not have done before you did the first two steps.

Resistance Exercises for the Ankle are exactly the same as the range-of-motion exercises, with one difference. You apply resistance with your hand. (For illustrations, see page 114, in *Quick Fix*). Place your fist under the ball of the foot, saying, "Press my fist down as you point your toe." If there is pain anywhere, spray as you work or have your subject spray. One thing to remember: people with pain can't be relied upon to report accurately just where it is. When the subject says, "Ouch! That hurts!" you say kindly, "I know; point to the spot and I'll see if I can fix it." The subject will be most obliging. Why? You believed him. You commiserated with him, so you don't think he's out of line on the ninny side. And you are following *his* directions. He is no longer "meat-on-the-hoof." He has your attention, and his opinion has value. When you have repeated the process and he says, "It still hurts," and you ask him where, more than likely he'll say, "In the same place." Then ask him to point to it, and ten to one it will be a different place. Spray that new place. When you got rid of one kink you uncovered a second, one that was probably "guarded" by the first. The body's trick of "guarding" explains why, when you first work over a chronic injury, you may find few trigger points, but the next time a flock of them.

Do the second exercise, *dorsiflexion*, by laying your fingers across the instep close to the toes, asking the subject to "pull my hand up toward your knee." Follow that with *inward rotation*, with your hand on the inside of the foot at the ball. Then *outward rotation*, with your hand against the outside edge of the foot. Watch for knee interference. You want the ankle to work, not the knee. Repeat the series four times, keeping in mind that you are trying to get the muscles to "squeeze" blood and other fluids back into circulation, not build strength. A *little* pressure will be enough at first.

Next comes "fun time." Your player or aunt has been sprained before. He or she knows what to expect. Moving will be painful, standing impossible and walking, are you crazy?! You know better, or will after the first time it works for you. Have the subject hold your hands and stand up with feet together, weight *evenly* distributed on each leg. Tell him or her to keep the knees together, bend them gently and concentrate on keeping

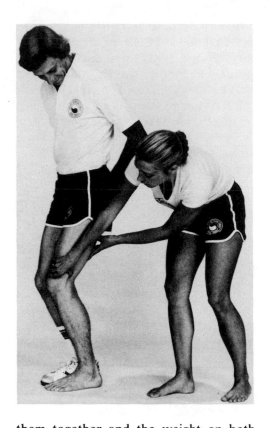

them together and the weight on both feet. That will interfere with the expectation of pain. It's hard to think of two things at the same time. You can't train a bead on a Canadian goose and pay attention to the terrier worrying your shoelace, giving equal concentration to both. Bend and straighten two or three times. Surprise will register. Agreeable surprise. That makes the next step easier. "Keep your heels tight together and go up on your toes." It will work. Just watch out for the overenthusiastic, who may think you mean *all the way*. A little way is just fine. It does a better "squeezing" job than hand resistance, any day. Do about four of those, and repeat both the knee bends and the toe rises again. If either action has induced pain anywhere, spray as you repeat the movement. Next, the walk. Still holding hands, walk backward, keeping to a rhythm, drawing the subject with you. If there is any pain, stop and spray as the subject stretches the muscle by bending the knee *without your assist-*

ing hands. Try again until the pain is gone and then say, "OK, walk by yourself and don't limp; you don't have to." You have just done a number of things. You have taken away expected pain (most of the time). You have said, "Walk," as though you knew it was possible. You have further added, "You don't have to limp," as though you knew what you were talking about. After about six of these successes you'll even *sound* as though you know, because you do.

This will have to be repeated every couple of hours until bedtime. When we were injured the day before an event, we used to stay up all night or at least set an alarm clock for sessions two hours apart. If you don't have anywhere you have to go, then get your sleep. The first session the next day will probably be as bad as the first session after the injury, maybe worse, because blood has had a chance to pool, but you can set things to rights in about fifteen minutes, and from then on it's easy.

Suppose it doesn't work? F-M is a diagnostic tool for many doctors, especially those who climb and ski in back country, where X rays are two or more days' hike away. If it does *not* relieve pain, look for a fracture or other anatomic pathology (even if the X rays show nothing). They may show one in a couple of weeks.

Suppose you are the athlete and no one will listen to you. You can follow the accepted way and see if it works. If it doesn't, there is always Myotherapy. It will take longer than if you started immediately, but it *will* work.

Most strains and sprains respond immediately, and in twenty-four hours, although they are surrealistic in color, they have full function, no pain and little or no swelling. Does that mean hop right back into your running shoes? That depends. What's at stake? Olympic medal? The chance at the bowl game? A match with the top-seeded player, a trip to Europe? I'd weigh it carefully, but now, you see, I am older. Once, I would have opted

to race, climb or try for whatever "it" was. Now, only the trip to Europe would interest me, but for that I'd do Myotherapy on the hour every hour until the plane left. It will be up to you, but your chances will be better with Myotherapy and retraining of muscles than they will be with a whirlpool bath, taping and injections of cortisone. Anyway, it's worth a try, and it *is* your ankle even if you are the aunt who fell over the Great Dane, especially if you are the aunt! Who wants to be "The Lady Who Came to Dinner"?

The *I* in M-I-C-E for certified Bonnie Prudden Myotherapists is the spray, but lacking the spray, which is quick, handy and easy, one can use the corner of an ice cube. It isn't as efficient, and it's not possible to carry one in your pack on an all-day hike or a canoe trip, but it's sometimes better than nothing.

Corrective Exercises

The *C* and *E* in M-I-C-E stands for corrective exercises. You have already learned the ones for the ankle. They are the same for the wrist, but the knee is a special joint. It is often a crying shame.

I was in Texas and on the same program as the man who said, "No more knee bends." My part of the program came first, and I was demonstrating the leg exercises learned by every Russian dancer and, I presume, the athletes as well, since their knees are excellent. I didn't understand the undercurrent of distress among No-Knees and his followers, but then, I didn't know what his paper was about and couldn't believe what I heard when I did. Skiing and climbing in Europe, as I did every year, I didn't know what sort of epidemic we had here with knee injuries. The Austrians and the Swiss didn't complain of such a problem, and it wasn't long before the testing revealed the extent and the cause of our national problem. We don't walk;

the Austrians, Swiss and Italians do, and from babyhood. We *could* change this situation, but I know human nature too well to think we will, at least in my lifetime. Those of you who hike and ski and climb with your children *are* inoculating them against knee injuries. The rest will have to take their chances, so we better cover that problem carefully.

If you can get to the person with a "trick knee" while it is merely complaining with cracking and banging and maybe a little pain off and on, so much the better. The pain usually takes you to the doctor for X rays, and the verdicts range from "*growing pains*" for the small-fry set, through Osgood-Schlatter disease and *chondromalacia patellae* for the teens and then right on through ligament tears and various forms of -itis, including tendinitis, until one comes to arthritis for the elderly (and not so elderly). Sometimes the diagnosis is right and sometimes it isn't. Sometimes it's right but the cause is wrong. All too often the real cause, trigger points in the *vastus lateralis*, *vastus medialis*, *rectus femoris*, *gastrocnemius* and *soleus*, are overlooked altogether. Before you consider a cast (it *may* come to that) or an operation, try a trigger-point hunt.

Have your subject supine on the table, and do quick fix for the groin and the two lines covering the *vastus medialis* and the *vastus lateralis* (see page 108), on either side of the leg. After you have done the *vastus* muscles, check out what you have accomplished by having the subject stand with feet together and do a half knee bend. There will be improvement, but that is good only for morale. Continue with your search and tackle the *rectus femoris*, down the front of the thigh.

Next have your subject flip over to a prone position. Start at the hip with the trigger points at circles 1, 2 and 3 and then down the center line to the *popliteal*, behind the knee. Do two or three trigger points on each of the three lines in the back of the upper leg (Fig. 50, on page

195), then the three lines in the lower leg. The knees themselves are usually innocent in knee pain, but again, like so many innocent bystanders, they run headlong into undeserved trouble. Test again with a few *half* knee bends and then do the stretch for the front of the thigh. Have the subject prone again and then bend the leg, bringing the heel toward the buttock as you press down on the ball of the foot. Do this slowly and carefully in order to avoid throwing the thigh muscles back into spasm. This also stretches the calf muscles. To get a stretch to the backs of the thighs, do flexibility bounces (page 221). If very painful, omit stretch.

When the knee feels a little better, and you need only a little improvement to start your exercise program, begin with isometric exercise.

Isometric means the muscle contracts but no movement ensues. Have the subject supine on bed or table. Contract the thigh muscles, the *quadriceps*. Even if all you see is a slight flutter, it's a start. Do several and go on.

Place a tightly rolled bath towel under the slightly bent knee. If it can't bend

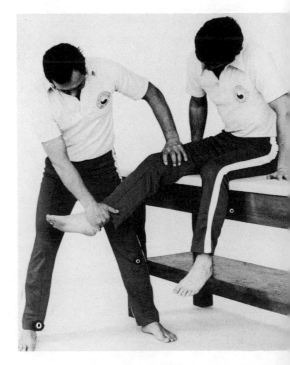

enough to accommodate a bath towel, use a smaller one, and if you have F-M use it over the most painful spot. Pick up the ankle so that the foot is about four inches off the table and ask the subject to hold it there if he can. Make the hold no longer than three seconds, then *you* lower the leg to rest. Do a few of these, until you see that the knee is tiring, and then allow about ten minutes rest.

Place your free hand above the knee to stabilize it, and with the other hand under the heel, raise it four inches above the table and ask the subject to *press the heel down*. You will be giving resistance while the *quadriceps muscles are lengthening, not contracting*. Do two or three. Do *not* ask the subject to raise the foot against resistance, whether it be manual or a weight. That resistance would come into play as the *quadriceps* muscle controlling the knee *is contracting*, or shortening. The first way, resistance while the muscle is lengthening, is far more efficient and gets better results.

Next lift the entire leg and hook it over your bent elbow. That will take the knee about ten or twelve inches above the table, with more room for the exercise. Keep your free hand under the heel and have the subject work against your resistance as the foot descends. Remember: here again you are "squeezing," so don't try to build strength at this point. Make your resistance featherlight and do several. As you work you will find the heel going lower and lower.

Next have the subject sit on the edge of the table with his leg hanging over. He may not be able to let it hang straight down at first, but never mind, that will come, and quickly. Stabilize the knee with your free hand and grasp the ankle as your prepare to give resistance when the subject lowers the foot against your *gentle* pressure. In a very short time there will be more strength and more range of motion. Try the half-knee-bend test again and see if there is less pain, a more secure feeling and a sense of looseness. You will

probably get an affirmative on all three. If not, there may be something cooking that is beyond Myotherapy.

If you are dealing with an athletic injury, you will be faced by someone asking *when* he can ski, play, fight, climb, etc. Conventional sports medicine says the athlete needs 95 percent of his or her strength back before engaging in competition. I would say that the injured joint should be stronger than the uninjured joint before going back into competition. And that's one reason for checking into a sports-medicine center. They have gadgets that can tell you exactly how strong the muscles are. I say that now because I have already come the long way that most of us travel, and I'm concerned with what happens if we overuse an injured joint. But, unlike a great many doctors, I have been a competing athlete and a world-class climber. I know people like I was. We will follow the injunction "*Carpe diem*" ("Seize the day"), and we will *carpe* any *diem* that is offered. Yes, it would be smarter to wait. Yes, it would be smarter to work longer than we are willing (or have time) to work. Yes, yes and yes, it might be better to sit on the sidelines for a week, a month, a season, forever. But who's going to do it? That's the way it is. And since that's the way it is, we might also *carpe diem* and use a possible way out to get that athlete back on the line as fast as possible. If Myotherapy works, why not use it?

Return to Strength

Of late we have depended to a great extent on machines, and where they work they should be used, but in rehabilitation of the athlete's knee, they leave much to be desired, and the knee is only one example. Any joint being put through full range of motion will have less strength as it starts its action and at the end. With the knee, the first third of the descent will require (and must receive) less resistance than the second third. The last third will also be weaker than the middle third. Another human being senses this far better than does a machine, which can be set for either the weaker thirds or the stronger. When you offer resistance to the subject with the leg hanging over the table edge, even though your resistance is light, make an adjustment to the thirds of power.

Follow the exercises done over the edge of the table with a kind of push-me-pull-you exercise, with the subject supine and grasping the edges of the table for support. If you are working on the subject's right leg, stand on that side and, placing his right foot against your shoulder, give him *light* resistance as he tries to push you away in a straight line along the side of the table. Guide the leg carefully in that straight line for the time being. At the full stretch, change your hands so that the left holds the muscle just below the knee and the right hand holds the heel. Resist lightly as he pulls the leg back to the starting position. If you are a strong person, you can probably give plenty of resistance at first with the hand holding the heel. If you are weaker, or later as the subject gains in strength, use the hand over the calf to help with resistance. Do only a few and then rest. As strength improves, use more repetitions and heavier resistance. This too should be done every couple of hours after injury. The knee will, like any joint, stiffen if ignored or forced to wait too long.

First injuries, 94 percent, respond best and fastest. Old injuries, 3 percent, take longer. First injuries that are not cared for properly with exercise and retraining become old injuries. If they are continually ignored they become chronic injuries, and you can hang up your jersey.

For additions to the program check out the section on *Self Center*.

Athletes want back into the game immediately. But if there are trigger points hiding out in muscles, they *know* it. They

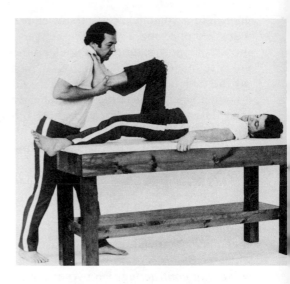

may not know *what* trigger points are or exactly where they are, but they know instinctively that something is not right *somewhere*. They go back to the game, but they start "guarding" the danger zones. It's hard enough to get back a sizzling first serve without worrying about the outside of your knee, taped or splinted as it may be. And there's something else. When a boxer opens up an opponent's eyebrow and blood is blinding him, that boxer is going to go for that bloody mess to make things more difficult. You expect that with boxers, right? But on a tennis court? The very same. If you walk out onto the court in a knee brace do you think for one minute your immaculately clad, perfectly coiffed opponent isn't going to watch like the predator she is (and you are too) for the stroke that causes trouble with that knee? Absolutely. It's called competition. No army would advertise a weak spot. Why do you? Get that knee free of spasm so you don't wear a sign.

You can't concentrate on catching a pass if your left ankle has been written up in all the sport pages and is now cracking like midafternoon on the fourth of July.

To say "concentrate" to a youngster on the balance beam (and most of them are youngsters) is ridiculous if the

Achilles tendon bears the diagnosis "torn" and her heel hurts when she lands on it. She will concentrate all right . . . on her heel.

Clean the trigger points for the recovered athlete *before* practice as well as after and you can prevent "guarding" as well as substitution.

Team-sport injuries usually happen to younger people, most of whom have had at least *some* presport training. It may not have been good, but it was action of some kind. Myotherapy has had phenomenal success with injuries to trained bodies. If the damage is to soft tissue, the results are usually immediate. In fractures it plays a part too, since it lessens swelling when used around the edges of casts. Even a full leg cast leaves the groin and hip free, famous for trigger points in athletes. In most arm casts, the shoulder and *axilla* are free for trigger-point work, as also are the upper back and chest, both of which influence the arm, and vice versa. Myotherapy is a tremendous aid *after* the cast is removed. Since the muscles have not been able to contract, there has been no flushing of the wounded area, and the soft tissue is in the same state as it was in before the cast was put on. While the bone healed, the soft tissue did not, and until it is cared for with mobilization work, trigger-point eradication, full-range-of-motion exercise and resistance exercise, recovery will be hindered.

If the fracture is in one of the areas handicapped by poor blood supply—the *carpal navicular* (in the wrist), the *ulna* (in the forearm) or the lower third of the *tibia* (the lower leg bone)—then extra effort should be made to increase the blood supply to those areas. How? Take out any trigger point you can reach leading to the arm or leg so that constricting spasm doesn't make the heart's job more difficult as it tries to pump blood to the extremities. Also, what gets the blood moving everywhere? A warm-up. You can do a fine warm-up in bed or a chair (see the pulley exercises on page 157 and the section on weight training in *Self Center*, page 275).

In my book *Pain Erasure: The Bonnie Prudden Way*, I went to great lengths about bed exercises done *for* the disabled person and into recovery via chair exercises and even with walkers and crutches. If you are hurt, you need such information. Don't just lie there, as I was forced to for three months with a smashed pelvis. If you do, you will lose muscle, strength, flexibility and coordination, and you will be weak as a newborn kitten. It's a long road back. *You* take responsibility for your body now that you know there's something to be done about it. Don't count on the doctor. He may be busy with other things. When I went in for my first hip replacement, thirteen years ago, the doctor told me he would operate in six weeks. I said I'd bring myself to the table in the best condition I could manage. "Don't bother; I'll make everything fine" was his reply, and so, since I didn't know about Myotherapy and every move was painful, I didn't do anything. I was *months* recovering. Three years ago I knew better, and when I went in for the other total I was in the best shape I could manage. I also started my program in my hospital room. It was many times harder and longer than the one offered by the PT department. In six weeks I was back on the gym floor teaching again. When I went in for my final checkup on the day a number of us were gathered for the doctor's OK, they were still gimping, while I was skipping. Was I special? No. I had a program and a reason. You certainly have a reason and you know there's a program.

One of the chief dangers that face all of us, not just the athletes, is that of falling for the name of the pain. Most problems labeled "bursitis" aren't "bursitis" at all, and that name can be pinned on any joint in the body. Before you start to worry, do your trigger points according to *Quick Fix*. If someone says you have "bursitis of the hip," hear only the word *hip* and take out the trigger points, do the side-lying stretch exercise and see if you still have it. That goes for all of them. Certainly *someone* will be so afflicted, but most of you will not. A good example is *"retrocalcaneal bursitis."* It sounds mighty impressive, but take the trigger points out of the foot (the whole foot) and the back of the leg and see if you still hurt.

"DeQuervain's wrist" and *"carpal tunnel syndrome"* sound nifty if you are looking for sounds, but do the upper back, chest, *axilla*, arm and hand and see what happens to your wrist.

"Chondromalacia patellae" and *"Osgood-Schlatter's disease"* roll off the tongue too. Start in the upper leg, all four sides, and then the lower leg. Stretch the muscles and then climb a flight of stairs. What does it feel like? One thing to remember, however: do your trigger-point work when you feel the *first* pain; don't wait until you are limping and every game is a nightmare.

Don't forget *"plantar fasciitis,"* long words for heel spurs. Look for trigger points in the calf and sole.

For sports injuries as a general rule, once you know you aren't busted, look at the muscle maps in this book and find the muscle that hurts. Note where it attaches and who its nearest neighbors are, for a quick fix. If your pain is relieved even slightly, turn to *Permanent Fix* and do the complete job.

If you are going to return to play after an injury, take precautions. Have someone make a tracing of the muscle map showing the muscles in your damaged area, locating all the trigger points you found. No matter how many years pass, *always* check those areas out before the game and afterward. That way, you will stay safe and play a better game.

Sports, both the serious variety and the weekend variety, which can be very serious indeed if you are a climber or a skier, backpacker, rider, cyclist, scuba diver, hang-glider pilot or parachutist,

should be fun. They should make you more attractive and interesting, and healthier. They can do all of that if you will use what you have learned here. And what's more, you'll be a far better athlete.

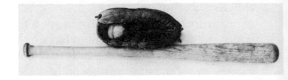

Baseball

Baseball takes its toll of elbows, shoulders and wrists, in that order for pitchers. Catching wounds fingers and hands. In addition, the squatting position injures knees. There is danger of contusions from fast balls, and in a slide to the base almost anything can happen. "Little League elbow" becomes "tennis elbow" as the athlete grows, and most of us who played any amount of baseball have at least one finger that looks as if it should be on the Crooked Man.

The training for baseball players is mostly baseball and more baseball, with little attention given to the strength or flexibility needed to back up the skill. Warm-ups should be done and, when the players are *hot*, stretch, especially for the shoulders, upper back and arms. The *axilla* is particularly vulnerable, but few baseball players recognize that there and on circle 13, the *scapula*, trigger points will be in clusters.

Use seeking massage (page 229) to find trouble before the game; be sure to cover the *pectorals*.

Rather than throw the ball constantly, use the weight bags through full range of motion for the arms, and as a matter of course do the neck stretches in *Quick Fix* (pages 55 and 56).

If a finger is injured, start with the *axilla* to first clear the arm, and end with the finger squeeze (page 81) *after* having checked the whole arm. For contusions, start your hunt at the *axilla* for the arm, and groin for the leg, and do the length of the extremity as well as all around the bruise.

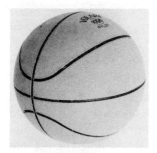

Basketball

In basketball the knees are most at risk. As in baseball, both strength and flexibility are overlooked as the players seek to hone their throwing skills. In addition, many basketball players have rounded shoulders, due to shortened *pectorals*.

A lay-up drill is *not* a warm-up. If the drill is the expected activity for a team coming onto the floor, then the trainer would be wise to warm up his team in the locker room. A player waiting to play is cooling off, and is then expected to take off like a ball of fire when he is sent in. Three minutes of warm-up with weight bags could prevent injury to a valued player.

Knee injuries for basketball players are not usually the result of a blow, as in football, but from a twisting action. The rubber sneaker offers just enough friction to hold the foot a little behind in a rotation. While the precipitating incident can be an awkward landing after a jump, the buildup of small tears and small scars has been going on for years as the legs have been pounding up and down the hardwood floor. If they have played on cement, it will be worse.

Always do seeking massage on both legs before a game or practice. Pay extra attention to the *quadriceps* and the calf muscles.

Using weight bags, do the snap-and-stretch exercise and the backstroke, on page 69, in *Quick Fix*, to loosen the shoulder girdle.

Legs can be strengthened with weighted stair climbs, just as the Austrians and Swiss use mountains (see *Self Center*, page 271).

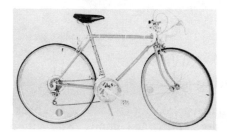

Bicycling

Cycling tightens the leg muscles, shortens the *pectorals* and, if the back is already injured, puts strain on its entire length. While it is excellent for cardiovascular training, the rest of the body needs a good stretch workout daily.

The position assumed by cyclists today in America, where cycling is thought of as a sport, rather than a means of transportation, shortens the arm muscles, which should be stretched daily with snap-and-stretch and backstroke (page 69 in *Quick Fix*).

The hamstrings may also be shortened, especially if the seat is too low. Do flexibility bounces, page 221, and have someone do the calf-muscle stretches for you (page 102). Do that whether seeking massage tells you you need it or not. You don't want to *need* it.

When you sit on a bike, your hands on the bars hold your torso rigid, facing forward. Do waist twists, page 218.

Every cyclist, especially the beginner or the long-distance rider, knows about sitzeritis: you can't sit on that thing another second; either you have pain or have gone numb. Do the hip rotations, page 219.

The real injuries in bicycling are usually head injuries. You can't prevent those, other than to wear a helmet; even then the fall often twists the neck. See neck exercises, pages 55 and 56.

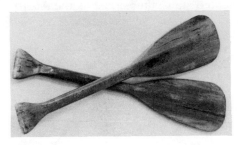

Boating

Canoeing calls for strength in the back, shoulders, arms and hands. Strengthen those as well as the abdominals *before* you take that Allagash trip. Spend some time stretching the upper back with stretches for round back and the door-pull stretch, page 73, in *Quick Fix*, and with the arm twists, page 76.

Rowing, whether it be a scull on the Charles River or a dory out of Gloucester, will develop a round back; the rower must guard against it with constant attention to the *pectorals*. Check with round back (page 164).

Sailing requires a nimble, agile body and a great deal of arm strength. Shoulder and back strains can be expected. Check both before a race and afterward.

Weight work for the arms, shoulders and back using all of the arm and torso exercises while carrying weight bags in the hands will strengthen, as will the dead lift, page 167, in *Permanent Fix*.

The worst trigger points are usually on the *scapula*, on Figure 33, page 153, *Permanent Fix*, at circle 13, but also check the *axilla* and *teres major* (circle 12). Even if the lower back does not contribute pain, figure that there *must* be trigger points at circles 1, 2 and 3, on Figure 40, in *Permanent Fix*, *and* the entire groin, on Figure 47, in *Permanent Fix*.

If boating is your sport, remember: it does little to nothing for legs, so add biking, hiking (with a pack), swimming and many deep knee bends.

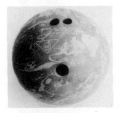

Bowling

Bowling is a lopsided sport if ever there was one. One trigger point in flare, and throwing even *one* small muscle into spasm can ruin your aim, so trigger-point hunts are a must. Every time you get that ball off, you stretch the muscles on the outside of the pelvis and leg on your right side. Check in the pelvis at circles 4, 5 and 6 (Figure 45, in *Permanent Fix*) and down the outside of the upper leg in the *vastus lateralis*, one of the notorious O'Quads. The left leg is your balancing point and the quads will be hard at work, since the knee is bent for the shot.

Bowlers often come up (or down) with "bowler's thumb," which as you now know means that the trouble may well start in the *axilla* and upper arm, or even on the *scapula*, at circle 13 (Figure 33, on page 153 in *Permanent Fix*). Do all of those trigger points before your team goes for the cup. You don't want to be the one to bring the score down.

Since bowling is so one-sided, you should use the weight-bag exercises with *both* arms and spend a lot of time on flexibility exercises. The arm twists, page 76, in *Quick Fix*, should be used before your turn.

Don't forget the warm-ups. One would not consider bowling a spike sport, but it is, one spike after another, and each one counts. Stay loose.

When you are in competition, have someone do the trigger points in your shoulders, chest and *both* arms before each game. There is nothing in bowling that works for endurance. Use the exercises on side one of my own record *Keep Fit—Be Happy*, Volume I, and the running on side two. You want to be the star player on your team? Prepare for the game before you pick up the ball, and it can all be done in your bedroom. You will find a complete program in my book *How to Keep Your Family Fit and Healthy* (see the *Sources* section). All you need is a bowling ball.

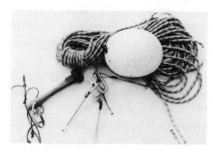

Climbing

Mountain climbing causes few injuries unless the climber is foolish, careless or just unlucky. Then the injury can be fatal. Falls don't come under sports, they are considered injuries, as are car crashes. Rocks falling usually damage heads, hands or shoulders, but they are just as rare. Where the mountain climber is also a rock climber, there is unseen, unnoticed and rarely felt injury daily, hourly and often from minute to minute, to the hands and arms. While this causes little or no diminution of skill while the climber is young, he or she often turns up with posttraumatic arthritis of the fingers and wrists around the age of sixty.

Would a climber stop climbing if told that? Not a chance. Climbers are truly addicted to their rocks, wildernesses, daring and triumph over fear. However, if care is given to the hands, arms, upperback, *axilla* and chest muscles, it may put off the evil day for a long time if not for always.

Climbing requires an excellent body, and the best training for it, strange as it may sound, is modern dance. Some climbers use brute strength, and while it certainly helps to be strong, being able to use the entire body, one part in opposition to another, as you hold yourself

in cracks and chimneys, makes the sport more like an elegant ballet than a wrestling match.

Chinning, especially with the hands facing out, which develops the triceps, is a good exercise. See *Self Center*. In addition, do the bent-knee sit-ups with hands clasped behind your head. See correctives on page 134 and use weight bags as suggested. When you can do ten sit-ups holding ten pounds of weight behind your head, you will be at a good level.

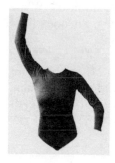

Dance

Dance, when it is done well, is one of the most difficult sports we have. It is also the best training for any sport and, begun at a young age, with the right teacher, it can make a good athlete into a star.

The dangers in dance are many, and mostly to the feet, legs, hips and groin. The back too will house multiple trigger points. Every dancer owes it to the art and to the self to have feet and legs checked with seeking massage before every class and performance, and afterward as well. The back should be given Myotherapy once a week at least, and so should the groin.

Shin splints and calf-muscle spasm are more numerous than knee problems, *but* if one of the *quadriceps* muscles goes into spasm, *because* it is so powerful the damage can be extreme.

Many dancers cause micro-injuries when they stretch cold muscles. They, like American athletes, think that stretch is all. It's half of all, but *when* we get it is at least as important as *that* we do. *Warm up before stretching* and avoid the worst injury of all, the one your own muscle does to itself. Wearing wilted wool leggings may be identifying, since only dancers use them, but they, like the silly socks worn by tennis players on their elbows, are like amulets worn on a cord around the neck. They don't really keep devils away. *You* have to do that, with warm-ups.

Use weight bags with as many movements with your arms as are in this book and any others you can think of. While dance is great for the legs, it does little for the arms and hands.

Keep in mind that if one muscle is in spasm it can throw you off so that your turns are incomplete and you may land wrong from a leap. One injury then leads to another and another.

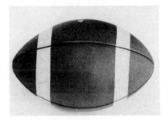

Football

Football is the sport that should make you remember what Arnold Schwarzenegger said: not "You *may* be injured," but "You *will* be injured." Knees and shoulders are most at risk in football. A way has not been found to protect the neck, either, and the helmet very often *causes* neck injuries.

Knees are best protected with trigger-point work to the *quadriceps* before and after every practice and game. Most injuries come at the beginning of the season, before strength is built, which should tell you *not* to lay off in summer, but get a job in a lumber camp.

Shoulder strains, sprains and separations are painful, and repeated injury to the weakened muscles will set you up for

an operation. *No* operation can give you back all of what you lost, so don't lose it in the first place. Flexibility is what football players do *not* have, and it is just as important as strength. If you have a child that looks as if he might turn out to be a football player, get him into a modern-dance class, where they'll stretch him into a pretzel, without damage. Then, when the pileup twists him into a larger pretzel, his muscles will give, and again, he'll emerge without damage.

The football player needs warm-ups and stretch, warm-ups and stretch, warm-ups and stretch, in that order.

If the neck is injured, unless it is fractured avoid the neck collar. A neck injury may not surface for a day or two after injury, so make the neck one of the parts getting regular seeking massage. Find the trigger point before it finds you as you snap off the winning (or losing) pass.

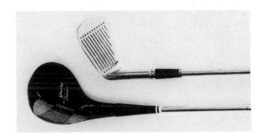

Golf

Golf is mostly played by the middle-aged and affluent, and quite often it is used as an office extension for business. Some of our young staff are excellent golfers, but not one of them goes into competition without warm-up. The reason? The first tee. The one just outside the clubhouse, where the crowd gathers and watches as you tee off. Tension (God, I hope I don't bomb!), plus a cold muscle in partial spasm from the fall on the ski slope last winter, can ruin the season and certainly cost you points. When you address the ball, you want to address the ball, not the kink in your back, shoulder, elbow or neck.

Since golf requires no extended effort, you need to use side two of the record *Keep Fit—Be Happy*, Volume I, the "running" bands. Since golf—like tennis, fencing and bowling—develops one side more and differently from the other side, you need all of the exercises on the record and the ones in this book that apply. You know which ones are easy and which require much effort. Do the first for fun and the second because you need them.

The trigger points that seem to be the worst in golf are at circle 11 in the mid back (Figure 40, page 178, in *Permanent Fix*). Do the waist twists, page 218, and many flexibility bounces, page 221.

The *pectorals* too need looking into and the *axilla*, especially the *axilla*. If you will do bent-knee sit-ups with weights held behind your neck (correctives, page 134), your abdominals will be strengthened and your drive improve. Putting may improve too if you will clear the arms and hands of trigger points. Your aim may be fine, but some muscle somewhere could be uncooperative.

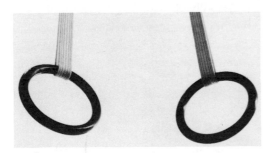

Gymnastics

Gymnastics is every bit as dangerous as football, and like many poorly prepared football players, the poorly prepared gymnasts fall by the wayside early on. They are out of gymnastics, but they aren't out of pain, and very often they are hurt so badly by their coaches that they can't go into anything else. I have seen arms that couldn't straighten, knees that couldn't bend and literally hundreds of shin splints, "heel spurs," back spasms and groin tears.

Gymnasts almost always "warm up" with stretches and very often rely on luck, rather than on coordination, to get them through a stunt. Weight training for the entire body should be part of the gymnast's training. The gymnast, like the rock climber, does a number on arms and hands. They as well as the shoulders should be checked with seeking massage before and after each session. Once a week *at least*, the gymnast should have a complete Myotherapy job done and any tightness worked free.

Fluori-Methane should be on hand at every competition, and the youngster should be checked for muscle spasm after *any* fall, even when she gets right back on the balance beam. If that's *your* child out there on the uneven parallel bars, be sure the coach sets the bar right for that child, not the one who went on before. A smash across the groin if the bar is only an inch higher than needed can cause all kinds of abdominal problems even when no organ is injured.

If you want your child to become a gymnast, don't wait for *her* to decide. You get her into a *good* dance class, where they work the whole body and where the teacher works every child, not just the stars. Or teach her yourself. Get the book *Fitness from Six to Twelve* (see *Sources* section) and get started *now*.

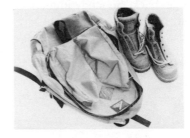

Hiking

Hiking is one of the best sports we have, since it can be done by all ages and its difficulty is controlled by the selection of terrain, distance and what you carry on your back.

Always carry something. It's excellent

for posture and for abdominal strengthening, and if it's tasty and thirst-quenching, everyone thinks you're great. You may run into trouble on the trail, and that trouble is usually some precipitating injury to the ankle or knee that had its origins many years before. Don't count on the years to protect you from old injuries. Do your seeking massage and clear the entire leg before you set out. Better make it both legs.

Knees too may be taxed on the trail, so clear the *quadriceps*. If you have had a bad back, ever, check that out too. It would be a shame to get to your feet after a trail lunch and find you couldn't straighten up.

To prepare for hiking, climb stairs as in *Self Center*.

Hiking is a strengthener for legs but, like dance, does little for arms, so use the weight bags in your hands as you do arm and shoulder exercises.

Hiking does *nothing* for flexibility, so you need plenty of stretch for the whole body as well as calisthenics for the whole body.

There is a danger in such sports as canoeing, climbing and hiking that is not connected to sports such as tennis, bowling or basketball. If you are injured on the court or in the lanes, you are where your help is. For the first three, you have to get back. So study immediate mobilization, page 231.

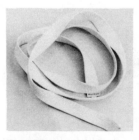

Martial Arts

The martial arts are fairly new to America but becoming ever more popular. For one thing, size doesn't matter, and it is size that keeps most boys off the football and basketball teams. Also, martial arts don't require a team of five, nine or eleven; one doesn't even need an opponent for a good workout. Lastly, martial arts do not discriminate against girls and women. The dangers are somewhat the same as for yoga. The American body is rarely flexible, nor do we recognize that fact. If Li can kick over his head, Leonard will try, usually without warm-up or training in flexibility exercise.

There are some forms that demand that the muscles take a beating to "harden" them. I have no proof of this, but I feel that such "work" may ultimately have the same effect as hanging from the cliffs by fingers: posttraumatic arthritis. I would take precautions, in any case, with trigger-point work to the *axilla*, the hands and arms, the legs and any spot that turns up an ache.

To the program add cross-country running (not on the road) or running with the record *Keep Fit—Be Happy*, Volume I. Also check with *Self Center* and mini-tramps.

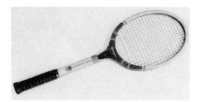

Racket Sports

Aside from the famous "tennis elbow," racket sports are also involved in "trick knees," sprained ankles, shoulder "bursitis," upper-back spasms, low-back pain, shin splints and calf-muscle spasm. And they can also give you a pain in the neck.

Why are they so lethal? Because the balls or birds are not predictable. In fact, if there's a way to return them at an impossible angle, the antagonists will do it. What causes "tennis elbow"? Usually a forehand that puts a lot of top spin on a ball. In other words, it is not a flat hit, but a slice that is accomplished when you rotate the arm inward. Do the arm, hand, *axilla*, chest and upper back. The exercises are the arm twists, in *Quick Fix*, page 76.

The shoulder gets its mock "bursitis" from serving, often with cold muscles. Same exercise and add the intercostal stretch with weights (page 155). Search the same muscles for trigger points as you did in the arm, and add the neck, especially the *sternocleidomastoid*. Your shoulder would profit from the pulley exercises, page 157, in *Permanent Fix*.

The knees run into trouble for the same reason the basketball player's knees do: rotation on a rubber sole that doesn't rotate as fast as the knee. Or trouble can result from a "charge" made on a weak leg. The *quadriceps* muscles will be damaged, and they run the knee. Do all the quads with Myotherapy and deep knee bends in your doorway gym (page 277, in *Self Center*). Follow those with the charges to the sides and forward and the groin stretch (page 220).

The low-back pain comes almost invariably from circles 1, 2 and 3, in the *gluteals*, and 4, 5 and 6, on the sides of the pelvis (also *gluteals*). With that information, get rid of the trigger points quartered under those circles. And also do the backs of the legs and the groin.

be at attention at all times. The constant motion of the horse works the *gluteals* and upper-back muscles. The rider on the English saddle must sit erect, with elbows "on." The western-style rider can be more relaxed, unless of course he or she actually is working cattle. Anyone riding a horse for the first time will be stiff and sore. A fall is usually forward, onto head, shoulder and arm. Check those areas for trigger points even twenty years later. And do *both* sides.

The *adductors* are dangerous, however. If they are loaded with trigger points from overwork gripping the horse, you could well develop back pain or even a "trick knee." Prevent both with Myotherapy.

Riding will develop strength but does nothing for flexibility, and the bent-knee position maintained when riding in the English saddle works against hamstring flexibility. The rest of the body will *be* moved by the horse, but only as that particular horse moves, which is limiting. You can ride a horse you are used to for three or four hours and not be stiff, but substitute another and you'll be sore all over again. Different gait, different adaptation of muscles.

Use the full exercise program, your doorway gym (page 277) and the record *Keep Fit—Be Happy*, Volume I, in conjunction with your riding. Keep in mind that, when riding, the *horse* really gets the workout.

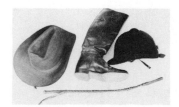

Riding

Riding a horse with an English saddle is very different from riding with western equipment. The former is for sport and the latter for work. Both require your adductors, on the insides of the thighs, to

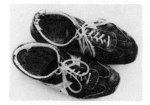

Running

If you have been stretching before warm-up, you need your legs, feet and back done thoroughly with Myotherapy. If you are running on the road, same thing. It's a lot harder to run cross-country, which means you wouldn't have to run as long to get the same workout, and you wouldn't be ruining your legs. The major injury areas are calf muscles and fronts of the lower legs, which complain of "shin splints." After a while you may have pain attributed to "heel spurs." Knees are next; they may get you off the road even before back pain starts.

Do seeking massage on your legs every time you run. Do a good warm-up *before* you run and your stretch afterward while you are still *hot*. Of the thirty million registered runners we had five years ago, fifteen million have given up the sport because of knee and other leg injuries. That's one out of two. Very poor odds.

Running does nothing for arms and works against flexibility. Don't think you've done your work for the day if you ran five miles in the dawn's early light. You need calisthenics and a lot of stretch exercise.

If you really like running and know how to protect yourself, do it every *other* day, and on your off days use calisthenics, weight training and a lot of bouncing on your mini-tramp for rhythm.

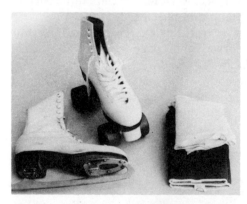

Skating: Figure and Roller

Figure skating calls for rhythm, balance, strength and flexibility.The injuries are usually to the knees and thigh muscles, especially on the inside, the *gracilis* and the *adductor*. The *quadriceps* muscles are constantly overworked, and in the beginning at least, many landings are made in an unbalanced manner. These bad landings injure, and sometimes the resulting spasm will hold off until the day of the Olympic Games, many years later. (See the information on the long second toe, on page 202.) This information also applies to speed skating.

Since ice is no more giving than cement, the leg is apt to develop "shin splints." A fall onto the *coccyx* can cause menstrual cramps, what feels like a spastic colon, and since the floor of the pelvis is in spasm, unsatisfactory coupling.

All of that applies to roller skating as well. The best preparation for such skating is modern dance. The flexibility series is a must *after* warm-up, and skating around the rink is *not* a warm-up. Use Volume I of *Keep Fit—Be Happy* and then proceed to Volume II.

The trigger points will be everywhere in the legs, but particularly bad on the line in the back of the thigh running down from circle 36. The groin too will be involved.

The hips, shifting weight, can pick up trigger points in the sides of the pelvis at circles 4, 5 and 6. *And* the *gluteals* often suffer with pain referred up from the legs. Skaters need a thorough Myotherapy search at least once a week and immediate Myotherapy to any ache or strain.

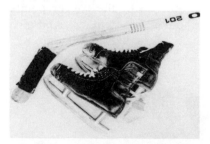

Skating: Speed and Hockey

Speed skating has the drawback of limited movement. The body assumes the bent-over racing posture and maintains that position throughout the race. The pull on the back is constant, and the powerfully pumping legs strain against the back of the pelvis. The groin is an anchor for the snatch-back as the reaching leg completes the farthest point of the stroke.

Power could be maintained between seasons with the weighted stair climb and the stretches, especially the low-back sitting exercise, page 227. Add to that the hurdler's stretch and the groin stretch, pages 226 and 227; also hamstring stretch, supine (page 227) and abdominal stretch, page 228. Finish with crotch stretch, page 228.

Hockey trigger points should be located with seeking massage before every practice or game. Warm-ups are needed *before* going out on the ice. Slow (or fast) skating around the course is *not* a warm-up.

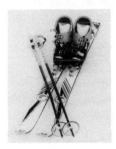

Skiing

If you consider that runaway skis can take you with them on a terrifying journey, if you realize that a hill with fifty people on it offers the neophyte forty-nine collisions and that every single tree along the side of the trail has your name on it, you'll be smart. And the second thing you will do is go to ski school. The first will be to get in shape to ski with all the exercises in this book, and I have some cassettes of ski exercises to be done *on* skis *in* the living room or the backyard.

Ski injuries used to occur to ankles and knees primarily, but with the new equipment the ankles are protected and the knees worse off. If your ski tips dig into a drift but you don't and keep going, you will pull tight hamstrings. If you "pinwheel," which is self-explanatory, your shoulders may be involved.

If you have a "trick knee," Myo the

quadriceps and do many knee bends, ride a bike, hike, climb and do stairs with weighted pack (see *Self Center*). If the hamstrings are tight, the Kraus-Weber minimum muscular fitness test, in *Permanent Fix*, will tell you. And don't even *think* of skiing if you fail the abdominal test, in fact *any* of the strength tests. In any case, warm up or climb up *before* you ski down.

Cross-country skiing is safer than downhill by a large margin, and cheaper by an even larger one, but you won't have much control on the down side of the hill if a hill you find—not for a while, anyway. The trigger points will be in the shoulders and arms more than in the legs. Check circles 12 and 13, on Figure 40, page 178, in *Permanent Fix*.

Skis keep the legs in a parallel position, so do additional things to maintain versatility, such as Volume I of *Keep Fit— Be Happy*, and jump rope, use a minitramp, work with weights and of course stretch.

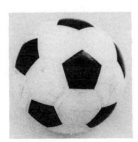

Soccer

Soccer is a game that has become "in" over the past several years. Played in 400 B.C. in China and A.D. 200 in Rome, it is now the major sport in many countries.

The most important thing to remember about soccer if you want to make it your game is that if you are injured, you can't go back into the game. Many soccer players play with injuries so they can finish. This occasionally finishes a career. Since soccer rarely stops once the game begins, enormous endurance is called for. Cross-country running is excellent preparation, since a level field surface is not as testing as hills and dales.

Of course there will be trigger points in legs, but if you watch soccer games on TV, you see far fewer knee bandages than you do for basketball. The constant running in practice as well as games strengthens the legs. So does a seeking massage in the legs, but don't neglect the chest and neck.

In soccer you may not use your hands or arms, but you may butt the ball with chest or knees or feet or head. The chest muscles are involved when *they* work or when the head butts. The neck supports the head. Look for trigger points in the neck, upper back and chest. The whole body needs flexibility, but the *pectorals* and neck are almost always overlooked unless there is pain, and if there is, R-I-C-E (rest, ice, compression and elevation) is sure to follow, with predictable results: a short season.

If there are trigger points in the legs, the stride may well be off and the speed reduced. Soccer is a speed game, and any inflexibility in the legs sets the player up for muscle tears and the team up for a lost match.

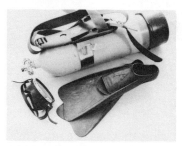

Swimming

Robert Kiphuth, the coach of Yale's famed swim team, put his swimmers on the gym floor for weeks *before* they got their feet wet. They were given calisthenics on top of calisthenics and stretch on top of stretch until the *whole* body was developed. This is especially important where the *abdominals* are concerned. That tells you where to start, with Volumes I and II of *Keep Fit—Be Happy*.

Add the weighted sit-ups and all the flexibility exercises. Swimmers must be as slinky as fish.

The trigger points for competitive swimmers are in the *pectorals*, *axilla*, arms, and upper back. We rarely see any in the legs of swimmers, but divers have them, and they also have all the trigger points suffered by dancers and gymnasts.

Skin and scuba divers who are using the sport for recreation rarely have pain connected with their sport, but the scuba diver who works for a living under water can develop it with whatever the particular job calls for. Check with occupations for the work that most resembles yours.

Snorkel and mask are wonderful for people who want to swim many laps for fitness but get cricks in their necks, red eyes from chlorine and a stuffed-up nose. Take out the neck trigger points and those in the *axilla*, which are particularly bad in swimmers and worst in those who compete in the breast stroke.

To make lap swimming pay off even more, wear fins. They work as resistance against water. Don't forget to stretch; a flexible body helps a swimmer in every way.

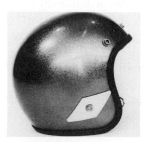

Trail Biking and Snowmobiling

Aside from the noise, the stink and the fact that hikers and cross-country skiers hate you, both are great fun. They get machine-bound people to places they could never make on foot . . . and back again. On the negative side, both can beat up on the back, groin, *pectorals*, arms and hands.

All those areas should be cleared of trigger points from time to time and always if an ache turns up. Remember what injury to the floor of the pelvis *can* do. I don't think you'd want to swap making love for riding a bike, so if you feel any pain at all in the groin or have hemorrhoid discomfort, clear the genital area and check both for spasm and the cause.

The lower back is another place that may well need trigger-point work. If suddenly you begin to urinate blood, don't panic, it's not the worst. And for goodness' sake don't go for a cystoscopy. Your bladder's all right, you've just been rattling your kidneys around too hard. Get off the bike or snowmobile and give them a rest and time to heal. In the meantime build up the muscles in your back with weighted exercise.

Neither machine does much for the body that could be called profitable, so calisthenics and stretch as well as strengthening exercises are a must if you want to hang on and enjoy. Take care of every muscle ache that comes along. The now is not as important as the later, when you are older and have swapped the bike for a boat and the snowmobile for scuba gear.

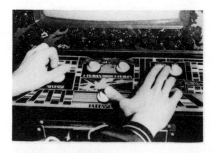

Video Games

Video games are played by millions of Americans *instead* of sport that involves the whole body, not just the hands. The thrill of competition is there and the hope of winning, but the physical outlet is missing. Consequently the tension builds in the shoulders and neck to surface years later when a long drive is called for—or even computer work, which is a form of the same thing.

The pain suffered in these games is felt in the wrists and thumb as a rule. The trigger points start in the *axilla* and the shoulders and go right down the arm. An Atari athlete will have the same trigger points as the person complaining of "tennis elbow." The exercises are the snap-and-stretch and the backstroke, pages 69 and 70, in *Quick Fix*, and the arm twists, page 76. You should probably use the stretches for the neck as well. They are on pages 55 and 56. If you have a budding champion in the family, hang a pulley on your chinning bar (see *Permanent Fix*, page 157).

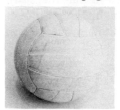

Volleyball

Volleyball is a great game when played with five on a side. When, as in many schools, it is played with fifteen or twenty to a side, it's a damn bore!

The trigger points are the same as in basketball and tennis, since it is a spike sport, with unpredictable moves and collisions. The hands take the beating, as in handball, and the constant blows injure the muscles in the palms and fingers. Be sure to clean the trigger points from the *axilla*, upper back, chest, arms and hands, even if there is no pain anywhere. The potential for injury is always there if the trigger points are there.

Running cross-country is good preparation, as is weight work for the arms. Who jumps highest gets the point, so climb the stairs with weighted pack. Stretch is essential here as in all other sports, since flexibility is the other half of the coin where coordination is concerned. To be strong but inflexible won't get you a place on the team . . . any team.

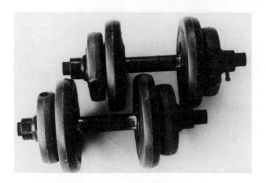

Weights

Weight training is essential in any sport if you want to be better than an amateur. The weight machines now available everywhere are limited in that there are just so many directions they can move. Barbells are similarly limited but less so.

Free weights, such as weight bags, have no such limitations. But if you enjoy the bells or the machines, go ahead *if* you know what you're doing. If you don't, get a good book or a good coach. In addition, use weight bags for both hands and feet in a calisthenic program.

Weight lifting shortens muscles unless you give almost equal time to flexibility. You can even use weights to help stretch yourself, as in the *axilla* stretch, page 275, in *Self Center*, or doing the dead lift, page 276, standing on a box or a chair.

The worst trigger points are almost always in the *axilla* and the *pectorals*, the upper back and the *gluteals*.

If you run, do weight training on your off days, but also add the calisthenics and the flexibility series.

Occupations and Hobbies

When you choose your occupation, you very often choose the pain you will suffer later in life. The connection is sometimes obvious, but more often there does not seem to be any at all. Birth sets some of us up for headaches due to trigger points laid down in the muscles under the scalp. Our sports and accidents have contributed a share here and there, and there is a fourth way to make trigger-point trouble for ourselves: with occupations. I've listed a number here, and if yours is not on the list, select the one that most closely resembles what you do most of the time.

Muscles that are overworked and constantly strained are loaded with trigger points, but so are muscles that are engaged in making micro-movements hour after hour. When muscles are damaged while doing heavy work repetitiously day after day, we understand what has happened. However, few realize that repititious *limited* movements, which never carry the muscle through full range of motion, can be equally damaging. When a patient is sent to one of our clinics, we ask eagerly about occupations, *all* his or her occupations.

One day at a Pain-Erasure Seminar like the ones I conduct all over the country, a middle-aged lady offered her painful right side for me to "fix." To my question

"What's your occupation?" she replied that she was a secretary. Strange, secretaries usually have stiff necks, headaches and painful shoulder girdles. I had never met one with a pain in her side. "Were you in an accident?" was the next question, but no, she never was. "What sports did you play when you were a youngster?" Actually she hadn't engaged in any, but she said she had walked a lot and still did. But walking doesn't cause side damage. However, when I asked her how long she had been a secretary she told me she'd only done that sort of work for two years. That explained the freedom from tightness in the neck and shoulders. It takes longer than two years as a secretary to throw those muscles into spasm. *"What did you do twenty years ago?"* She thought for a minute and then laughed. "Oh, heavens! I was a drill-press operator in a munitions factory and did this all day." As she spoke she gave a demonstration of how she reached up to pull a lever down, over and over. I didn't have to tell her a thing. The minute she reached up, her side hurt.

Now it is you who will retrace your steps. Go back over your life and make a list of all your occupations and also your hobbies. A hobby for one person is fun but could be an occupation for another, depending on remuneration and the number of hours required. I read a lot for fun; a proofreader reads a lot too, but it's a livelihood and is rarely fun. I won't suffer from the activity, but the proofreader may well develop a stiff neck. I like to ride horses and do it for pleasure, but one summer I worked on a ranch and rode many hours every day. I was buttweary every night. I like to play the piano when I'm in the mood, and it never tires me. Two of my patients are pianists and for years have complained of back pain and one has numb fingers. Five hours at the piano every day is *work*. I like to drive sports cars too, and I need no supporting cushion or ten minutes to straighten up when I get out or a handful of aspirin at my destination. A friend of mine does. He's a salesman for a pharmaceutical house with a two-state territory, a car and a quota to meet. He also has two sons in college!

When you make a list of your occupations, try to remember how many hours a week they consumed and do the same for your hobbies. Several things are possible. One, your hobby, which was active (skiing, for example), balanced out your sedentary job as an accountant. Or your active hobby was seasonal, sailing, but you sat out the winter and often ached. You thought it was the cold weather. Or you may find you have stepped over the line somehow and turned a delightful and relaxing hobby into a must-do-it occupation.

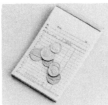

Accountants

To begin with, the accountant is a perfectionist. He directs, orders and controls figures all day, every day. Accountants are accountable. They have enormous responsibilities and pressure. They don't move out of their chairs, and they are usually bent over their troops of numbers, which represent a very important ingredient in our lives: money.

Bookkeepers have many of the same personality traits as accountants. They are certainly tied to their chairs and they hate payroll day.

Accountants and bookkeepers and others like them do close work in responsible positions, allowing little latitude for error. They suffer from headaches, stiff necks, and shoulder and arm tension that often takes in their writing hands. They can, of course, get low-back pain if their abdominals are weak and their back and hamstring muscles tight. So can anybody.

Take the Kraus-Weber minimum muscular fitness test, on page 131, in *Permanent Fix*, so you will have an idea as to where you must start. If you are a weekend athlete, it's not enough. The other five days you are in irons. Myotherapy can get rid of the headaches, the stiffness and the pain in the neck, shoulders and arms, but you need a good exercise program on a regular daily basis. Read up on the *Self Center* and decide how you will go about getting fifteen minutes of concentrated exercise a day. Do snap-and-stretch and backstroke exercises, pages 69 and 70, often throughout the day and shrug your shoulders between clients. Check your posture for round back, and if yours has begun to round, check in the *Posture* section. Do the same for a potbelly.

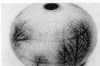

Arts and Crafts People

Arts and crafts people often suffer from some of the same characteristics as accountants. They too are perfectionists, but theirs is monitored from within, whereas the accountant is monitored by his balance sheets. If the figures come out right, the accountant can relax and the tensions are off. The artist (like the writer) usually wants to do the work over immediately, because it's not *quite* what was envisioned. That is the "never-satisfied syndrome."

Potters develop round backs, and if they turn their wheels with pedals, pain will eventually attack both the leg and the lower back. Since the chest is rarely stretched, they take in less oxygen than they need. Painters who stand at easels all day often develop low-back and leg pain. They blame the latter on varicose veins. Standing also brings on hemorrhoids. Those who do miniatures are like the jewelers in their neck, shoulder and hand pain. The sculptor who works with hammer and chisel injures his hands with micro-damage all day.

Arts and crafts people often ignore sports altogether, since their psyches are fed by the creativity in their work, *but* who can create well when hands are either twisted with pain or numb? What potter can turn out a lovely vase if he can't stand up straight anymore and is tired all the time from a lack of oxygen and the strain of holding spasmed muscles even partially in line? For that matter, wouldn't it have been better for Renoir to be free of the pain of arthritis, which forced him to work with brushes tied to his crippled fingers in his later years? Perhaps he would not have painted better, but most certainly he would have enjoyed it more.

Since the artist expresses himself or herself through work, it would be a good thing to read *Self Center*, on page 267, and remember that you yourself are a world and from that world comes the beauty so needed in the world of us others. If you will move your body to rhythm it will show in your work. I once did an experiment with children, who are not notorious for drawing well-proportioned figures. Each was given a crayon and a piece of paper and told to draw a portrait of a friend. After a few minutes I col-

lected the papers and began an exercise class to music. At the end of an hour, during which we ran, jumped, skipped, swung, twirled, rolled and tumbled, I repeated the drawing request. Then I compared the first with the second drawings. They were *all* bigger, freer and better proportioned. *You* might try a vigorous warm-up followed by some stretching exercises and see what it does for *your* arms and hands . . . and your work.

Use the same exercises needed by sitters: snap-and-stretch and the backstroke, pages 69 and 70, in *Quick Fix*. They are really quick fixes for stressed arms, hands, upper backs, shoulders and chests.

Check the surface on which you stand all day. Is it tile over cement? Can you substitute wood?

Most arts and crafts do not of themselves provide releasing movement; quite the opposite, and concentration often builds up to cause unbearable tension in the back and shoulders. The pain and disability, however, may show only in the hands and wrists. Don't wait for pain to signal a problem. You *have* a problem if you have been at your work for more than a few years. Use Myotherapy to tell you where your trigger points are hiding, and get rid of them. Follow with the stretching and strengthening exercises and a daily fifteen-minute program designed by you for you. Keep in mind that for you it would be better to exercise for three minutes five times a day than a straight fifteen minutes. Then watch what your new regime does for your art.

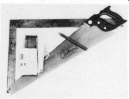

Carpenters

Carpenters represent the many builders of our world. Most of them too are perfectionists, for when they are less, nothing fits. The carpenter is luckier, however, than, say, the mechanic and the mason, because the craft requires him to use many muscles in various ways, and you certainly can't build a house while sitting in a chair. The job has a built-in physical-fitness program.

When the carpenter does hurt, however, it is usually his shoulder, lower back or legs. Myotherapy should become part of his life, every ache and pain followed up, giving special attention to the legs. Deep knee bends should be done often during the workday to keep the legs strong and well flushed. If one must stand long hours, blood has a tendency to pool in the legs. The results of poor circulation can be seen in ugly, crusty toenails, swollen ankles and slow healing.

Since the carpenter works for strength all day, but does nothing for flexibility, a good fifteen minutes will be needed for warm-up and stretch. Running in place with the record *Keep Fit—Be Happy*, Volume I, side two, would help with endurance. None of the carpenter's work causes increased heartbeat rate or hard work for the lungs.

It is usually the carpenter's back that is strained and hands that are injured. Keep the arms, chest and upper back free of trigger points, so that should an injury be sustained, healing will be fast and pain kept to a minimum. The points for the carpenter's low back are usually under circles 1, 2 and 3, with extra attention to 11.

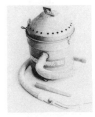

Cleaners

Cleaners, whether they be house-cleaners or commercial cleaners, have a better shake in one way than those who sit for their work. They *have* to move. The living creature fares better when it moves than when it is sedentary, whether the reason be occupation, hobby, age or condition. One old gentleman who was living in an old soldiers' home told me he got up every morning and went for a long walk so they wouldn't think he was dead and bury him. If you have ever visited a nursing home, you know that there is a very real possibility of that happening.

The dangers in cleaning jobs come from having to move furniture *if the back is already a refuge for trigger points*. If you get up from a kneeling position and put your hands in the small of your back praying for "quittin' time," you brought the problem *to* the job, you didn't get it there. Remember: the "precipitating incident" is rarely the original cause of the pain. Check your whole body with seeking massage and get your trigger points erased, and then set up a fifteen-minute-a-day exercise program using the exercises shown here or on the record *Keep Fit—Be Happy*, Volume I. The work will become easier and you will have strength left over to do some of the things you've always wanted to do.

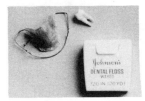

Dentists

Now, here is an occupation that's a killer. Dentists and violinists have the same trigger-point patterns, because they assume similar awkward postures for their work. Both hold those positions for many hours a day. Both do very fine work requiring enormous concentration. The violinist is better off, however, because no one is afraid of him.

The dentist stands next to his chair or half leans on a stool, and the blood pools in his legs. This gives his heart an extra load. His back is strained and so are his neck, arms, wrists and hands. Many dentists complain of wrist pain so bad it could lead to the operation for "carpal tunnel syndrome," which rarely gets rid of the pain, because that wasn't the trouble in the first place.

The dentist will have trigger points at the back of the head under circles 66, the *splenius capitis*, and right down the back of the neck on each side to where those muscles attach to the vertebrae, at circles 18. They will be in the shoulders under circles 14, 15, 16 and 17. Follow that with work all over Grid D, giving special attention to circle 13.

Then the chest will need work, for, like the potter, the dentist contracts the *pectorals*. The low-back pain is no different from anyone else's low-back pain. The trouble will be in the gluteals *and* the groin.

The dentist's arms and neck will need doing, but the arms of the *dental hygienist* will be even worse than his, because she constantly rotates the lower arm as she scales teeth, roughly between ten and thirty-two to a customer.

Both of these professionals need to do deep knee bends between patients, and waist twists and flexibility bounces whenever they leave the office for *any* reason (pages 218 and 221).

Walking would be a great help to offset standing or leaning all day; the least they can settle for is fifteen minutes of calisthenics (see *Self Center*).

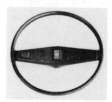

Drivers

In America everyone is, was or wants to be a driver of something. Sometimes the only machine available is a lawn mower, in which case keep your fingers out of the machinery. A lot of fingers are lost to lawn mowers and if that happened, do Myotherapy on the upper back, the *axilla*, the chest, the arms and *then* the painful stumps of the fingers. Do a lot of arm stretches, because fingers begin in the armpits and shoulders, even the fingers that aren't there anymore but hurt as though they were. The pain that accompanies amputations is called *phantom limb pain*; all too often the sufferer is fluffed off with "It's all in your head." I'm reminded of the doctor who saw me after I'd broken some ribs falling into Luncheon Rocks one spring in Tuckerman's Ravine. I told him I could get through the days just fine but the nights were pretty grim. He said I'd be fine in six weeks. It took eight. Two years later he fell on a climb and broke two of his ribs. To his surprise he found he could get through the days all right, but the nights were grim. He took pills. Now all his rib fracturers get pills for sleeping. I sent him the following:

> There was a faith healer of Deal
> Who said, "Although pain isn't real,
> If I sit on a pin
> And it punctures my skin
> I dislike what I fancy I feel."
>
> Anonymous

People who drive cars for an occupation and sit long hours with one foot on the pedal get low-back pain and "sciatica." Truck drivers who sit with one foot on the pedal and the other on the clutch shifting up and down all day, get low-back pain and "sciatica." Both have shoulder tension and, quite often, stiff necks. Give most occupational drivers the range test, under Passive Stretch, for the neck, on page 53, and you will discover that they have very limited range of motion even though they don't have pain . . . yet. (You know what to do about stiff necks using trigger-point hunts. Your work should include the neck, the upper back, the *axilla*, *pectorals*, arms and hands.) If you do it for them when they get in from the trip and again before they take off, you can help a lot. *They* will have to do the exercises, and if you can get them to do exercises for one week *often* during the day, they may feel so good they won't need a nursemaid asking if they've done their exercises. That's like saying, "Have you done your homework?" In addition, give them a bodo to keep next to the flashlight. Both are for emergencies.

Low-back pain and "sciatica" need back, groin and leg work. Leave out one of the triad and the pain will be back the next day before you can drive to the first customer.

Pilots belong in a class with cab drivers and bus drivers. They are all locked in, they all deal with the public and there is danger in all their jobs. All three develop low-back pain and shoulder pain, but the bus driver who uses a door lever every few blocks ruins his upper back first.

For all these people, trigger-point work is essential, as is a bodo handy should a trigger point heat up while en route. Warm-ups from time to time or even a few partial warm-ups would help. Waist twists (page 218), snap-and-stretch and backstroke (pages 69 and 70), flexibility bounces (page 221), and deep knee bends (page 280) are essential. The person who sits all day hinders circulation as much as the one who stands. The thighs are squeezed, the legs work mostly from the groin and, while the *gluteals* are contracted over and over, they are never stretched. Nor is anything else.

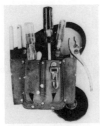

Electricians

These people are in a very risky business for one special reason: the screwdriver. The electrician moves around a lot, but the moves his hands and arms make are small, usually screwing and unscrewing fixtures. Sometimes there is so much spasm in the electrician's arms that he cannot straighten them at the elbows. Start the trigger-point work in the chest, upper back and *axilla*.

Move down the arms when you have finished those areas. The every-day-and-often exercises are snap-and-stretch and backstroke, pages 69 and 70, in *Quick Fix*.

Most electricians, like most men, are very inflexible, and while it did not seem to matter to their P.E. teachers, it will matter very much to the man who develops a back pain and still has two houses to wire before his assistant gets back from vacation. Female electricians are usually more flexible, as are women in general, but their arms will be in exactly the same danger.

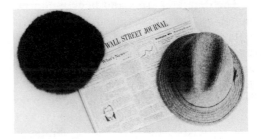

Executives

Mr. and Ms. Executive have all kinds of pressure, which makes them tense, and tense muscles shorten. The corporate gym has been discussed before. You can work out on the machines, which consist of weights, treadmills, stationary bikes and rowing machines. Nothing, however, is done for the three very real needs: flexibility, rhythm and relaxation. Read *Self Center* carefully and start looking after the most important executive you know.

Take to the stairs when you can, and walk when you can. Ask yourself if you can take some time off, and if yourself says, "No way," call a meeting. Get yourselves all together, you the executive, you the woman or man, you the decision maker . . . and look across the table at you the tense, tired, overweight or drawn worker with the backache, weekly migraines, "tennis elbow" that ruined your game . . . and exhaustion. What's it all for?

If your life is sedentary, prepare for a sport with *Self Center*. If you do play golf, know that it's not enough. Tennis tightens muscles, and so you need both calisthenics and stretch. If you jog, get off the road. If you ride horseback, your legs need stretch and your lungs and heart a different workout. If you must stay in there pitching, then be physically fit for the fight. If you aren't, something else may give and it could be your *joie de vivre*.

One thing more: the fit person is usually aggressive. Does your job call for the aggressive approach? You bet it does.

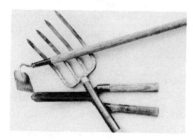

Farmers

Farmers' work is never done, and that's the crux of their problem. They strain backs lifting feed sacks, they wrench shoulders trying to get stubborn cows to git-on-out or -in. Every part of them gets rattled on the tractor, and their hands are bruised from wrist to fingertip. The trouble is, there's no way they can stop what they are doing, because every day there's sunup; Nature doesn't take vacations.

Farmers are usually inflexible too and have been that way since childhood chores started their muscles into tight patterns. Warm-ups should be followed by lots of stretch exercise. Farmers' problems could be anywhere and everywhere, and while the job keeps them

moving and strong, they do need (like the weight lifter) to stretch after each chore. Do the flexibility bounces (page 221, in *Quick Fix*) and the snap-and-stretch plus backstroke, pages 69 and 70.

Many farmers have shortened pectorals from overwork, and consequently, rounded backs. Check with round back in *Posture*.

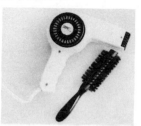

Hairdressers

Hairdressers combine the worst of three jobs: psychology, dentistry and arts and crafts. They stand at an awkward lean all day. Their craft will be judged within the hour, *every* hour. And women pour their troubles, hopes, fears and angers all over them. The barber is better off; all he hears are the game scores.

For the awkward stance there is one help: get a chair that goes up and down. For the conversation, there's really nothing, but at least know how valuable you are. Better by far than Valium, and without you there would be many more suicides. You are often the only one who appears to listen and the only one who really looks and then says a kind word. I know a hairdresser who says, "Well, you're good for another thousand miles . . ." *every* time he finishes a client. They could shoot him, and sooner or later they go elsewhere. I also know one who never forgets what her clients say. She knows their worries and all about their loves, where they are going and who's coming to dinner. They *all* want her to do their hair . . . or is it their hearts? But it *is* exhausting, and for it you need strength, a good back and good legs. Don't forget: the hairdresser has an artist's hands.

The hairdresser of either sex needs fifteen minutes a day for calisthenics to music (see *Self Center*). In addition, do deep knee bends between clients. The body is held erect all day facing straight forward and needs waist twists (page 218, in *Sports*). Every time you go for supplies, do the flexibility bounces, page 221.

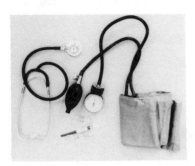

Medicos

The word covers a lot of people. Surgeons stand all day on cement doing concentrated work often under pressure. They get backaches. The anesthetist is either bored to death or in a panic. Some of the worst catastrophes in surgery happen when the anesthetist pulls the wrong plug. They all know it and live with the anxiety. They also wear heavy lead aprons to protect them against X rays. An anesthetist's days are very sedentary indeed.

One shortcut to better health is to leave the elevators to the patients. You need at least a half hour a day of exercise to offset your job.

Nurses often have to lift heavy patients; that means back pain for most. They walk on cement all day every day: leg pain. They stand on cement and their feet hurt. They came out of high school, where they had no P.E., and right into nursing school, where the administration is not one bit smarter than the one in the high school and there is no thought given to physical improvement. When we tested nurses with the Kraus-Weber minimum muscular fitness test, over 50 percent couldn't pass.

The nurse needs a daily exercise pro-

gram. And stay away from "aerobic dance" unless you want to add insult to injury plus shin splints. Weight training could give the edge necessary for lifting. This is especially important for those working with the handicapped, who have very unpredictable movement patterns.

Then there is the X-ray technician, who lifts patients all day long and also walks and stands on cement; the psychiatrist, who sits in a chair all day; the pathologist, who peers into microscopes; and the hematologist, who does the same thing. If you run the gamut of medical personnel, you find that they are even more at risk than many of their patients. Their record of drug addiction, alcoholism and suicide speaks eloquently of unbearable stress. One of the best ways to lower stress levels is with physical outlets. Medical schools, too, have been criminally negligent about the young people within their halls. It is almost as though they have not yet discovered that the body is in league with the brain for good or evil.

Read *Self Center* with *yourself*, not your patients, in mind. See if the most important doctor, nurse or technician in your world doesn't deserve a little care and pampering. The only patient who can't do without you is **you**.

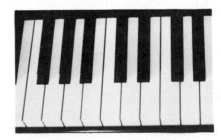

Musicians

Musicians are a very special breed. They are artists, with all the discontent of the artists; they seek perfection, like the accountant; they are the athletes of the art world, and they are sinned against by ignorant teachers from the very start. There is no physical education provided for the musician in the American school system. The musician dares not use valuable, highly trained fingers for the games of baseball, basketball or football. Even something as dull as volleyball with twenty to a side (the usual fare) has the potential for ruining a hand. And that is usually the extent of the program.

Music schools are no better when it comes to caring for the young artists than schools for nurses and doctors. So, from the start, the students lack full range of motion, so necessary for health *and* art.

If you have youngsters in your family who show promise as musicians, start now to provide physical outlets. They can walk, hike, swim, run (cross-country, not on the road, or you'll do in their legs and backs), bike, dance and do exercises to music. They can jump on the mini-tramps and they can jump rope. Get *How to Keep Your Child Fit from Birth to Six* if you have a little Mozart around. If the youngster has already passed the six mark, get *Fitness from Six to Twelve*. If he or she has reached the teens, *Teenage Fitness*, as well as what you will find in this book.

If you are the artist, remember: full range of motion every day for every muscle and joint. *No* traction and *no* slings unless Myotherapy fails, which it has not done so far with musicians. Since a well-known pianist was returned to the concert stage by Myotherapy, we have had hundreds of musicians flocking to our clinics. They want to save their careers and they want to play without pain. *You* are the only one who can do that for you.

Most music teachers, like too many doctors, do not realize that the *whole* body is involved and that the entire body is interdependent. The *whole* child comes for a music lesson, and the *whole* artist shows up for rehearsal. The whole artist plays the concert too and just a little weakness in merely two little fingers is as good as a death knell.

If you are the teacher, read this with a finger pointed straight at yourself. If you

are good enough and the right pupil comes to you, you may develop a Rubenstein. Many artists in the past lost their art to muscle spasms. *Their* teachers were no help in saving them. But you, the teacher, can take precautions and help your students. Teach them that the body is not composed merely of hands. Teach them to exercise it, to care for it and to keep the muscles free of spasm. Each of them is and has an Amati, the whole beautifully fashioned, strung and tuned body. The *only* instrument that is really and truly one's own.

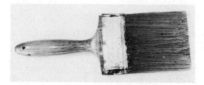

Painters

Painters have innumerable danger areas. When they paint overhead, they damage the shoulder, upper back, *axilla* and arm. Simply holding the paintbrush constantly in the same hand and using it the same way over and over again injures many muscles with micro-damage over the years. Painters rarely, if ever, sit down; worse, not only do they stand up, they stand on ladders. Ask anyone who has balanced on ladders for a lifetime of work, what the fronts of his legs are like. If they look all right when you ask, question further: "Did you ever have sores or calluses on the fronts of your shins?" Of course he did. How else but by putting pressure on the tipped down-feet and the rung-supported lower leg can he stand up there? The *anterior tibialis* will have plenty of trigger points and may well be causing the leg pain he's had for ten years. Then there's the lean-out from the pelvis and the lean-over supported by one leg and the opposite hand. All of it is strain. *Intermittent* strain the healthy body can usually stand. *Constant* strain is different; it's like Selye's stress. He says that stress is like carrying a pail of water in one hand. At first the body adapts. It rearranges its normally balanced self to accommodate the uneven strain. For a while it *seems* to do fairly well, but actually isn't doing well at all. Here and there, parts break down and ultimately exhaustion sets in. Shortly after that, if nothing is done to relieve the stress, the organism dies of exhaustion. The painter hangs out, in and over for years.

Then there's the back. Very few painters survive without at least one encounter with a runaway ladder. The ladder runs away when it is being moved a few feet along a wall or around a corner. The taller the ladder the better the chance for a runaway. The base is lifted from the ground for the move while the upper end of the ladder is pulled away from the roof. All it takes is a misstep, an errant breeze or an error in judgment as to the angle, and the ladder can tip, sideways or over backward, or, worst of all, start to swing around in either direction. Sometimes the tired back can't interrupt the tip or swing. It's exactly the same as trying to keep the car on the road to prevent an accident. The holding can tear up the back, especially at circle 11. Such damage can be far worse than what might happen if the car rolled into the ditch. When checking the painter's back, spend lots of time on circles 1, 5, 11 and 13.

Painters need stretch, and while they probably think calisthenics are for the birds or ballet . dancers, they often do them very well and come to enjoy the swinging movements. If you watch them paint, many of them keep time to the radio as they work.

Do trigger points on painters as you would for a professional athlete, always when the one comes off the field and the other off the house. Always too when either complains of an ache anywhere. Watch for substitution. That's when they begin to make awkward movements, trying to do the job with an arm that won't reach full range anymore or, heaven forbid! a hand that can't hold on. You may not see it on the job, but check when teeth are brushed in the morning or hair is combed.

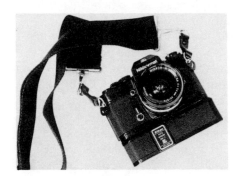

Photographers

Most photographers do two terrible things to themselves: they take pictures, and they develop them. In order to take pictures, they need equipment, and the equipment today is even heavier than in ancient times, when it consisted of a tripod, a black sheet, a box and plates. The camera man who is afflicted with a Mini-Cam, such as news photographers carry on one shoulder, is like the "aerobic dancer" and the football player. He can't say to himself, "*If* I get hurt"; he has to say, "*When* I get hurt."

Camera people have deadlines, and they may get only one chance at the shot. Those are both causes for tension. Where will the tension hit? Since he or she stands on cement, or tile over cement, most of the time, it's bound to be legs and back. But then there is the problem of carrying a heavy weight over one shoulder for hours each day. That pain could be shoulder, arm, neck, ear, jaw, hand or upper, mid or lower back . . . or groin.

The good thing about taking pictures is the many angles the body is forced into and out of in search of still better angles for shots.

Photographers need some other activity besides carrying a camera case with four special lenses and enough film for any emergency. He or she, and most of the time she is more flexible than he but just as vulnerable, needs calisthenics, mini-tramp, jumping rope, stretch exercises and a dear friend who will "do" the back after "one of those days."

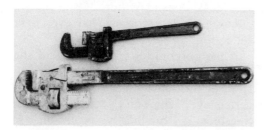

Plumbers

Plumbers do a lot of things designed to hurt the human frame. They thread pipes and strain the *pectorals*. They turn themselves into pretzels and crawl around hot pipes. They run into live steam and wrestle heavy conduit, they slip on wet or greasy floors, they take pratfalls with machines in their arms and fall off of unsteady platforms. When a plumber is called on in an emergency, it's usually due to a valve that's already under four feet of water or every pipe in the house is frozen and the toilet bowl is cracked.

The plumber, whatever else hurts, will have trigger points in the *pectorals*, the *trapezius*, the *axilla*, both arms, both hands and the small of his back. I know there are female plumbers these days and they will hurt in all the same places. It isn't the sex that determines the pain, it's the job. Condition does matter, however, and the weak or inflexible plumber who gets hurt all the time should take up another profession. There's no such thing as a weak plumber—only ex-weak plumbers.

To be safe, clear the danger areas of trigger points. Build strength with weight bags used in every direction, not just the limited motion found at a weight center. You can get that kind of exercise on the job. Don't forget warm-ups and *stretch*.

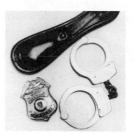

Police

"A policeman's lot is not an 'appy one . . . ," according to Gilbert and Sullivan, and I know several policemen (and -women too) who would agree. They sit, most of their days, patrolling in cars. When action is called for they have to start from a sitting position after perhaps hours of almost total inaction. The action is often dangerous, scary and extreme. Such action tears up cold muscles, although in the heat of the chase, they may not discover the injury. This is true also of soldiers in battle. The most incredible deeds are done with severely wounded muscles, and then later, when the danger is past, the pain sets in and one is made to "notice" that something has happened. In the case of the policeman there may be a Charley horse to contend with and then, a few days later, it will be forgotten. Forgotten by the policeman or -woman, *but not by the muscles*. They don't forget anything. Years later, a slip, even a trip, and the back goes into extreme spasm, hospital-bed kind, called "clinical."

Police of either sex are not happy with their image, any more than dentists are. I'm scared of the dentist before I even get there. I am also scared when I hear that siren. Most of the time, neither of them mean me any ill, but I can't get something inside to accept that. Both of them know this, and while I've known a couple of cops who reveled in it, most would rather be what was once called "the cop on the beat." He was the one the kids loved. (There's no way for the average dentist to develop a sweet, loving image, not with that drill, needle, ice pick in his hand.) The frightening image bothers some cops, and then of course there's that gun at his side and the billy club and all those stories. Police don't like those, either. They are very aware that some nut could end everything for them, *and what salary is worth that?* There's a lot of tension and not much respect or remuneration. Small injuries and tense situations unite to cause much-more-serious injury, with pain to match.

Finding *potentially painful spots* in seemingly OK muscles would help. How do you know where the potentially painful spots are? You use seeking massage (see page 229).

The physical buildup at the police academy was good, but then what? Did you keep it up? Are you in good enough shape to handle most things? If not, there are plenty of exercises in here. Do them with weights and don't forget that other side of weight training: stretch.

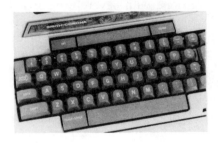

Secretaries

Secretaries have a good image, but rarely the one they want or deserve, and this takes a toll. Secretaries work at a desk sitting in the same position hour after hour, making little letters fall in line as accountants make figures come out even. They too are perfectionists or they lose their jobs. If they lose too many jobs they have no references. They are underpaid for what they do most of the time, and their days are *so* predictable. As Pearl Bailey once said, "Living from day to day is so *daily*." But that's the emotional side. The physical side comes in two words joined with a hyphen: *microtrauma*.

If you type away hour after hour, you use one set of muscles only, and you use them in only one way. There is never any stretch to offset the constant contractions. If the secretary copies material, she *always* turns her head in the same direction. The desks are built that way. Her chair allows for no change of position. Her desk doesn't either. If she uses a computer video terminal, her eyes fight reflection.

If the corporation has a gym and she goes, she will almost certainly be bored. It wasn't meant for her. If she is "of a certain age," she won't go near the place. She feels it's for the "younger set," in the shorts and tight T-shirts. She's probably right. Few go for fitness, and if they did they probably wouldn't find too much of it.

But what's a secretary to do? Read *Self Center* and set up one in your house. Don't say anything about it to the "younger set," just go home and do it. If there is another secretary with similar interests ask her to join you. Then bet theater tickets on which of you gets the first question: "You look *different*; what are you doing?" If you *are* the "younger set" you can avoid the neck, shoulder and arm pain said to be "arthritis," if you will do the same thing. Make the same bet with your crowd and you'll work harder.

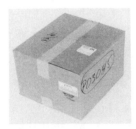

Shippers

Shippers, receivers, UPS men, movers, deliverers and all the rest who keep commerce, the economy and our lives going right along, very often suffer (eventually if not right away) from back pain. This is especially true if you were injured or seriously ill at some time earlier in your life. Lifting will heat up the trigger points and there you are.

If lifting hurts, get another job. Some bodies are wrong for the job but would be fine in another. Learn to listen to yours and *obey* it. If you insist on doing what hurts day after day, ask yourself why. Do you think your employer is going to like it? Nope. He's going to be annoyed when you are out with a bad back, "trick knee," "bursitis," "tennis elbow," or stiff neck.

If you really are stuck (usually in a family business that needs you), then think trigger points, full range of motion with weights, and stretch.

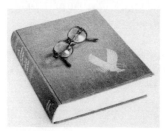

Teachers

The teacher who wants respect is teaching in the wrong country; he or she should be in China; *there* they respect teachers, but the salaries are so low you couldn't live on them and you'd have to be older than a Supreme Court justice to get a really top-ranking position. You haven't time for that.

Teachers are born, not made. If you aren't a teacher, but you thought it would be a good-paying job, you already know that that's far from the case, even in America. You might be able to stand the disadvantages if you were a born teacher, but for money!? And not much money!? "I'd rather hoe beets . . ." as I've heard one not-born teacher say. The trouble is that once you find teaching isn't for you, it's hard to start over. If you have a family it could be impossible. What's the matter with teaching, no matter who teaches? *Energy.* Kids have *so* much energy, *and they bombard you with it all day long.*

And the system being what it is, you really can't teach unless you fight it, and that's exhausting too. Since you can't teach, you get frustrated; the youngsters aren't learning a lot, so they too are frustrated. What happens then? Riots.

Teachers have back pain, shoulder and neck pain, and headaches. They should not be allowed to leave the teachers' room with any one of them; the pain will only get worse. Teachers need the *Self Center*, warm-ups, and stretch exercise, and since they are not only the last hope of most kids—they are the *only* hope— they should learn what is happening to the children. They have only to meet most parents to realize why they are like they are, but then, the parents are the way they are because they too came through our schools. Before children can be taught much of anything, they need good bodies, good nutrition, and nature. Not much of any of that around. I know a Latin teacher who has his class decline verbs to flexibility bounces. His class thinks he's great. Sitting *hurts* kids. I know a first-grade teacher who teaches spelling doing knee bends; she also has a self center in the classroom and teaches Myotherapy, exercises to do with old people, and massage. Her pupils are six and they know every muscle you read about in this book—where it is, how to say it even without front teeth, and what it makes hurt when in spasm. Her class thinks she's terrific. The nursing homes they visit in order to exercise with "adopted grandparents" think *they* are terrific. If you need a good program for the children in your care, get *How to Keep Your Child Fit from Birth to Six, Fitness from Six to Twelve,* or *Teenage Fitness.*

The world is changing, and teachers are going to have to change. New thoughts are loose in the world, and one of the things a teacher (the born one) must not be is a casualty. Keep your body and your sense of humor in good shape. The children need you.

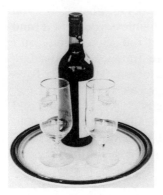

Waiters and Waitresses, Busboys and Bus Girls, Bartenders, Keepers of Food Stands, Cooks, Cooks' Helpers, Dishwashers, Countermen and -women, etc.

These are the people who feed us, and no one who has read this book will ever again watch with equanimity a tiny, five-foot-three woman shoulder a tray full of dirty dishes on one small hand and, bending like a new moon, stagger toward the kitchen. Think about the cooks, often sliding around in greasy kitchens, which are also steamy and as full of pressure as the pots they cook in. The next time you try to drown your sorrows (or the supervisor's voice) in a bar product, think of the server's legs.

Of all the jobs, the most thankless are the above, and we should here include the stewardess, who not only serves, but from a moving platform. So, exposed constantly to physical strain, a grumpy public and often bosses who aren't so great either . . . you have shoulder pain, back pain, leg pain, and all too often a pain in the you-know-what just sat down at your table.

Learn to do trigger points on each other. If no one is around, keep a bodo handy and do them on yourself. Stay fit with your own self center and check the section on the long second toe, page 202. Maybe you need pads in your shoes and trigger points out of the *tibialis anterior*, the outside front of your lower leg . . . and your feet.

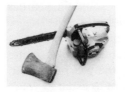

Woodsmen

Woodsmen are asked to spare trees, but they rarely spare themselves. Woodsmen in this book stands for all those who labor to keep the rest of us warm and safe, with telephone wires that are connected at both ends, trees that fell down carted away, frost heaves flattened out, floods kept back or the debris cleaned up; they cart away garbage, tow away cars, swing the levers in factories, dig the coal, pump the oil . . . do the hard work of the world.

By Friday the most they can think of is a beer and TV. *And most of them hurt somewhere all the time*. The woodsman and his ilk are rarely weak. They wouldn't last. But they are inflexible, so test and find out where. Do warm-ups *before* the beer and TV so that you can stretch too. Do a little of that every day and I think you will find you have more strength and more energy. *Get rid of the trigger points* that cause *little* aches, the kind you *could* ignore. If you don't, they'll gitcha in the end, and which end will it be? Neck, shoulder, low back, knee, foot? Keep a bodo handy if you work alone; you might have to do immediate mobilization. I have a friend who was digging postholes with a machine and it caught on some barbed-wire fencing. Before she knew what was happening, the wire had pulled loose, coiled around her thigh and twisted right through, compound-fracturing the femur, the huge thighbone. She did trigger-point work all the way to the hospital so the leg would be ready for the emergency operation she knew was coming. A few months later she was out digging postholes again with a well-functioning leg. Her doctors were amazed.

Self Center

The Sochi Palace

When someone has been smart enough to improve on what we have, whatever it is, we really ought to find out what's different and why what they have is better. Then, it seems to me, we ought to copy it and improve on it. After all, Americans have always been an ingenious people. For many years, Russia has had the jump on us when it comes to the care of important people. All *we* can think of is the yearly physical (which is more than suspect), the stress test and the executive gym. Some use it to advantage and others use it as a step up the corporate ladder. Still others use it to excess, which is easy, since its scope is so limited. Let me tell you about the palaces in Sochi.

In the Soviet Union, if a key person is found to be flagging at work, the government comes to the rescue. It has very selfish, sensible reasons for doing that. Key people are hard to come by and it takes a long time to train them (the reasons for our executive gyms). When Ivan is seen to be dropping into a slump, which here we call burnout, he is removed from the workplace *and* his home and sent to a sanatorium for *renewal*. The places the government provides for this important work are usually the palaces "liberated"

from the nobles; many are in Sochi, on the Black Sea. Ivan (and in Russia as in most of the world the one to be saved is Ivan, not Olga) will be evaluated thoroughly both physically and emotionally.

Once the tests are in, a nutritionist will provide a diet. That does not necessarily mean a thinning diet; rather, one designed for his particular needs. One such sanatorium serves two hundred different diets a day.

Ivan's other physical needs will be served in a variety of ways, and *all* of his programs will be suited to *his* condition as it is found to be right then . . . and jogging would be the last thing suggested, if at all.

WALKING. Ivan will be given a map of the territory surrounding the sanatorium. Every road and trail is listed and rated according to difficulty and length. He will probably start on trail A, which is both short and level. As his stamina improves (and he will be checked constantly), he will be directed to longer trails, covering more rugged terrain.

AIR BATHS. Most Americans would ask, "What's an air bath?" Just that. Ivan takes off his clothes and lets the air circulate all around his body while he rests. This "airing" of the skin would not be important for the bikini crowd, but while they are ubiquitous in Madison Avenue's publications, most of the rest of the world is wrapped up or stuffed into camouflaging garments from burnouses to Brooks Brothers' best.

SUNBATHS. These are more understandable to us, since most Americans go to the shore not to swim but to get a tan that makes them *look* as though they were swimmers, tennis players, or at least outdoorsy. Ivan goes to the roof, where in summer he can lie on the men's side of the canvas and tan himself all over. In the winter, sunlamps are provided.

MASSAGE is nothing new to Ivan; it never went out of style in Europe and Russia. Granted, massage could be had in America if you were of the upper classes, which were used to getting them in other countries when they traveled or lived abroad. For the most part, however, America, plagued by leftover pockets of Puritanism (the naked body was never to be viewed even by its owner, and in the orphanage we *babies* wore *bathgowns* in the tub!), shunned massage. Then, in a savage swing of the pendulum, we threw off all restraints and launched our sexual revolution. However, we were so uneducated physically that we had no idea what real massage was or what it was for. As a result, we linked it to sexual stimulation, and the rash of "adult books" did nothing to disabuse us of this thinking. So for years it was relegated to back streets, upstairs in places with red wall paper called "massage parlors." Today its practitioners are licensed in *massage*, and it is called "massage therapy"; we are beginning to accept what other countries and cultures never lost. Ivan will be given a complete massage every day while he is in sojourn.

EXERCISE. Ivan will not be asked to play volleyball, but will be given a specially designed exercise program, which he will do under the watchful eye of a trained instructor. That program, like his walks, will be gradually stepped up as his health and energy improve. At all times there will be someone in attendance ex-pected to note his progress and compliment him on it.

SWIMMING. Ivan's lap swimming will be carefully monitored so that he will not tax himself unduly even if he would like to overdo. He will be reminded at that time that he has a duty to Mother Russia to take care of his valuable self.

BICYCLING. Ivan will have a bike at his disposal if the weather is clement, and he will be able to use it on paths where cars are forbidden.

REST. At stipulated hours throughout the day Ivan will return to his room to rest, and in the evening there will be quiet entertainment. It will not be violence on TV or raucous music. Ivan is a cog in the national machine, and as such it is his duty to be healed, not stressed. Tension and noise are both forms of stress.

At no time will the stress of business or of home be permitted to intrude until he is well, his energy normal and his level of stress tolerance high. He knows someone will call him if there is a real emergency, so he can proceed on the assumption that no news is good news, and relax, taking each day as it comes.

In a very short time Ivan is slimmer, harder, tanner and better-looking. That much he can see in the mirror. His exercise work has become easier and he is doing more advanced work. He knows that from his coach; besides he *feels* totally different. Feeling good often means ready. His libido will have improved and with it his self-confidence and interest in sex, which to his horror had flagged along with the rest of him. His rested mind will soon be able to handle problems efficiently again, and efficiently means easily, without strain. Since he has had ample time to think about himself and even to talk with others of his kind who are on lifesaving programs, he may have even discovered that his primary stress was home-based. He may have already made the decision to change it. In a few more weeks he will have the stamina necessary for implementation.

"Good for the Russians," you say. "At least they're doing *something* right. But what has that to do with me? My government, or boss either, wouldn't know if I were dropping dead in the front office or the backyard." But this has *everything* to do with you.

Each life is a whole world. No one has ever read the books you have read exactly as you have read them. No one has really heard the music as you heard it, nor even seen the sky as you see it. No one knows all that you know or even a small part. No one has loved as you have, or suffered either. So who is the most important person in your world? You. Who runs your world (though you may wonder at times)? You do. You are both government and boss. If the government of your world cared about you (and it better) is there somewhere it could send you? Is there a program for just you, and could you get away? And after you got there, will the government pick up the tab? There *will* be such a place, and we will call it "self center." If you want it you can have it, and you can have all the Sochi sanatorium gave Ivan. Yes, there is effort involved, but the prize, believe me because I went to one, is worth every cent and every minute.

Actually, most of us don't have too much choice if we want to save ourselves from exhaustion, obesity, a nervous collapse and the results of unprotected aging. The places we can go don't give us value and often injure us, and if we are so situated that we can't go anywhere, there goes hope for a better life. Where, then, do you find your self center? *You make it yourself.* Where do you put such a thing? You put it in the basement, in the garage or even in your own bedroom (that's where mine is). All the directions are here and all the checks and counterchecks. In the section on *Aging*, you will write a list of things you would change if you didn't think they couldn't be changed. You may not think things can be changed because the most important

person in your world is tired. You don't have to be old to be tired. My most tiring years were as a young mother/housewife/cook/cleaning woman/chauffeur/shopper/gardner/house painter/laundress/nurse/canner/scout leader/Red Cross worker/first-aid instructor/community-chest organizer/ski-patrol leader/skier/climber in Westchester, New York. And I did those things all in the same week and often many of them in the same day. You can be tired at any age and for many or just a few reasons. Perhaps the most important person in your world hurts too much to change things. Try quick fix and permanent fix. Perhaps that person is desperately unhappy. Unhappiness, unless it is embraced, can be very temporary indeed. Only death is permanent. Happiness never comes when you chase after it as though it were a rainbow. It is a byproduct of many things, and you can't be quite sure which things, so don't get bogged down too deep in one. Keep the door open and you'll be surprised. Whatever your excuse for not saving the most important person in your world from pain, misery, illness and aging, forget them and join me in your self center, which we will build together.

First, what has Ivan got that you don't have right now? His introduction to the sanatorium was an evaluation. On page 131 you will find the Kraus-Weber minimum muscular fitness test and the record sheet. That's your first evaluation, and as you give, take and record it, keep in mind that you are now the most important person in *your* world. You are the government that cares enough to send you for help, and you are the helper, the coach, the doctor and the nutritionist. You are getting to be quite a crowd.

DIET. There's a poser. There are so many, and most of them are so *dumb*. You can take care of your own with common sense and some time spent reading some nonfad diet books, or you can go to a nutritionist for a special program. I do the former, but a good many people are finding the latter very helpful. It doesn't work, though, if you don't, and do have a care. If the nutritionist is for real, he or she went to a good college and has a degree in it. The world is full of quacks, and you should be aware. If they start prescribing unicorn oil, leave.

THE EXERCISE PROGRAM. Here's where the fun comes in. You need some equipment. Here is where the cost comes in, so suit your pocketbook. Your government can't afford to go into debt over this, because debt is stress.

WALKING. Decide on how long you should walk at the start; it may be a block or it may be a mile or it may be half an hour. If you know it's half a mile to the bus stop, your mile is measured for the day. If you want to walk for half an hour, take off briskly in any direction after checking your watch. After fifteen minutes start home again and don't be lured on, block after block or field after forest, the first week. Give yourself a chance. See how you feel. If merely a little tired you are doing fine. If exhausted enough to require a nap, you overdid it. You are in worse shape than you thought. Cut back to half and work up.

EXERCISE EQUIPMENT. You already have the best piece of exercise equipment to be found almost anywhere: your stairs. But you need something more: a cassette player and earphones or a record player. You need one or the other for almost any exercise if you want to make it fun, so invest. Most people have light packs these days, but if you don't, that's your next purchase.

STAIR CLIMBING. Evaluate your ability to climb stairs by which stair on which flight you *feel* your legs. There are fifteen stairs in my self center, and if I have not been climbing anything for a while I will feel it on the top stair of the second trip, the thirtieth stair. There was a time when I felt it on the fifth! One flight may be all you are good for at first. Accept it and in a way be glad. Where you are at the start doesn't matter; it's where

you are in a month that counts. If you are on the bottom you won't have to work so hard to improve. After a week add a couple of flights. *Listen* to your legs and your breathing and to how you feel. Patients, if they are allowed, will tell the doctor exactly what is wrong with them. Bodies will tell their owners what's right and what's wrong—if those owners will but listen and look for *good* as well as bad. Keep track of your progress, which means you now need another gadget; a stopwatch.

Every year now I go to Barbados for mid-winter vacation. By the time I get to my room overlooking the sea I am usually exhausted from work and what seems to be endless travel, endless people and endless problems. For two days I don't *do* anything except read. Then I walk all the way to the third cove; it takes half an hour. The water is always warm in Barbados, and I am tempted to mill around in it, nothing more. The fourth day I add stairs. There are two stories to my hotel, so the first day of "training" myself back to health, I walk them eleven times, slowly, with my stopwatch running. If someone stops me on the way I click it off until I can resume. Why did I choose eleven? Because when I counted the stairs, which are seven inches high, eleven flights brought me close enough to two hundred feet to call it that. A week later I double my climb to four hundred feet and the following week I get it up to six hundred feet a day, but that isn't all. My stopwatch tells me I have cut down on the time as well. Then I start skipping one stair step on each of the three sets of stairs per flight. That can go on and on, but by the second week my walk is encompassing five coves and taking over one hour. Three of those coves are just right for a cool-off swim, but by then I am running in place in the water. I start with two hundred steps per cove and add fifty a day. One beach is loaded with sunbathers, so I either walk in shoulder-high water or swim that quarter mile. The walk is harder. By the second week I have added my record *Keep Fit—Be Happy,* Volume I, for twenty minutes.

The third week I add Volume II and weight bags and kung fu exercises. By the fourth week I'm human again and dangerous. As soon as I get back to Massachusetts I conduct a really wicked exercise class for the students at my school. They exercise every day for a couple of hours and I check the success of my crash program against how they feel when it's over. That's *one* way to get into shape without pain and injury, but the smart thing is to keep the level up *after* you get back in the saddle. And you can do that without pain in your self center.

Stairs

Stairs are the mountain in your house, whatever mountain you want it to be. If climbing stairs were your only exercise and you took only two hundred feet at a time, but you did it five times a day it would take you only three days to climb Greylock, here in Massachusetts. You could do a little better in five days over in New York State climbing Marcy. It would take six to climb Grandfather Mountain, in North Carolina, a week for Harney, in South Dakota, a week and a day for the fabulous Mount Olympus, in Washington, a week and two days for Guadalupe Peak, in Texas, and two weeks for Longs Peak, in Colorado, or Whitney, in California. Climb your first mountain free, but as soon as you feel fit for it, start adding a pack and weight bags. Keep the pace slow and steady. Mountain climbers average about a thousand feet an hour.

One trouble with jogging on the road is the sameness of the stride, the angle of the foot and the weight. Use the stairs to exercise *all* the muscles in your legs. Wear a light pack or carry weights in your hands. Vary the weight each day. Turn the feet in as you climb and you will feel

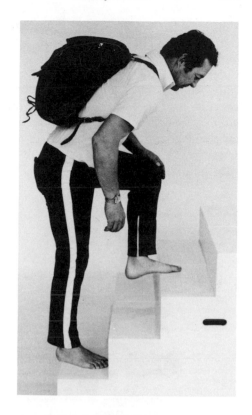

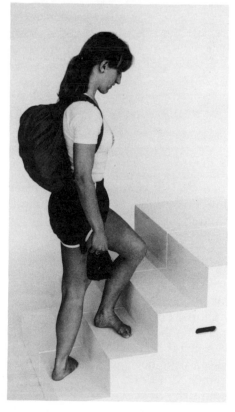

your muscles working very differently from your straight climb. This works the *tibialis anterior* and is particularly good if you have flat feet or are practicing for figure skating. When you walk back down the stairs turn your feet way out and your *quadriceps* will talk to you. The second time you go up, reverse the positions, climbing with the toes out and descending with them turned in.

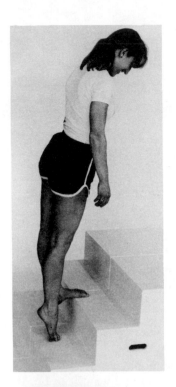

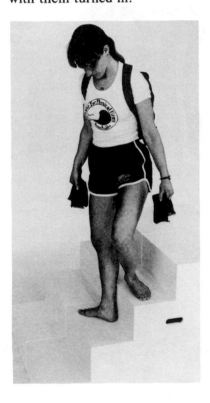

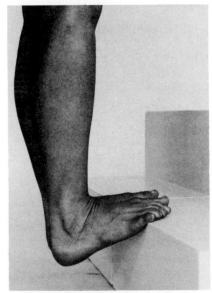

To stretch the front of the leg, use two slow counts for each step. On the first count mount the step but leave the toe of the following leg on the step below. Point it sharply and maintain the touch as you consciously straighten both knees *hard*. Hold that for the second count. Come down in a relaxed walk.

On the next trip step up with one foot and bring the second to a parallel position with just the balls of the feet on the stair. Allow your heels to hang down as you bounce four times. Use the other foot to mount the next stair so that they alter-

nate. Come down in a relaxed walk. This is important, because as the exercises become more difficult you want to have a pause in between and yet not stop to rest.

Going up and down stairs backward is a whole new world to your feet and legs.

Excellent it is but easy it isn't. Hang on to the banister until you get the hang of it, but don't use it other than for balance.

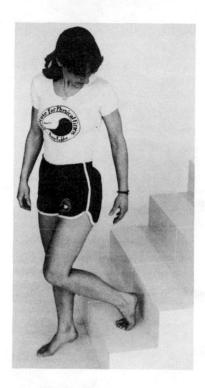

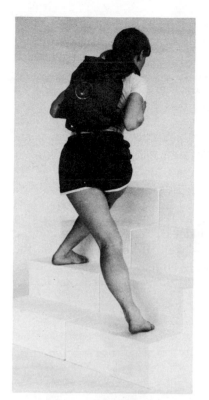

Crossing over going up and down is a great test of the *quadriceps* muscles and therefore the knees. Be sure yours are free of trigger points before you do this one. Just step the mounting foot across the stair as far as you can comfortably reach. After my hips were replaced with two total hip replacements I could reach across only twelve inches. I'm up to twenty-two now, with eight more to go to match what I could do before my hips began to hurt, eighteen years ago.

The side step is really a triple exercise. Face the banister. At first use it for balance, and soon, not at all. Leave your arms free as a second aid in balance, and finally, when you are sure of yourself, put your hands behind your back. Mount with the following leg crossing in front and be careful not to turn your body. Come down in the same manner. On the

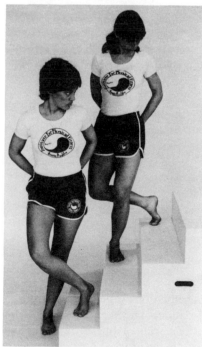

second trip cross the following leg in back. The third time do the grapevine step, which is to alternate back crossing with front crossing.

The seat climb. All this time, your legs have been getting the workout but little is happening to the arms, back or abdomen. That's another of the lacks in jogging. Sit on the bottom stair and reach back to lay both hands on the stair above. Lift your seat to that stair and continue to the top. Walk down. On the next ascent place your hands *two* stairs up, but move your seat only one. The third time place the hands two steps up and move the seat two steps as well. You will be surprised at the workout you will give your shoulder girdle. After a time add the descent as well. If your legs are on the short side, you may have to help on the two-step seat lift with alternating feet.

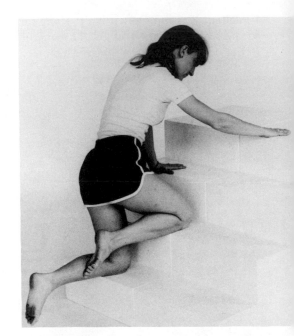

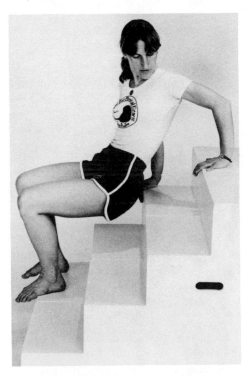

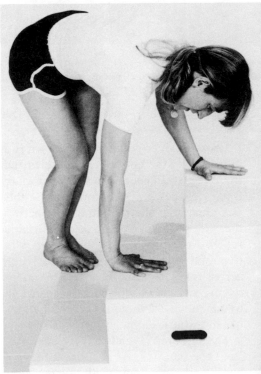

The knee crawl is really a hip exercise and should be done on carpeted stairs or on well-padded knees. Knees were not meant to be walked on. In my convent days all of us hated what happened to our knees. They had great big calluses the size of quarters from kneeling at prayers. You wouldn't want them. Get down on hands and knees and crawl upstairs, keeping the lower leg parallel to the stair below.

The hand walk/foot jump requires considerable practice and should be done very slowly at first. Learn what your feet are supposed to do by jumping them from side to side to a good beat. Then kneel at the first step and make your hands mark time on the next. Follow that by standing on the floor and walking your hands up five or six steps. When you *think* you can put both together, walk your hands to the same beat as you jump your feet from side to side.

The wheelbarrow requires an assistant, and since the assistant will be working as hard as you, change off after each ascent. The ''wheelbarrow'' places both hands on the bottom step and raises first one leg and then the other, which are then grasped *at the thighs*, not the ankles, by the ''laborer.'' Together they proceed up the stairs.

The headfirst descent is not for beginners; even when you are pretty sure of yourself you would be wiser to start with your hands three steps up from the bottom, to get the feel. At no time bring your feet closer than two steps from the bottom hand. If you are a long person, make that three.

There! you didn't have to buy anything special except a stopwatch, which you will use all through your program but could also do without. You need music for the whole program, but you *could* do without it. I couldn't, because my motor runs on it.

Add stairs to your day wherever you

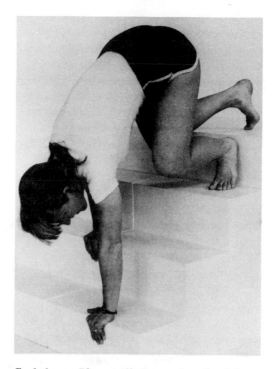

find them. If you climb two hundred feet with or without a pack, multiply your own weight by two hundred. If your weight is one hundred and fifty pounds, *each of your legs will lift fifteen thousand foot-pounds.* No mean feat in *any* program.

Weight Training

On page 166 you have the directions for making weight bags. The total cost will be a few dollars, and if you want to save even those, use sand instead of lead shot. Weight bags are very versatile: you can use them with almost every exercise, including walking and stairs as you have just seen. Just raising them overhead works arms, back, chest and shoulders. If you lie on the floor and with straight arms carry the weights from your thighs to the floor above your head, the arms, upper back, chest and abdomen get a workout.

Move yourself up onto a table or a bed and allow the weights to hang down over the edge for your starting position. Re-

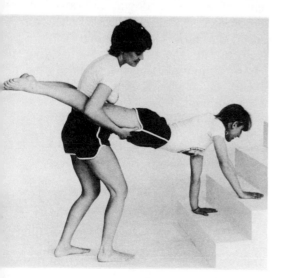

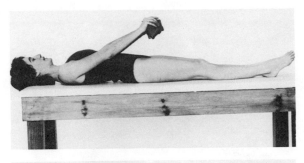

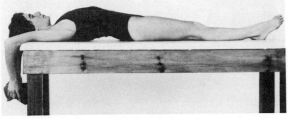

peat the same exercise and you will also stretch the *axilla*, which is *always* in need of a good stretch. You can also stretch the *pectorals* if your table is narrow enough to allow you to stretch both arms out to the side into a hang-down position. An inexpensive pectoral stretcher is a bookshelf resting on a few volumes of your encyclopedia, a couple of boxes or two chairs.

Legs can be worked in all directions while bearing weight bags. The prone leg lifts strengthen (and slim) the *gluteals* and the backs of the legs. One way is to do the leg lifts with the legs parallel. Just lift the weight bags high enough to clear the table. The *slower* you lift and lower, the harder and better the workout. Next, spread the legs wide and repeat the lifts. A good way to start any of the weight exercises is with a set of light weights, going through all of them (and any others you would like to add) with a minimum of repetitions. If it all seems terribly easy,

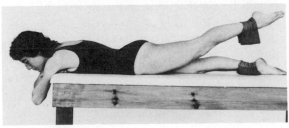

add weight and double the repetitions. When you find you tire, stop, but remember when you stopped and try to surpass that by just a little the next time.

The bicycle is another multiple exercise. Start on your back, resting on your elbows. With the weights on your ankles, do the conventional bicycle for eight repetitions. Then, keeping both elbows tight to the floor or table, roll over onto the right hip and bike for eight. Next, the left hip and finally the forward position. As you improve, add the spread-leg bike, in which you take the starting position and bike but with the legs spread. The *dernier cri* is the no-hands bike. For this one you *really* need abdominals. Start as before, but as you begin your leg movements, lift your arms from the floor. If you can, do the exercise to the left and right as well.

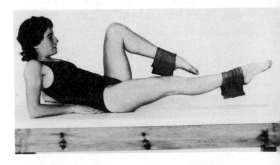

The dead lift is a must for those with round backs. Put your weights on either end of a wand, dowel or sawed-off broomstick (thirty-six inches). Lean over from the hips and, keeping the legs straight, lift the weighted bar to your chest without altering the angle of your back, which should be almost parallel with the floor. Do only a few repetitions at first and with light weights. Increase both weight and repetitions as you improve.

Deep knee bends. Put the bar across your shoulders and do *two* knee bends as a start. Go as far down as you can, but remember, you have to come back up. That may mean you have to begin your knee bends in the doorway gym, which follows. Do *not* be discouraged if at first

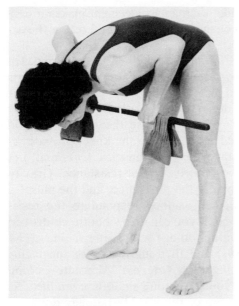

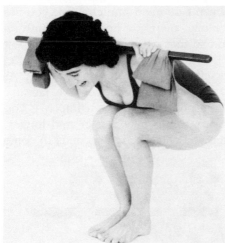

you seem to be a third-grader when it comes to exercise. Even the finest of athletes was once a third-grader, and it won't take you a year to get into fourth grade.

The Doorway Gym

The doorway gym can cost practically nothing if you know a carpenter or a handy person or are willing to buy a chinning bar at the sporting-goods store. There's a catch to the boughten ones, though: they have suction cups on each end so they can be made to fit any door-way, metal or wooden. Those cups are totally unreliable; what you don't need is to fall on your bent knees or *coccyx*. To make the suction cups safe, use little angle irons, which can be picked up in the hardware store. For metal doorframes you can add an inner frame. Since you are not merely going to do chin-ups on your doorway gym, it *must* be secure.

FIG. 56: ANGLE IRON

To make your gym versatile indeed, you will need to put two bar supports (Fig. 58) two inches off the floor, twenty inches off the floor, thirty-six inches off the floor, as well as four inches down from the top of the doorway. The lowest pair holds the bar just off the floor for your bent-knee sit-ups and backward rolls, in which you lie supine holding on to the bar and roll your legs up and over to touch the floor on the other side of the doorway. For the lowest pair, turn the supports on their sides.

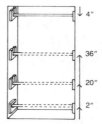

FIG. 57: DOOR FRAME

You can rest your bookshelf on the bar at the twenty-inch level for the weight work on page 275, and if you tie a noose around the upper end of the shelf you can slip your feet under it and do your bent-knee sit-ups at a slant. If you want to rest with your head lower than your body, you can lie on it. Just be sure that your board is strong enough to support your weight. If you are going to buy one, get half-inch plywood. It won't break, but pine could.

At the thirty-six-inch level, your kids can skin the cat or do pinwheels (so can you and so should you). When you skin the cat, you hang by both hands and kick your feet through the space between them to land on the floor behind you. Then you pull back through, leading with your seat. Pinwheels are easier: Stand facing and holding on to the bar with your hands spaced apart so they are close to your sides. Lean forward and over the bar, allowing your legs to roll over to land on the other side of the doorway. Of *course* you remember doing those. Well, if you could once, you can again and should try again. What you don't use, you lose, remember? You may not think you lose much by not tumbling any more, but you do. You lose proprioception: you aren't as good at knowing where you are in space and at handling yourself in space. That might be a disadvantage in a fall. Also, the physically *educated* body should be able to sing more than one song.

The top line holds the chinning bar at the highest point, and as you will see, offers unlimited exercise; chinning is the least of it.

In my nursery school we have many bars—at least six or seven. The frames are of wood, and instead of one expensive, suction-cupped chinning bar we use several pieces of galvanized pipe so that we have a ladder as well as several supports for slanting boards for crawling up *and down*. It's the *down* that builds arms and chests. The supports are of three-quarter-inch plywood and support the pipe length at levels ten inches apart. Aside from making the gym more versatile, such an arrangement makes it easy to change the level and therefore the action.

Chin-ups are a cinch for well-muscled boys, and an impossibility for most girls and even boys who lack physical training or do no manual work. But they are easy to master. You use the same trick you used to strengthen the knee: provide resistance as the muscles *lengthen*. Let *down* slowly against resistance. Gravity provides the resistance, and the muscles lengthen as they respond to the resistance. If you can do a smooth, controlled chin-up, do one with palms facing in (*biceps*) and then another with the palms facing away (*triceps*). Alternate as long as you are getting smooth, even lifts. At the top of the lift, start *slowly* down. If you can't do even one chin-up, you are not alone, merely a beginner. Climb on a box so that you can start at the *top* of the lift with your chin above the bar. Let yourself *slowly* down inch by inch. At first you will come down like laundry down a chute, but as you improve you will be able to take longer and longer. When you can take ten seconds to come

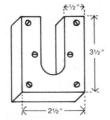

FIG. 58: BAR SUPPORT

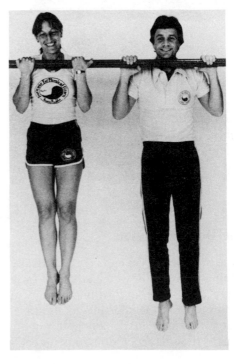

down, you should have the strength to go up at least once.

Rubber-Strap Stretches

For abdominal strengthening without having to get down on the floor, and also a handy exercise gadget that is available all day long, use two lengths of rubber inner tubing, forty inches long and three quarters of an inch wide. Where do you get it? At a garage. Ask for an old inner tube, cut it open with a razor, a knife or scissors, and drop it into a pail of water laced with Spic and Span or a reasonable facsimile. Used inner tubes are filthy. When it is clean, cut it into strips. There's a whole gym for the whole family right there in your hands. Tie one forty-inch strip near each end of the bar. If you don't want that bother, buy surgical tubing at a medical supply store.

Wrap the other ends of the straps once or twice around each hand and, standing with legs straight and well apart, pull the straps toward the floor. As you get stronger and go down farther, take an-

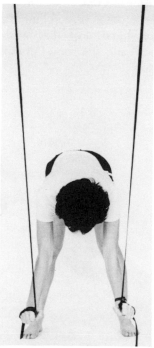

other turn in the wrapping, to make it harder. Do eight for starters and get into the habit of stopping as you go through that particular door. Do eight every time. Eight takes fifteen seconds, so if you go through that door four times you will have done thirty-two exercises without even noticing the used time. Besides, what have you got to do that's more important than care for yourself?

Rotated Stretch

Keeping the feet apart and standing inside the room close to the doorframe, do the same abdominal exercise but twisted first to one side and then to the other. Do eight to a side for a set. As you improve, stand farther from the doorframe and increase the number of sets.

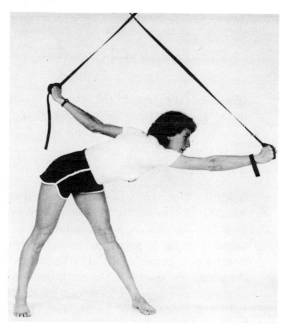

Shoulder and Chest Stretch

Standing first inside the doorway and then outside, bend forward from the hips to stretch the hamstrings. Wrap the straps around your hands until they are short enough to put your chest muscles on the stretch. Lean forward with arms out-

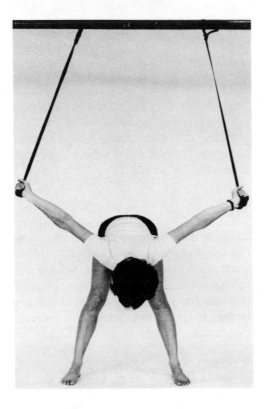

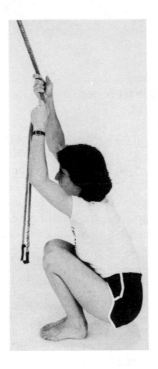

Rope Climb, Easy

stretched, first with the palms facing down and then up. Alternate for eight.

The Rope Tricks

First of all, if you leave your rope hanging in the middle of your doorway, you can't go through without being reminded to do at least one exercise, the deep knee bend. Even if you haven't done one in years (for shame!), the rope makes it easy. A fourteen-foot length of half-inch nylon would be fine for adults. If your children are around, add two feet. One deep knee bend is good at the start, but add one each week for a month. *Be sure your heels stay on the floor.* When you are doing four every time you go through the door you will be expending eight seconds a trip. Five times a day that would be twenty knee bends. Could you do that many easily? If you can, you don't need a rope.

Lie down on the floor with legs spread. The rope should hang directly above your upward-stretched arms. Keeping your body stiff, see if you can lift off the floor and hold for three seconds. When you can hold for ten seconds, try to climb the rope, hand over hand. For that, slide through the door until the rope falls toward your ankles.

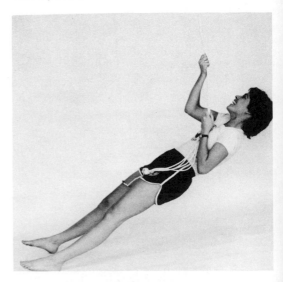

Rope Climb, Difficult

Have your partner grasp you at the thighs while you are lying on the floor. He places your feet on his thighs as he stands in a somewhat bent position with legs spread and knees slightly bent. You will be carrying most of your body weight when you climb the first two feet.

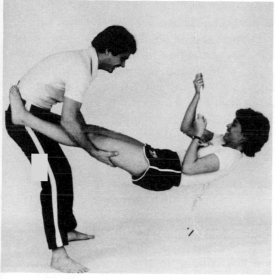

Waist Stretches

You can use a partner for help, or brace your feet against the sill or another bar at the two-inch level. With feet spread wide and hands grasping the two separated ropes, lean away first toward one side and then the other. Do eight.

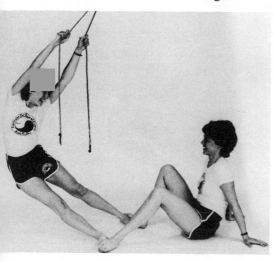

Forward and Back Leans

With feet stabilized and arms outstretched, lean forward on spread straight legs to stretch the chest and then backward as you bring the hands together to stretch the upper back. On the backward stretch, round the back and drop the head. Do not break at the waist.

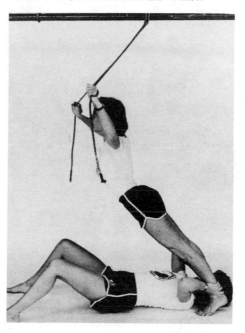

The Almost Impossible Climb-and-Reverse Chin-Up

From the lying position reach up to grasp the rope at arm's length. Swing both legs up to grasp the rope with your feet. Lift your weight from your shoulders and hold for a few seconds. As you find that easy, add seconds. When you can hang easily for ten seconds, try to chin yourself once, then twice and then three times. When you can do that, see if you can climb a little way up the rope *and back down again.*

Abdominal Curl

Grasp your chinning bar with both hands, arms stretched straight. Lift your feet from the floor by bending your knees.

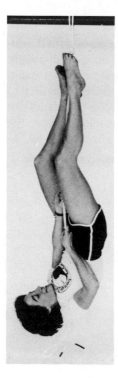

Almost Impossible
Climb-and-Reverse
Chin-Up

Jumping Rope

This is one of the best exercises for endurance and aerobic development there is. Years and years ago, Dr. Kaare Rodahl, at Lenkenau Hospital, in Pennsylvania, did a study that proved that just minutes of rope jumping every day could do wonders for the heart and lungs, and if you don't do it on cement it won't give you a backache, either.

Put on a record you like and jump rope any way you enjoy for *one third of that record*, or about one minute. That's enough if you are just starting. Little by little, stay with it longer until you can do the whole record. Running in place for the same length of time is not nearly as taxing, so take it slow. Some people do a kind of two-step when they jump. One jump goes over the rope and the other is a kind of space filler in between jumps while the rope goes over the head. As soon as you can, replace the "two-step" with the "one-step" that boxers use, in which alternating feet go over every turn of the rope. Finally, shorten the rope and try bent-knee jumps.

How high can you bring your knees toward your chest? Just off the floor? That's a start. Try to hold them off for three seconds and build up slowly to ten. Little by little, once you can hold for ten seconds, you will find them rising higher and higher. Home base happens when you touch your chest, then hold that for ten seconds. Follow that success with two and then three curls.

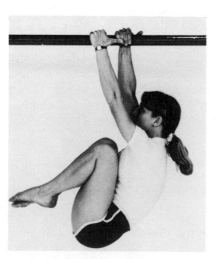

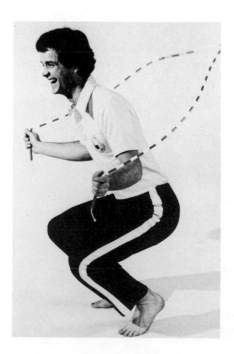

Bicycling

Biking is good exercise if you can do it safely, but after automobiles bikes produce the greatest number of accidents. A stationary bike is something else again. You can bike to music, which is a little like skating, skiing or swimming to music. You can watch the news if you are pressed for time, or read the paper. No matter what you do, your legs will keep on pumping and burning up the miles and calories. You can even watch it rain, sleet or snow as you cruise all warm and dry. In summer, turn on a fan.

Every year, I'm asked to say good things about some piece of equipment, and in my entire life I think I've named four. One was a piece of isometric equipment that I turned around and made into a gadget that could be used for isotonic exercise. Another I talked about in my book *How to Be Slender and Fit After Thirty*, two poles like ski poles anchored to a base for leaning into. You can do the same thing with the double rope in this chapter. The third is the stationary bike, but choose a *good* one with the pedals as close to under the seat as possible, not set so that the legs are thrust out in front.

The stationary bike should become a habit, and the only way to make a habit is to do it and do it and do it. But if you are too ambitious at the start, it will take too much effort or time. Either way, you will quit. A habit is *every day*, and at the same time if possible. Start with no more than two minutes, but those minutes must become sacred. You can get back on later, and later again if you want to, but *the* minutes vary only by increasing the time, and that but a little each week. Peddling for two minutes at twenty-five miles an hour isn't slow, so don't turn up the tension on the wheel for a while. If you add a minute to the time each week, you will be biking three minutes a day the following week. Increase only one minute a week from the original two minutes and it will take a month to get

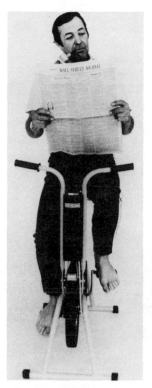

through the five-minute stage. If you are just tolerating your required ride, stick at five minutes a day. If you like, start upping a minute a week again. If you are crazy about it, double the time, *but* there is no one exercise that does everything, and if you don't do calisthenics, your body will be stuck at breakfast. Others will enjoy lunch and dinner, but your palate will know only oatmeal. Biking must not take too much time. Ivan would not be allowed it.

The Mini-Trampoline

The fourth piece of equipment I have found useful and fun is a circular jumper, a mini-trampoline. I have one called The Sun Dancer. It's more expensive than most of the others, but it's a good one, and you usually get what you pay for. I have four in my own gym, and we have ten more at my school. One is usually sufficient, unless you have closet space and a few friends.

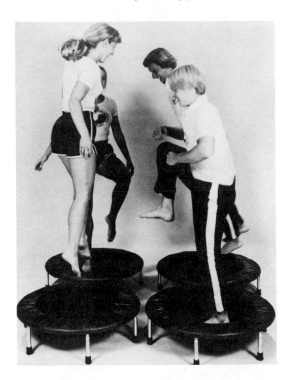

Use music and you can run, jump rope and dance on yours. I keep a stopwatch nearby and the mini-tramp, like the bike, is a must, for one minute every time I have to leave my office; that's about ten times a day. Action is like calories: both are cumulative. You do *not* have to do all your exercises in an hour, two hours or more, without stopping. If you believe that's a must, you will never start.

A massage table is a useful item and can be expensive or not, as you wish. The expensive variety is portable and can be ordered at a surgical supply store. The inexpensive variety is your everyday kitchen table, a desk or an old door across two sawhorses. If you are going to use Myotherapy to any extent, you will want one or the other.

The sun is the light and the life giver of our corner of the universe, and for many of you, whether you know it or not, the sun is the health giver of that world where you reign. The caucasoid ethnic division, or the whites of our many worlds, used to avoid the sun under mantles and hats, and some had good reason. The peoples of the British Isles, for example, seem to lack the protective pigmentation that those of browner skins revel in today, but there was a time when a brown skin meant either peasant or soldier. The first was despised, as was the second unless the soldier was a captain or better. Sailors, too, were weathered, and they too were low on the social ladder unless captains, or better yet, admirals. Times and fads change, and today a white skin usually spells three things to brainwashed America: unhealthy, indoors and unfit.

So you need a tan. How do you get one? You lie, work or play in the sun. For me it's easy. In me, my father's Indian blood shows up in an hour with a pale glow, and in three days I'm dark. Not so my sister. Her glow isn't pale; it is angry red. So what does a golden girl do when her genes have determined that she be blue of eye, fair of skin and blistered every June? Madison Avenue says *sunscreen*, and it comes in every grade from one (that doesn't *do* anything much but costs a lot) to ten, which screens out almost all the ultraviolet, which is what

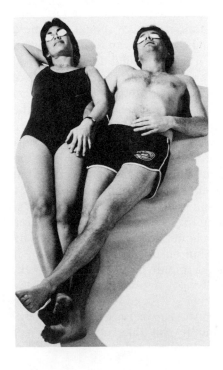

the sun-hungry skin is looking for. Any cream that screens out *all* ultraviolet rays is working against you as well as the tan. Vitamin D is what your body is looking for too, and it is absorbed from the skin oils, both yours and any you put on. It takes four hours for the absorption, however, so don't be so quick to shower.

Since you want some ultraviolet but no burn, how do you get it? You take it easy at first. If your skin is dry, baby oil is helpful but screens nothing. If you have the patience to build up your tan little by little, you can get a good safe one going starting any time. Move the furniture away from whatever window in your house gives you the best sun from eleven to one. If you are one of those unfortunates who doesn't have a sunny room ever, you will need the alternative: two sunlamps.

Glass also screens out the ultraviolet rays which tan, so you will have to open the window wide and let the sun shine on your face and chest (and whatever else will fit in the sunny spot). Fine in fine weather in spring, summer and fall, but what about winter in the higher latitudes? There is plastic that does not screen out ultraviolet, so have a frame made to fit your window and tack the plastic to it. To multiply the sun's rays, get one of those reflector "blankets" and hang it over a couple of chairs behind you to turn the warmth of the sun back toward you.

If you can, take all your clothes off for your sunbath. It clears up the skin blemishes caused by some materials, lack of air and constriction, such as that caused by girdles, bras and even tight jeans. Sun should be brought to the genitals, but watch out for sunburn. The skin is as tender as that covering your eyes.

When you buy sunlamps get good ones that will actually tan you. Two are usually enough for an allover tan, but pay the same attention to time as you would on the beach in Barbados. Read the instructions and if they say you should start with one minute, believe them, at least until

you can prove otherwise with no pinking at all. Use oil to augment what you provide naturally and give yourself time to absorb the vitamin D.

What else do you need for your self center? You need a couple of exercise records. I recommend the two I mentioned earlier: *Keep Fit—Be Happy*, Volumes I and II. Volume I is easy and great for a start. Volume II is hard, but if you have mastered the first, you can handle most of the second except for the Russian leg exercises. That will take time. On Volume I there is a good run; on II, both a tumbling routine and a weight-lifting series. If you want a book that will give you some insight into yourself and your friends, get *How to Be Slender and Fit After Thirty*. It doesn't say so in the title, but it will do the same thing for you after forty, fifty or sixty, or even seventy.

Pennies in the Bathroom

This is a trick to remind you to do *some* exercises at intervals all day long and also to drink more water. Take a guess at how many times you will be in the bathroom any given day, starting with toothbrush time. Put that number of pennies next to a small container every morning. Decide on *three* and no more than three exercises that you will do every time you use the bathroom. Each time you complete them, drop a penny in the container and drink a glass of water, which will assure your return fairly often. One can ignore a lunch break, but not a bathroom break. Two minutes' worth of exercise would be ample.

Swim Gear

If a pool is available, get yourself a mask, snorkel and fins and swim face down, which will not strain even the violinist's neck. The mask will protect your eyes from the chemicals. Check yourself as you did on the stairs. Can you get *across* the pool without feeling it? How about one length? When *do* you feel it? Be sure you make a record of your improvement. Every summer, I conduct two five-day workshops, one at Amherst College, in the East, and one at Western State, in Colorado. The "Aqua-Ex" portion comes on the last day, after five wild days of exercises all day long. This year, a lady came up to me all but dancing across the water. "Before the workshop I could hardly get *across* the pool and I just swam two full *lengths*! Look at me, I'm not even breathing hard." That's how fast you can improve.

Clothes

You need only one more thing to complete your self center: the outfit. Go out and buy yourself the snappiest warm-up suit you can find, but one that can breathe. Nothing shiny and waterproof . . . and avoid outfits designed to make you sweat. Some are called sauna suits. You won't *need*, in fact shouldn't wear, gym shoes, but get a good-looking, comfortable pair anyway, just to go with the outfit. You may want to do your walking in them. If you are going to go in for fitness, you might as well take the credit and admiration for it. One thing more: a warm-up suit creates the image of fitness. Most leotards do not. Old gray sweat suits are all wrong, washed-out shorts and shapeless T-shirts aren't in, and jeans are too tight. It's fashionable to be (look) fit. Ride with it and I don't care what shape you are in or what age you are.

So you have decided to try to make the life of the most important person in your world better, happier, healthier and more fun. As director, you have outfitted your self center with whatever you felt was necessary for the program you the coach will set up. As most important person (MIP), you have prepared your calendar

as you would had you planned a vacation or a business trip. The things that could not await your return are done and, since tomorrow is the big day, you are all packed. You have your warm-up suit, shorts, T-shirts, shoes, parka and gloves if it's cold. You have bought your very own stopwatch and a notebook just in case you get any good ideas while you are away.

Meanwhile, at the self center you the coach have decided what your new MIP will follow. You do know something about him or her since you have been privy to the brain while this book was being read. You do know if the person is young, middle or older, tall, short, over- or underweight, in shape looking for better or out of shape looking for something. You have decided what pieces of equipment to try out the first week and what besides the things that *must* be done, might please. The *musts* are warm-ups, calisthenics, stretch, and *some* endurance. You have already determined whether this is to be an all-out effort like a five-day workshop, or an hour a day. You know whether your MIP can get the hour all at once or piecemeal. Tomorrow you two will meet and both the dialogue and the action will begin, as will your records of improvement.

You the MIP should lay out your exercise clothes the night before, especially if it's Friday night and you intend a fitness weekend. Of course you the coach will see to it that you are busy all day Saturday and Sunday, but will give you the MIP "homework" for the other five days. Nothing should be haphazard, hit-or-miss. You are too important.

First Day at Your Self Center

Weigh in on your accurate scale and enter your weight on the weight chart you were given by the front office, where you the receptionist gave you the MIP your charts before you met yourself the certified Bonnie Prudden Myotherapist, who took your history (page 119). The psychologist who lives in your head gave you your stress test (page 290), and you have the results of that in your folder.

After breakfast, take your folder and meet you the coach, who will measure you and give you the minimum muscular fitness test and check your vital capacity with a tape measure (page 156).

You the MIP and you the coach will do the warm-ups together, some weight work, stair work and stretch *when you are very warm*. Everything will be recorded so you the coach can design the future program from how well or poorly you the MIP do on the first day.

You go through Volume I and do the walks on Volume II of *Keep Fit—Be Happy* and change to your warm-up suit and go for your walk. If the streets are out of bounds for any reason, do your walk up and down the hall. The air won't be fresh, but it won't be full of carbon monoxide, either.

If you are trying to lose weight, make out an eat sheet and list everything you put in your mouth. Don't let a slice of toast or a cracker go unnoticed and unrecorded.

Russia looks out for the Ivans who haven't time to go to the Black Sea. Those are moved out of their homes too, but just over to the other side of town. They leave the office every day at three and go for their programs. And they don't go back to the office until ten the next morning. That allows them at least five hours for workout, swim, massage, walk and some quiet. Can you scrape up that much time for your most important person? Don't tell me too many people depend on you. What would they do if you weren't there? Nobody is indispensable, not even you. *Except to your own world.* There you are indispensable and there would be no world without you.

Always keep in mind that in that world you are the *only* really important person and you deserve the very best that's available. Just what will be available depends on your government: you. Haven't you thought for years that an eighth-grader could do a better job of running the United States than almost anyone doing it? Well, here's your chance. How are *you* going to run *your* world? Parsimoniously? Wastefully? Or wisely and compassionately?

Moments You Will Never Miss

When you have to go upstairs for any reason, go twice and the second time use one of the stair exercises.

If the phone rings in the kitchen go upstairs to answer it.

Always do a chin-up or a let-*down* as you go through the doorway with the chinning bar. After chinning, do five deep knee bends holding onto your rope as you go *into* the room. As you leave, do ten abdominal strengtheners with the rubber straps. If you have a cranky back, *always* do the limbering series (page 185) before you get out of bed and before turning in at night.

Do *toe rises* at the sink while brushing teeth.

Half knee bends in the shower or while preparing a meal.

Pelvic tighteners at board meetings and anywhere else you *have* to sit or stand. See the limbering series.

Moments You Wouldn't Miss for Anything

Walking along trails in October.

Cross-country skiing in January.

Buying clothes two sizes slimmer.

Having people say, "What are you doing these days? You look great!"

Skin diving in the Caribbean.

Climbing Mount Washington in August.

Taking a bike trip through Ireland, a

pack trip in Wyoming, canoeing on the Allagash.

Having your kids look at you and say . . . "Wow!"

Some of you will have friends to do this with, but some others of you will have to go it alone. That's not easy, but it can be done and it always gets the wanted results. Just try to keep in mind: *I am the most important person in my world. I owe it to my world to be as healthy and fit as possible.* All Ivan has to concern himself with is a single country: Russia. You have a whole world.

Aging

Aging happens to everyone who manages to stay alive any length of time, and one of the problems that goes with it fits the song that goes:

And always remember, the longer you live, the sooner you're going to die.

It's a no-win situation, and hard enough to face when *you* are saying it to yourself. What is really irritating is when others start saying it by telling you to "slow down," "take it easy," "slack off," "act your age," and "be sure to check your insurance." Then you are faced with the disquieting suspicion that you may not have time to finish what you have started. When Katharine Hepburn was asked how she felt, she answered, "Fine, unless you ask for particulars." That's another aspect of getting older: small inconveniences like not being able to find your glasses without your glasses.

Aging is at best a nuisance, but it's not nearly as bad as adolescence. *Nothing* in life equals adolescence, even when everything else is great, which it never is. Adolescence is awful because you can't prepare for it. In your prepubescent ignorance you can't even imagine what it will be like. One day you are a kid, happy with your Girl Scout cookies and cookouts, and the next day you wouldn't be caught dead with either. You think you know what you *don't* want, but you haven't a clue as to what you do. You

have acne, menstrual cramps or "growing pains." You want to love somebody, but whom? Your teachers are dopes, your siblings "creeps" and your parents *embarrassing*. You know you'll die before the dance, and you'd just as soon nobody asks you or says no when *you* ask. Fortunately it only lasts a few endless years.

Aging is different. You *can* prepare for it, and you begin by accepting the fact that only you are responsible for you. The old saw about youth being wasted on the young isn't right. It isn't wasted. It's all the poor little things have. The individual who has chalked up fifty or sixty years has accumulated a lot of experience, know-how and, let's hope, common sense. The trick lies in using all three to keep the vintage body cared for, polished and going.

Not long ago during the question period after one of my lectures on fitness, a hand went up. It was a gentleman who ran ten miles a day and he'd been waiting all evening for a word that would tell him he was doing great things for himself. "I've listened for two hours and you never once mentioned the heart." True, I hadn't. For one thing I think there has been enough cardiovascular twaddle going around to last for years even if the heart wasn't mentioned in the next three. The whole evening, I'd been talking about the *body*, the one that carries the heart. What's the good of preserving the passenger if the coach is allowed to deteriorate to the point where it breaks down and rolls into the ditch? In these last years we haven't merely neglected the body while attending the heart, we have in many instances broken it.

Everybody ages all the time, and for the adolescent it's a good thing, too. Imagine being stuck in *that* age for a lifetime! Aging begins to work against you toward the midpoint, and that's when you ought to—*must*—take a hand. To prepare for aging, take stock now, right this minute. Ask yourself some very important questions which may *sound* like some you asked back in *Permanent Fix*, but they are different, because now you are asking from a different perspective, with the future rather than the past in mind. They are questions a lot of people don't want to ask, let alone answer. Do it anyway.

Stress History Number 2

STRESS QUESTIONS
1. What am I doing with my life?
2. Do I like what I'm doing?
3. Am I where I want to be?
4. If not, where *do* I want to be?
5. Am I with people I like?
6. If not, what kind of people *do* I like?
7. Is there something bothering me? A lot?
8. *Who* bothers me?
9. What would I change tomorrow?
10. What would I change if I didn't think it can't be changed?

THEN ON THE PHYSICAL
11. How old am I?
12. What do I weigh?
13. Using the measuring chart on page 131, add up my inches; what is the total?
14. What chronic pain do I have?
15. What intermittent pain do I have?
16. What is my general condition now?

17. If I go on as I am now, what can I expect to be like in ten years?
18. Should I change what I'm doing now with my life?
19. What should I change?
20. How could I go about it?

AND ON PLEASURE
21. What do I do for pleasure now?
22. What physical recreation do I enjoy?
23. What do I do for physical fitness, whether I enjoy it or not?
24. What would I do for physical fitness if I could?
25. What's stopping me?

Ten years ago there was a very definite ceiling on what older people could do, where they could go and what they could take up or slough off. The limiting factors were pain and infirmity. Since 95 percent of pain can be erased or controlled, one of those factors has disappeared. In the case of infirmity, once pain has been banished, many infirmities also can be taken care of. A still-limiting factor might not even have been recognized as such before, because pain and disability clamored for first attention. What still remains is to be found in the stress questionnaire.

Check your answers, and if you find a few negatives just set them aside for now, all but number ten. Write yourself a letter putting down all the ways you would change your life if you had a magic ring that made all things possible. Then put the letter away. Before you can change one thing you think impossible to alter, you must change or reinforce what *is* possible. Your physical self.

1. Your *age* can't be changed (except by waiting), nor can the way most people *see* age. In America there are only a few acceptable years. Roughly twenty. At the one end is miserable adolescence and at the other miserable senescence. Do you remember the shouted slogan of the sixties "Don't trust anyone over thirty"? How arrogant! And how amused I was

when the shouters approached and then passed that critical age and then approached and passed forty. No, you, as they, are stuck with the *age* you are, but you can maintain or attain the strength, flexibility and coordination that make up a youthful appearance. You can raise your level of energy to the one attributed to the young. You can protect yourself against the inroads made by neglect but attributed to aging.

2. What do I weigh? is a serious question. Weight does play a part in how you look, act and feel about yourself, and diet isn't enough. Check with the weight chart on page 130, Figure 21, and stick one just like it on your bathroom wall near the new scale you are going to buy. If you can swing it, get the latest: a digital scale. Accuracy is paramount. So is weighing in *daily*.

There are plenty of diets around, but don't go for a yo-yo diet. A yo-yo diet is one that promises you the moon and dishes up disappointment. *You* know what to eat and not to eat, but there's a good way to make both a diet and an exercise program work for you. A way in which *you* take responsibility and the credit. Knowing what you weigh and eat daily as well as just how many minutes you exercise will give you a baseline for a program.

Make yourself an eat sheet. Also list whatever you do for your exercise program. *What* you do is as important as how long it takes. Once a week, check your measurements.

If your inches diminish as your weight comes down, great, you're doing fine. If your inches diminish but your weight is stubborn, still great. Your exercise program is replacing fat with muscle. *But* if your weight and inches remain constant, you are eating too much and/or exercising too little. You can attack the problem one of two ways, or both. Look over the eat sheets and subtract one item, let's say bread. Just wipe it off the list and for the

present out of your life. Or you can up your exercise program. Let's say you add five flights of stairs a day. You need not do them all at once, but do them. Check your charts and see if you have made a starting dent. It is said, "Eat it today, wear it tomorrow," but I think that's too soon to get an accurate result. If you splurge, write in "splurge" on your chart and check for a week to see what happened.

3. About pain. There is enough information in this book to enable you to get rid of most pain—yours and that of your friends. Check with the section on disease and see what you can do about yours. Dis'-ease means lack of ease. It also means discomfort, and even a backache fits that description.

As to your general condition, it could take a full year to attain the level that satisfies you, and *then* you will be fit enough to change things, the things you wrote about in your letter. Get it out and choose one thing that needs to be different if you are to have less stress. Change it. You can now.

That may sound like a tall order, but it isn't. When you look in the mirror and see a strong, attractive body, know that others see the same thing. When you get up in the morning feeling fine and ready for whatever the day brings, others get that message. When you feel good about *you*, something happens *in* you and *to* others. You are the same person they've always known, and yet you aren't. When what you have always accepted becomes unacceptable and you set about changing things, there will be some unrest, but, for a wonder, it won't upset *you*. Not at all. And if someone you love is in trouble, you will be strong enough for two.

Start preparing for aging while it is still unthinkable, while you are young. Start building the strength you will need later on *before* accumulating years can undermine you. Start finding out now what it is you want from life while you still have leeway and could take a different path, career, partner or way of life if you were of a mind to do it. Old, old people become set in their ways because they have pain and they lack strength. You can't use that excuse, nor should you want to.

The Self-Image

The self-image is how you see yourself, accurate or not. The trouble is, we can't see what kind of habits we have laid on ourselves. Instead of trying to see yourself at first, look at everyone else around you. You will see a lot. Your friends who wear bifocals all of the time will approach the top of every staircase with hesitation. They will do the same at the curbstones. Use bifocals when you do handwork in front of TV or when you drive. In both instances you need to see near and far in quick succession. You don't need that when you are walking around the house or the streets. Bifocals make *anybody* move old. Watch.

Look at the shoulders of older people and see how they have rounded. Only you can stop yours with trigger-point work in the chest, *axilla*, arms and upper back and then the exercises.

Notice the walks of older people. They have shortened their steps because of trigger points in the hips, groin and legs. The spasms are in effect, not enough to cause more than a little ache from time to time, but enough to keep shortening steps and develop both a bad habit and a poor image. When you walk, swing right along, and if something hurts, fix it.

The safest exercise program I know is the one I put on the record *Keep Fit—Be Happy*, Volume I. On side one there are nineteen minutes of exercise, starting with an easy warm-up. Do the whole first band and then do *part* of each of the others until you come to the relaxation at the end. Do all of that. Each day, as you improve, do a little more. Check the *Self Center* section and see what parts of it would suit your living quarters and lifestyle. You don't have to go outside your own house to get fit, but it is more fun to work with company, so invite some friends to join you in your program. Test each other, take out each other's trigger points, encourage each other and admire each other's results.

When life in America was different and we were forced by circumstances to use our bodies in everyday labors, we didn't have to worry all that much about staying in shape. It wasn't even mentioned. We tend to ignore the things we have. Today in order to stay alive on the highways we drive defensively. To be physically fit, healthy and comfortable, we are going to have to *live* defensively, thinking about what we eat, drink or take for any reason. We are going to have to keep ourselves pain free, with good posture and a minimum of stress. If we don't take care of us, who will?

Disease

Disease isn't the end of the world. It happens all the time and to some of the nicest people. Once you're sure what it is you've got, ask yourself four questions:

1. What is the name of what I've got?
2. What does that mean to me now and in the future? The first answer you can judge for yourself, since you are suffering from it now. The second is only the doctor's guesswork, so don't settle for it unless it is positive. Keep in mind the prognosis I got: a limp, no sports . . . and no babies.
3. What part of me needs the most work?
4. How do I go about it? That answer is in this book.

First, no matter what the disease, you must keep moving, at least part of you. You must keep as many joints as possible going in full range of motion, and you must keep up your rhythm. The last problem is the easiest to solve. Get a tape player and the kind of music you like and move *something* to it as often as possible, even if it's only your eyes, one thumb and your big toe. Play music of various tempos, sometimes slow, sometimes fast—and sometimes discordant. Play some happy music, some dreamy and some sexy. Like life.

Next, you need to know what *you* can move and what needs passive exercise and the help of another person. See the double-bed exercise, in *Pain Erasure the Bonnie Prudden Way*. As your strength

improves, take over some of the passive exercise and be sure that *after warm-up* (you may need a heating pad for that), you let someone stretch you. If the muscles hurt, use trigger-point work. Intermittent exercise is better by far than a program delivered all at once as it is in hospitals via physiotherapy. Five minutes before your bath, five midmorning, five before lunch, five midafternoon, five before supper and five before bed will work miracles. First of all you won't get so *tired*. Lying in bed is *tiresome*. Not only that, but bed rest, no matter how necessary, starts calcium leaching out of your bones. You will need more calcium than you could drink if you owned a cow, so get the tablets made from oyster shells. I'm not vitamin-smart, but Dr. Travell is. She says bonemeal isn't a good idea, because it could have come from polluted sources. A horse accustomed to cropping grass along the highway and absorbing lead, for example. Dolomite, another source of calcium, also may come from polluted areas. Oysters are safest.

Moving is what keeps your circulation going, and bed rest is one of the things which, like trigger points causing spasm, slows you down. When you get your rehab in the morning for roughly half an hour, which is what we just suggested be spread over a whole day, you have to wait lying immobile for twenty-three and one half hours for another range-of-motion period. By that time the range may have shortened imperceptibly, and if you add days, weeks and often months together, that's a lot of shortening. You can't afford to lose any ground.

Stay out of bed as much as possible. You dare not get to like the ceiling. When I was strung up like a Christian on the rack for three months, I wept for a chance at the window, only half a room away. Nobody, including me, thought to move the bed over there, not because they didn't love me, but just because they'd never spent more than a day in bed, ever. So how could they know about the ceiling? As for me, I felt I was trouble enough without asking for favors. Get out even if all you can do is lie across the bed with your feet or knees on the floor. It's a different *feel*, it's a different view and your back is exposed. Wonderful, wonderful. Forget *effleurage massage*; that's a kind of gentle stroking that makes you want to scream, "Get at it or forget it." Have someone go after every trigger point they can reach and then do deep, kneading massage, not one that hurts but one that says to the newly relaxed muscles, "Don't you dare go back into spasm." Stretch whatever muscles you can.

When they get you up into a chair, don't settle for one, get three. One of them should be a rocker. The object is to make you use your muscles differently. Changing from one chair to another, lying across the bed prone, kneeling as you rest on it, rolling over on it, and all of these changes happening at regular intervals, will improve range of motion, circulation, and your point of view. There may be a certain amount of grumbling from those who have to do these things for you, but if you assure them that it will cut your inactive and nonproductive days short and get you back to whatever you want to do, sooner, they may take heart. At least *you* aren't grumbling. If they help you, you won't even feel like it.

Have a doorway gym built in your room (see *Self Center*, page 277).

In the section on pulleys (page 157), there is a great set of exercises for arms just in case your legs aren't working at the moment. You can use those while you are still in bed, as you can the weights (page 166).

Cerebral Palsy. There are diseases you can bring with you when you are born, or pick up on the way or as a result of accidents. A prime example is cerebral palsy. My first meeting with cerebral palsy was on our block when I was little. She sat all day in a wheelchair and had as much trouble with English as I was having trouble speaking German to my Fräulein. She had beautiful hair, I thought, pigeon toes and apparently a sore throat. Fräulein didn't understand a word she said, and I understood every one. That's the way most little children see people with a problem like that or advanced age unless someone tells them different.

My next meeting with someone with the disease was eight years ago. The young woman came to one of our five-day workshops and started in with the exercise program. Within two years she was so improved in strength, flexibility and coordination she could run as fast as anyone in the gym and was soon running the physical-fitness programs at the state school for the handicapped in Laconia, New Hampshire. She did wonderful things for the residents. Things no one ever thought could be done.

Then, two years ago, Corbett was brought to a one-day pain-erasure clinic in Minnesota. She was one year old and so still she was like a small mummy. In fifteen minutes we were able to give her parents an idea of Myotherapy, plus a map showing Corbett's trigger points and the exercises she would need. A year later her parents brought her all the way to Stockbridge. She had made wonderful progress and could now sit happily astride her mother's hip. But Corbett could still not stand alone, and when she did stand with help she was a tippy-toer. That means her heel cords were too tight to permit the foot to rest on the full sole. Her parents knew of another little toe-walking girl of the same age who had been operated on to lengthen the stretch at the back of her leg. After the operation, that child could not even stand up, let alone walk. When the same operation had been suggested for Corbett, her parents, having seen that sad example, came East to us instead. It took only half an hour to get Corbett's heels on the floor and teach the parents how to keep up the program. Corbett hadn't been able to use her hands; they were like stiff mittens. Another half hour and she would feed herself for the first time and even pick up an errant piece of spaghetti. With half an hour a day, within a week Corbett was a different little girl. Her parents went back to Chicago, sold their business and moved to Minneapolis to be near one of our certified Bonnie Prudden Myotherapists. Corbett continues to improve, loves her exercise and tolerates Myotherapy. Try to find Myotherapy *before* you cut. A cut muscle is rarely as good as a whole one.

Muscular Dystrophy. So far, our only experience with muscular dystrophy has been with profoundly affected children who have been so long in wheelchairs that their arms and legs are painfully bent. Both arms and legs responded well to Myotherapy and exercise, but the shortened muscles would have benefited far more if the work and exercise program had been begun at once, when the disease was discovered. The trigger points were numerous and sensitive at first, but less so as the circulation improved. If it can do nothing else, Myotherapy can prevent the aches and pains brought on by immobility.

There are cyclic diseases, such as rheumatoid arthritis, lupus erythematosus and multiple sclerosis, which go into "flare" and cause havoc with the organism. After doing all kinds of vandalism, they go into remission for longer or shorter intervals. Then begins the long, painful climb back to as near normalcy

as possible. During remission the patient can feel fine and wonder if perhaps he or she has escaped a terrible fate. Then, without warning, the vandal strikes again. The trouble with these diseases, aside from their debilitating effects, is the medication used to keep the person's pain within bearable limits. Sometimes their effects are worse than the disease, but the patient in agony has little choice. The trick to using them with a modicum of safety lies in the dosage. If nothing is done for the patient other than the medication, the dosage will rise until it reaches unacceptable levels, then another drug will be used, and so on ad infinitum, which isn't so far off. We have found that if Myotherapy is used with an exercise program, passive at first and then active, pain can be kept to a minimum during "flare" and away altogether during remission. This allows for a concentrated buildup of fitness in preparation for the next attack. Even then the patient can get away with far less medication, as is the case with insulin for diabetics. Exercise is the key, but if you can't move without groaning, exercise is out of reach. A *little* poison if it helps is acceptable when it makes the key aid possible.

Multiple Sclerosis is the disease with which we have had the most experience, and it responds beautifully to Myotherapy *if* it is used early on. When the patient is terminal, Myotherapy cannot do much beyond relieve pain, but in the early stages it helps with both weakness and balance. We have trained nine-year-old girls whose mothers have developed multiple sclerosis to work on them with Myotherapy. They have been able to keep their mothers on their feet and at work with neither pain nor lack of balance. And they have done it on two half hours a week.

Diabetes affects the feet and eyes when circulation is impaired. That can mean pain, ulcers and ultimately amputations. Blindness is a very real danger. Myotherapy can keep the spasms out of the muscles in the legs and around the eyes, face, head and neck. Exercise has proved very beneficial as long as it is not of the eye-bulging, face-purpling, breath-holding variety engaged in by the denizens of the weight-training emporia. Stick to sports like tennis, skiing, boating, hiking, rope and mini-tramp jumping, dancing, swimming and riding.

Hearts. It wasn't until the fifties that heart patients were given a new lease on life with exercise. Before that they were like today's Valium addicts: crippled by prescription. Bed rest was the only answer, and the injured heart became so flabby and weak that it fluttered at the slightest exertion, like that of a Victorian maiden when marriage was proposed. The men, told to "take it easy," did so in fear and trembling and destroyed their business lives, their home lives, their sex lives and their own lives.

True, you don't start your exercise program the day you pay your hospital bill, any more than you would start to exercise the day your baby was born. In both cases, you would wait a day!

Read the *Self Center* section and have your coach write up a ridiculously easy program . . . at least you the most important person would call it that. But you the coach, who have read the information through a coach's eyes, will say, "There, there, just humor me." Your coach may even let you do your one-minute program every half hour instead of every hour or two hours, depending on how weak you are. Use a timer so you don't miss the chance to exercise because you became interested in the newspaper. The news will keep. For the next few days listen to your heart and lungs. Notice what your legs are saying to you. *You* the coach will know when to up the program and what to add.

Less fatigue, increased circulation,

better balance, a better appetite, more interest in what goes on around you and a far more cheerful outlook are only a few of the pluses your exercise program will bring you. If your attack has left trigger points in your chest and upper back, get rid of them. The damaged heart lit up the trigger points in your chest muscles, and probably the attack added a few new ones. Get rid of the mechanism that could throw your chest muscles into spasm and possibly trigger some retaliation from the heart itself.

Get out of pajamas and into warm-ups as quickly as you can get to a phone and order them. Dressing gowns and slippers reek of invalidism, and that's bad for your self-image. You don't want to come out of this with a sinecure, you want to be back at the old stand, or a better one. Tan and fit (see *Self Center*) on your return to the office, you will confound the wolves gathering for the feast of your old job. *Never* advertise weakness, illness, inadequacy or fear. Your demeanor says instead: "Relax, fellows, the time is not yet, go back to your lairs." But while you are claiming to be master of your own ship, be master and not slave. Read over your own histories on the physical and on the stresses in this book, and ask yourself what your ticker was trying to tell you. Is it worth it? If not, forget victory over the wolves and get out while the going is good. You've been told the alternative. You may not be able to live as high off the hog as before, but is high off the hog really what you want? And is it worth open-heart surgery? That isn't known for increasing the life span, and it is painful and expensive. Plus there is that danger from the anesthesia. I've seen some of that when it went wrong, and *nothing* is worth brain damage.

What's to do? Build your self center, buy snappy walking shoes, get the trigger points out of chest, upper back, arms, neck, head, back, groin and legs. Your legs, when they are working, act as an auxiliary pump aiding the heart. You want all the help you can get from *healthy* legs. Spend a lot of time out of doors and on yourself, love some and laugh a lot. Enjoy your life, don't just live it. A heart attack can save your life if you're smart. Be smart!

Cancer is the scare word of our time and often lives up to its reputation. Whatever its duration, short, long or terminal, its very presence is stressful. Muscle pain accompanies many types of cancer, and chemotherapy plus the medication given to allay pain and anxiety compound the pain and misery. Myotherapy helps both the pain and the edema, and exercise, whether passive or active, can be of enormous help, especially for the bedridden.

Spondorondos. Spondo comes from the Greek word *spondylos*, meaning spine, and rondo, or rondeau, is a musical composition having a refrain that occurs at least three times in its original key. So when I say "spondorondo," I refer to backache of any kind except that caused by fracture, tumor or other anatomic pathology. The rondo part of the word refers to the rounds we embark on when first we begin with back pain. It is the rare sufferer who sees less than the required three repetitions of the original refrain, number one, the general practitioner or an internist, number two, his friend the orthopedist, and number three, the neurologist. The plural refers to the second round, the psychologist or psychiatrist, the osteopath and finally the chiropractor. From the thousands of letters I received after my first book on pain came out, four years ago, I learned that millions of others have equaled my own odyssey in frustration, additional pain and lack of success in the search for help. What was left for me was injections until we found Myotherapy. Now we find that, of all the pains reported by suffering humanity, back pain is the easiest to fix with Myotherapy and keep away with exercise.

What do you need? A friend or a bodo. What must you do? Check with your histories and get rid of your trigger points. That must be followed for the rest of your life with the limbering series, page 185 and with the exercise for back and hamstring flexibility, page 221, in *Sports*. In addition, there must be a "sports program" and you can make a "sport" out of chair exercises if you are very elderly (see *Pain Erasure: The Bonnie Prudden Way*) or a stair climb if less so. Your weights can weigh half a pound and still be of value. Your walk can start to the bathroom. That's already a great big plus. It can continue on to the kitchen. Now you are beginning to take control of your life. A little more every day, once your trigger points have been cleared and the stretch exercises begun. Do not be taken in by the additions made to spondo. Itis, schmitis, unless there is pathology, it's just a backache.

Disease usually comes in on little cat feet, softly, silently until a claw comes out and we are aware of something wrong. Then we discover that disease is not a little cat; it very often turns into a huge, fiery dragon and you have two choices: slay it or succumb to it. Of course you might ride on it for a long time, unable to either ride comfortably or get off, but that requires enormous effort, concentration and perseverance.

While you are engaged in enduring, everyone else goes on without you. The best course is to steer clear of dragons entirely by staying as fit as possible, paying attention to what goes into your body and setting a watch on just how much you use that body without thought to rest and recreation. If you do have the misfortune to fall ill, try Myotherapy for pain, exercise for maintenance and a daily dose of outdoors, fun and laughter. Are you where you want to be? Are you with the people who please you and like you too? If not, why don't you get fit and then *do* something about it?

Posture

Your posture is as personal to you as your fingerprints. It is as recognizable to others as your ID card, your Social Security number or your passport. It is every bit as revealing as a candid camera shot. It also exposes what you are like *inside* and what is going on *inside*. And just as your life changes from day to day, so does your posture. If most of what happens to you is good for you, your posture will say so. However, if you become ill or emotionally overstressed, you will wear the information for all to see, with your posture.

Posture is described in the dictionary as "being a position or attitude of the body or bodily parts." Posture begins to take shape in the womb, and as the fetus grows in that confined space, it makes its first acquaintance with the three major postural faults suffered by humankind: round back, soft abdominals and inflexibility of the hamstrings. If Mama, the hostess, doesn't know much about nutrition, or smokes, or lives in close association with drugs (*any* drugs) or alcohol, the fetus's posture may suffer because of the poor nutrition or the pollution. From the moment of birth, depending on where the stork or Easter Bunny has dropped you, posture can improve or go off in any of a dozen other directions, none of them good.

If you land in a *relaxed*, welcoming household in which healthy people care about babies *and* themselves, you too will be relaxed and usually healthy and certainly cared for. If the household is tense, you will have "known" it since conception. You too will be tense, and it will show on your natal day. Healthy, relaxed babies are very different from the other kind, and you can see it in the hospital nurseries. Later, tense children develop a kind of "turtle back" stance, which is evidenced by raised and rounded shoulders and a shrinking into them by the head and neck. This is a kind of armored protection against physical abuse, verbal abuse or the tension that may exist where frustration, anger and hatred hold sway, but where no one ever gives an outward sign of the roiling within. Armoring when donned for protection is one thing, while armoring manufactured by the body itself in the form of tight muscles is another. You can remove and abandon the first, but you *live* in the second. Getting rid of such armoring takes know-how and work plus understanding as to the cause. One can rebuild and reshape a child's posture *only* if the builder understands what is at the bottom of the anomaly and is in a position to help. An hour or two a week of exercise, even several hours, can never offset twenty-four hours a day of sorrow, fear and often physical battering.

Since posture problems begin early, they show up early if the observer is aware of what to look for and what various signs mean. The best time to take care of them is early, while the muscles are pliable and the bones easily influenced. If you wait too long (and the teens are close to too long), you will find that the muscles under tension have shortened, have become very inflexible and are housing a raft of trigger points. We are now seeing little people, only six and seven, who cannot bring their fingertips within nine inches of the floor in the Kraus-Weber minimum muscular fitness test, and they are only forty inches tall themselves. If you or your child fails the flexibility test, you or he or she will in all probability develop poor posture or suffer with back pain. If the abdominals are weak, pain is almost a certainty.

Flat Back. In this condition the whole spine is flattened by inadequate curves. Looking at people with *flat backs* from the rear you will see that both pants and skirts seem to be painted on a stiff sheet of cardboard.

Round Back, or Round Shoulders are so named because that's what they look like. In extreme form, the condition is called *kyphosis* and is an abnormal rearward curvature of the spine. The cause of a rounding back is usually tight *pectoral* muscles, in the chest. There are often very tight arm muscles and trigger points in both arms and chest and in the *axilla*. The upper back is often weak and overstretched.

Scoliosis is an abnormal lateral curve, or series of compensating lateral curves, of the spine (page 167).

Lordosis, commonly called "swayback," is an excessive inward or downward curve of the spine. It *usually* makes its appearance at puberty but can be seen earlier if the watcher has a discerning eye and concern for the child. It *usually* "sets" at around seventeen, and the curve does not increase. To find out if you or someone else has one, use the test on page 183.

Those are only the four horsemen of posture. There are dozens of other posture anomalies. Best known are *pigeon toes*, in which the toes turn in, usually because of trigger points on the inner sides of the legs and in the hips. The *turned-out walk*, in which the feet would point to ten past ten on a clock dial, are usually due to trigger points on the outsides of the legs, in the outside line of the pelvis (circles 4, 5 and 6 on Figure 10, page 91), and in both *gluteals* and groin. The *forward head* accompanies a round back, and with *scoliosis*, there are *uneven hips and shoulders. Uneven skeletal development, knock knees, wry neck, flat feet* and the "hurry syndrome" are all posture problems; most of them influence and abet each other to the detriment of the host or hostess.

All posture problems involve muscles and bones, but since bones don't go anywhere on their own, what must we blame? Muscles and nerves. Occasionally there is an interruption in the communication somewhere along the nerve pathways as in paralysis, but such cases are very few compared to the population as a whole. Most of us have the other kind of problem: poor posture due to muscle damage, massive or micro. Muscle damage is also due to psychic damage, the kind that pulls shoulders into a protecting shell that cannot really protect but can cause very real injury of its own.

Habit is often an enemy of the people. Take something as simple and seemingly necessary as bifocal lenses. Watch people who wear them all of the time when they step off curbs or down a stair. The head tips down and the chin pulls in. The trigger points will be all through the neck, the upper back, face and jaw.

The *forward head* is developed when the person with the round back tries to look straight ahead. Since the cervical spine is a continuation of the rounding thoracic spine, the rounding should continue, but then vision is impaired so the round-backed person raises his face to improve sight. This severely strains the back of the neck, the upper back and the jaw, and trigger points will abound in all those places.

Trigger points in one area can produce posture problems in others. The "hurry syndrome," in which the person leans forward as though he or she were constantly pushing into a high wind, is an example. The trigger points are usually to be found in groin, *quadricepses*, *psoai* and *abdominals*. As with flat back, few people would say, "So-and-so has a posture problem"; even fewer would say, "Groin pull is causing that tiring lean." When the person with the anomaly has it long enough, groin pain may develop, or what feels like a spastic colon. Trouble may come in the form of menstrual cramps, constipation, or even diarrhea. Keep in mind that when there are trigger points in the front, its opposite, the back, will house them too.

Injuries can contribute to posture anomalies, and the whiplash of the vulnerable neck is one with almost universal examples. Almost everyone snaps the neck at some time or another, resulting in pain and stiffness. When conventional healing is used, it may take forever to get better. Counterirritants, which heat the area; traction, which stretches it; collars to hold the head in place; and analgesics—none of these gets at the cause: trigger points in the neck, head, face, chest, upper back and arms. If the sufferer already has a *forward head*, so much the worse. The neck was already stressed and injured and cannot be brought back to health until the round back has been improved.

A bent arm causes special problems in addition to its own limitation. A bent arm isn't a good arm, and when possible should be straightened. Many people who have suffered strokes have paralyzed arms and arms that are spastic. The bent and paralyzed appendage swinging unbidden at half mast across the chest wreaks havoc with the self-image. In time the muscles shorten irreparably, and even if the cause is removed and the arm regains its ability to move as directed, it will not be able to straighten. Start in the *axilla*, chest and upper back *before* checking out the arm and hand.

A short leg is indeed a posture problem, but just how short is short? Many people have sides that don't match, but a good many more have sides that would match perfectly. Consider this. After my second hip was replaced, the affected leg was a full inch longer than the other. My back often felt as though there were a steel rod in it somewhere, and I developed the "hurry syndrome." After two years I had a most fortunate "accident." I leaned forward at an awkward angle to pick up a piece of Kleenex from the floor, tripped, lost my balance and fell forward. Long years of gymnastic practice threw me instinctively into a forward shoulder roll like the ones you see on football fields. I had thought I couldn't do that anymore, but it turned out I could. When I stood up, my legs were even and I could stand straight *without effort*. Why had I not found the restricting band of muscle? I was looking in the wrong place. Since I was being pulled forward, I'd been hunting in the groin and abdominals and lower back. Mid and upper back did not come into it, I thought. After all, it was hip that had caused the problem. Pay careful attention in *Quick Fix* and *Permanent Fix* to the zones and how they affect each other. Don't do as I had done, be taken in by cause rather than relations. Before you allow your mind to think, "Put a lift in the shoe," think trigger points and make your search a real dragnet.

Kyphosis, *scoliosis*, *lordosis* and flat

back are all caused by misbehaving muscles, and muscles are like misbehaving children. Most of the time, there's a reason. They can be overtired, overstressed, or overwhelmed by changes such as beginnings or endings. The ending of a love affair can make kids (and adults) act in very strange ways. It can also cause backache and tension headaches. The beginning of a new job can tighten muscles to the screaming point, and it can also turn even a grown man into a nervous wreck until he gets the hang of it. Nursery school for little kids is sometimes so traumatic they vomit and wet their pants. Not exactly misbehavior, but not something you want to clean up, either. Changes are good for many kinds of "misbehavior": "I don't want to move to Cincinnati. I'll divorce you first." But it turns out to be perfect. "I'll never leave my school and my friends; I'll run away first." He does run away, overnight, finds out it's scary out there, and his new school turns out to be exactly what the old one was, only better. Change from a desk job to a field job and see what that kind of change does for your leg, foot and back muscles . . . and your sex life.

Bad beginnings also come along with breasts or beatings. One blossoming pubescent girl lifts her chest, presses back her shoulders and presents her lovely changes to the world. A second, for whatever reason, folds her arms across her chest to hide what she thinks of as her ridiculous growths. The first stands well, looks well and feels well. The other is negative all the way and ends up with the habit of hiding behind crossed arms, causing a round back, forward head, shortened chest muscles and a protruding abdomen. After a while the offending breasts will droop to her waist and she'll have another problem.

The battered child begins a guarding posture early on and develops a "cringe." Sometimes the beaten child takes the opposite stance, chest out, fists balled and a look that says, "I can and

will lick anybody." His and her unfortunate predicament is that they become a little schizy, taking out terrible fear and anxiety on peers by doing battle on any and all occasions. Then, in the presence of their tormentors, their bodies retreat behind the guarding. This posture is then donned in the presence of all adults and later of all people with authority. Their muscles reflect their uncertainty with unpredictable movement patterns.

Anger, hatred, frustration, fury, sorrow, dejection, rejection (even the fear of it) show through posture, the body's language. Joy, exhilaration, excitement, sexual tension and expectation show through posture. You have often heard the expression "All the world loves a lover." How do you suppose all the world knows who's a lover and who isn't? The news is in the walk, in the lifted head, in the arm and shoulder swing. It's in every move, and it's catching. One doesn't have to love some special person; loving life is enough. Enough isn't the right word. A better one would be "heavenly."

Then there is the opposite of loving life: the blue funk. How do we know who are in a blue funk? We know by the way they sit, stand and carry themselves. They don't have to say a single word, but virtually everyone knows they are the ones to avoid.

I used to phone a man I knew just to hear him say, "Hello." It was a warm and welcoming sound, which at the time I needed badly. There are houses I like to visit as much for the ambience as for the joyous greetings. There are people I can't bear to call on the phone and houses I wouldn't enter if I were caught out in a blizzard in my pajamas. Madison Avenue has nothing on us when it comes to advertising. Watch your own posture for a while.

Feet are funny, especially *flat feet*, which paddle, rather than walk. They often turn outward, and the prints they leave in the sand resemble those of Bigfoot's baby. I've never seen a flat foot grow an arch, but if you strengthen the *anterior tibialis* with the wolf-in-the-garden exercise, below, and the stair exercises in *Self Center*, those feet will serve you well. For the turnout, look for trigger points on the outsides of the legs and in the *gluteals*.

The turnout is also called the "duck walk"; it produces a rather pompous waddle. It often accompanies a sway-back. It could be *caused* by a swayback, but on the other hand it could *cause* a swayback. One cannot afford to ignore one problem in favor of another. Fail to fix both and both problems will return.

Slumping in a chair is often frowned upon, but why shouldn't you slump if you are in a slump chair? A straight-backed chair would make a slump inappropriate, so the real question is, Can you sit comfortably in a straight-backed chair with your back straight? If you can't, you need to work on pelvic tilts to loosen your groin and dead lifts to strengthen the upper back.

When you see a child beginning to develop knock knees or bowed legs, your first thought should be about diet and weight. Then comes the trigger-point hunt. For knock knees, the outsides of the legs and pelvis should be checked for trigger points causing *weakness*, the insides for trigger points causing spasm strong enough to pull bones out of line. Be sure to clear the feet and the groin and *gluteals*. For bowed legs, the opposite. Then the exercise program: stairs, stairs, stairs and more stairs and deep knee bends.

Babyhood is the time to start worrying about legs and feet. They form the base for successful childhood work, which is play. A child cannot build good legs without exercise of every kind, climbing and descending hills, climbing up and down rock, walking on fences, stealing bases, shinnying up trees, wading in stony brooks, riding bikes, roller skating, ice skating, skiing and sliding, running,

jumping and rolling down sand dunes. It starts with "Come, take my hand and we'll go for a walk." It moves up through "Here, I'll time you while you run all the way around the house," "Last one to the house is a rotten egg," to "Anyone for a run on the golf course this morning?" If you try to begin with the last, you will be in for a disappointment: "Naw, I gotta see 'Star Trek.'"

If your child's feet do "funny" things, fix them. If he tiptoes when barefoot, look for the trigger points in the calves and the backs of the thighs. If he turns in or has flat feet, do wolf in the garden: Have the child sit in a deep, comfortable chair holding onto the arms. Have him turn his toes inward until they touch to form the closed garden gate. Put your fist inside the gate because you are the wolf who is not to be let out. Pull with just enough force to make the little legs work keeping you inside. Hold your pull for a few seconds and then relax. Do this five or six times each day until the child is strong enough to keep the gate shut as you pull him around the kitchen floor.

The Kraus-Weber minimum muscular fitness test (page 131) is an absolute must. Bring the children to passing with the correctives provided. Kids copy everything you do and everything you say, even the way you say it. If a neighbor's kid whines, listen to its mother. If that kid clobbers your kid for no reason, wonder who clobbers whom in that house. If your kid clobbers, also without cause, wonder about you. There is a cause somewhere. If the bad behavior is really just due to a lousy disposition (some kids are born on the wrong side of the delivery table), discipline and constancy are your only hope. Swatting is no answer; constancy is. Even a mean horse can be controlled, but not by a confused rider.

You'll never know how you walk, sit or stand unless someone tells you or you see it yourself on film. If a friend tells you, "You walk like a football player," that's a tactless way of saying that you walk like your older brother. Why shouldn't you? You adored him. "You mince" is a way of saying you take tight, careful, overcontrolled steps. Get into a modern-dance class or a good exercise class (not at the spas and not "aerobics"). Or you can do it for yourself with Volume II of the record *Keep Fit—Be Happy after* you find Volume I easy. "You walk with a waddle" (there *are* people who would say that just that way). Check to see if you walk on two parallel lines that are several inches apart. Seek trigger points in hips, groin and outsides of the legs. Lay down a line of tape somewhere and walk its length, often crossing each foot over to the other side of the line to pull the feet closer together. If you or the child has duck feet (toes turned out), do the cross with the toes turned in. For pigeon toes, the same walk but with the toes turned way out.

When someone says, "You run like a girl," that's awful, even for a girl! It means you flip your feet out as your legs come forward. There may be trigger points anywhere, but especially in the outside of the lower leg, the *extensor digitorum longus* and the *peroneus longus*. Do also the outside of the upper leg, the *vastus lateralis* and the *iliotibial tract*. Include circles 4, 5 and 6, on the pelvis (Fig. 10, page 91), and circles 1, 2 and 3, in the *gluteals* (Fig. 9, page 181).

If you can find someone to videotape your standing, sitting, walking and running posture *before* you start your program, you will be able to note your progress with your eyes as well as how you feel. Be honest when you are taped. Don't try to be right. How do you know what is *right*, anyway? Some folks' *right* turns out to be stiff. If checking is easy because the equipment is available, do so monthly. If checking is difficult or expensive, try for quarterly. You will be delightfully surprised *if* you work at it, and you will quietly cause a sensation.

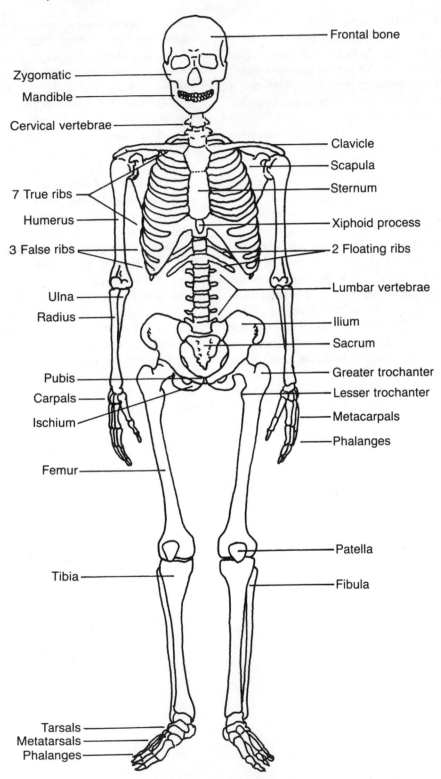

Frontal bone

Zygomatic

Mandible

Cervical vertebrae

Clavicle

Scapula

7 True ribs

Sternum

Humerus

Xiphoid process

3 False ribs

2 Floating ribs

Ulna

Lumbar vertebrae

Radius

Ilium

Sacrum

Pubis

Greater trochanter

Carpals

Lesser trochanter

Ischium

Metacarpals

Phalanges

Femur

Patella

Tibia

Fibula

Tarsals
Metatarsals
Phalanges

FIG. 59: FRONT VIEW

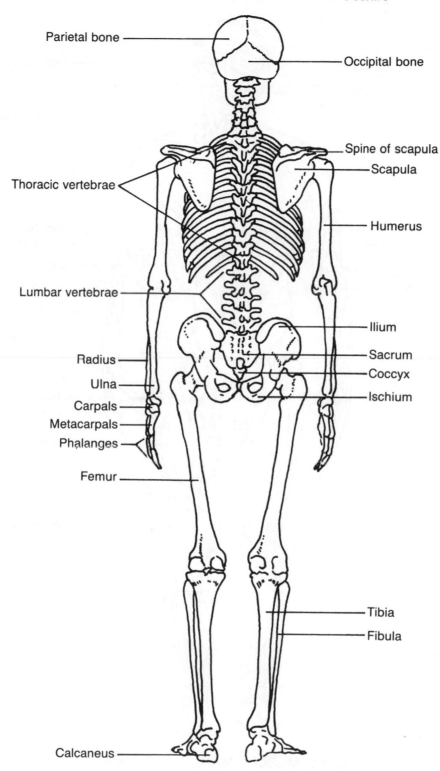

FIG. 60: SKELETON, BACK VIEW

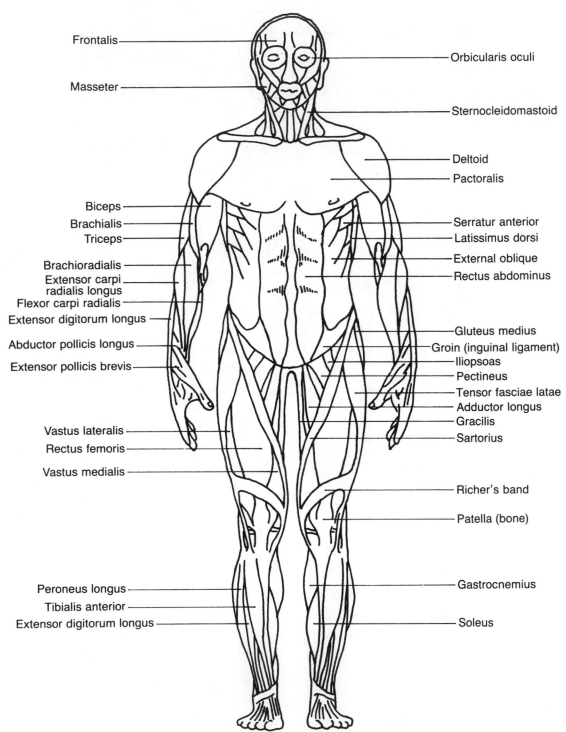

Frontalis

Orbicularis oculi

Masseter

Sternocleidomastoid

Deltoid

Pactoralis

Biceps

Brachialis

Triceps

Serratur anterior

Latissimus dorsi

External oblique

Rectus abdominus

Brachioradialis

Extensor carpi
radialis longus

Flexor carpi radialis

Extensor digitorum longus

Gluteus medius

Abductor pollicis longus

Groin (inguinal ligament)

Iliopsoas

Extensor pollicis brevis

Pectineus

Tensor fasciae latae

Adductor longus

Gracilis

Vastus lateralis

Sartorius

Rectus femoris

Vastus medialis

Richer's band

Patella (bone)

Peroneus longus

Gastrocnemius

Tibialis anterior

Extensor digitorum longus

Soleus

FIG. 61: MUSCLE MAN, FRONT VIEW

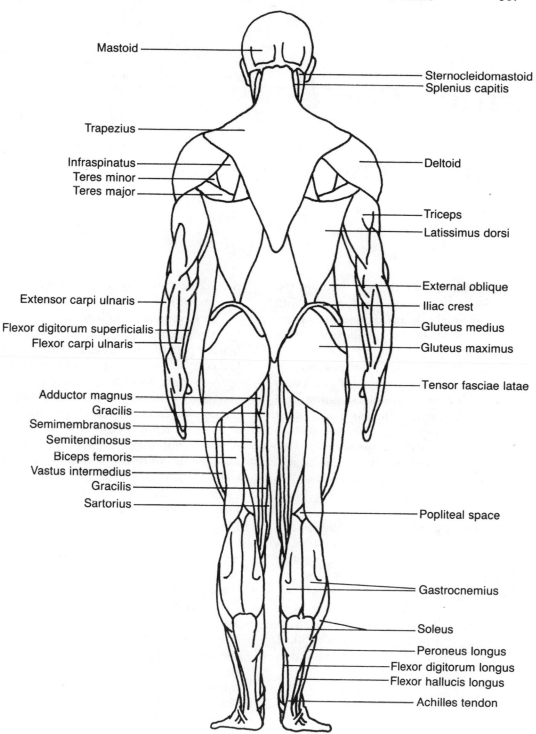

Mastoid

Sternocleidomastoid
Splenius capitis

Trapezius

Infraspinatus
Teres minor
Teres major

Deltoid

Triceps
Latissimus dorsi

Extensor carpi ulnaris

External oblique
Iliac crest

Flexor digitorum superficialis
Flexor carpi ulnaris

Gluteus medius
Gluteus maximus

Tensor fasciae latae

Adductor magnus
Gracilis
Semimembranosus
Semitendinosus
Biceps femoris
Vastus intermedius
Gracilis
Sartorius

Popliteal space

Gastrocnemius

Soleus

Peroneus longus
Flexor digitorum longus
Flexor hallucis longus
Achilles tendon

FIG. 62: MUSCLE MAN, BACK VIEW

Afterword

by Desmond Tivy, M.B., B.S.
University of London

The subject of Myotherapy involves the interaction of structure and function, with a strong emphasis on function; thus inevitably it involves the complexities of an incompletely understood cybernetic[1] system. The past history of comparable therapies has been one of semantic obfuscation and misunderstanding, and there is danger that the same will occur with this therapy. The feedback portion of the cybernetic loop involves the kinesthetic[2] sense; therefore mere words, unless wielded by a poet, cannot suffice to promote comprehension—but I will try!

Essentially, Myotherapy relieves certain disorders of musculoskeletal (strictly neuromuscular) function, and cannot influence structure. It can, predictably, relieve trigger points, which are the basis of the fibrositic (or fibromyalgia) syndrome. The hypothesis behind the fibrositic syndrome is that areas of localized dystonia[3] develop, on a multifactorial basis, throwing the neurovascular system "off balance," so to speak.

The fibromyalgia syndrome has been well documented and delineated, with the familiar patterns of pain and stiffness, and less consistently, of depression, and subjective symptoms of temperature changes and/or numbness. Among the multiple factors that can precipitate it are personality, disordered sleep patterns, occupation, hobbies, injuries, posture, weather and so forth. It would seem that trigger points are probably a lot commoner than we have realized and are by no means confined to full-blown cases of fibrositis.

Myotherapy involves (1) temporary erasure (using cold and local pressure) of whatever neuromuscular circuitry causes a trigger point, and (2) reprogramming said circuitry[4] with stretching exercises. Faith, enthusiasm, hope, etc., are all helpful adjuncts and motivators to the therapy (as in *all* therapies but are more important in the treatment of trigger points than, say, appendicitis, since a sense of well-being favorably affects muscle tone and because the treatment is done more *by* the patient than *for* him).

---

[1]Cybernetic = pertaining to control systems.

[2]Kinesthetic = pertaining to the feeling or sensation of movement.

[3]Dystonia = improper or painful tone. A paradox in the dystonia theory can be overcome if the "tone" part of "dystonia" is thought of as "tension," thus allowing the presence of trigger points in tendinous, fascial and aponeurotic tissue, which, being noncontractile, cannot strictly have tone. But local tension in the mechanical sense should not be confused with the generalized "tension" seen in a "tense" person (though the two often coexist).

[4]"Said circuitry" probably involves the "gate," and probably involves endorphins (at what may be a general as well as a local level), and almost certainly involves sympathetic pathways (including vasomotor ones) at the spinal level.

Other ways (manipulation, injections, acupuncture, TENS, vibration, biofeedback, etc.) have been used successfully by others for trigger-point erasure, whereas Myotherapy uses pressure, which has high convenience and availability and low side effect and cost compared with most other methods—in a word its merit is simplicity. But such simplicity can also be a demerit if it leads a patient to suppose that short cuts in the treatment will give the same results.

Other ways have also been used for reprogramming after pain alleviation, ways that attempt, as does Myotherapy, to teach the system how to "balance" itself—i.e., restore proper local, as well as general, muscle tone. It is my impression that the exercises used in Myotherapy clinics are more effective than others I have come across. Whether the patient is sufficiently motivated to do them is another matter!

Reprogramming (learning) proper muscle tone and balance (defined as that which promotes a pain-free existence) can seemingly be achieved in three possible ways, alone or in combination: (1) avoidance of pain-producing postures and movements; (2) strengthening of muscles that allow pain because they are weak; and (3) muscle-efficiency promotion by relief of trigger points contained therein, with subsequent muscle stretching. It is this third method that is used in Myotherapy, although the patient may, coincidentally or unconsciously, use a certain amount of the other two methods as well.

Bonnie Prudden rediscovered and developed and has promoted this therapy, using nonoriginal techniques in an original way. To my mind, her key contribution has been the discovery of many more places in which to look for trigger points than have hitherto been noted—places that if left untouched preclude the sought-after erasure of pain. That such a multitude of places exists is hardly to be wondered at if one reflects on the total functional interconnection of our neuromuscular cybernetic system. Which is not to say that all trigger points are of equal practical importance: some can be ignored; others are effect, not cause.

The side effects of Myotherapy are noted in the Afterword that I contributed to Bonnie Prudden's *Pain Erasure*[5] and also are included in the text of the present work. I can think of few therapeutic modalities at my command with fewer side effects than those of Myotherapy.

Who might try Myotherapy?

a) Those whose head, neck, torso, or limb pain does not seem to have a direct structural origin. The implication that the problem is functional may be derived from the history, or from the absence of objective physical findings.

b) Those whose structural problems, such as arthritis, have been controlled physically (e.g., by medication) as well as possible but who continue to have pain for reasons that may be functional.

c) Those with probable structural problems such as suspected lumbar disk prolapse that may be potentially treatable by surgery, to whom the patient or physician exhibits reluctance to embark on an irreversible procedure in a less than ideal setting. (Should Myotherapy happen to work, surgery will have been avoided. Should Myotherapy fail, the lack of side effects ensures that little has been lost: indeed, resolve toward surgery has now been strengthened, which may be for the better.)

d) Those with unknown diagnosis but whose bias against medical diagnostic workup (for any number of good or bad reasons) precludes such workup. (The same comments apply here as in c): for "surgery," read "workup.")

[5]Evans, 1980 (hardcover); Ballantine, 1982 (paperback).

Who should *not* try Myotherapy?

a) Those whose problems are better treated by medication or by correction of anatomic fault.

b) The poor. (Myotherapy is not inexpensive and is often not covered by insurance.)

c) The unmotivated. (Myotherapy requires patient cooperation and effort. And, probably, also understanding.)

d) The anticoagulated. (Myotherapy may cause bruising to unacceptable, though probably not dangerous, degree.)

The key to *treating* trigger-point syndromes is the ability to visualize them anatomically. But the key to *understanding* them is the ability to conceptualize them functionally. The function of muscle, whether eufunctional or dysfunctional, seldom has much to do with the muscle itself: rather, it concerns its environment, and in particular its neural connections that allow robotic control to occur. Though any part of the cybernetic loop can misfire, it is the whole series of interconnecting loops that may be conceptualized at any one moment: for, like a chain, it works or fails as a whole, while dependent on the integrity of its component links.

It is the interconnections, both near and distant, that help explain the characteristics of fibrositic syndromes; and especially explain the reasons for the successes and failures of various treatments that have been used for their correction—in particular, the connection to "memory." Since all habituated muscle movements are memorized, whether those of speech or walking or whatever learned physical skill, then it follows that muscle tension (or its consequence, fascial tension), whether local or general, can be a response to either a *present* sensory input or a *past* one. Thus a muscle contracts when stimulated; withdrawal of the stimulus allows relaxation again; repetitive stimuli can produce a persistent muscle contraction due to conditioning. Subsequent muscle relaxation may require an erasure procedure to "clear the circuit" and also will require a subsequent ambience that does not retrigger the memory.

It is when one thinks this way that it becomes quite clear why psychological factors are so important in all syndromes in which function is at least as important as structure. And it is quite clear why slow, persistent reeducational techniques are so vital to success and why therapies that treat only one part of the system tend to fail, compared with those that deal with wider areas or with more "links in the chain." Thus psychotherapy, while often helpful, is too limited an approach to be the sole one, or even the best one. And thus pain erasure by, say, manipulation, is often useless unless reeducative steps are taken. And thus injections to localized areas in, say, the back, may fail unless treatment is also directed to, perhaps, the neck or the legs.

I find that computer programmers and electrical engineers understand neuromuscular function better than most; it is so close to the subject of their work that it seems intellectually self-evident to them. And I find that musicians, dancers and athletes also understand neuromuscular function—not intellectually (visually), but because they "feel" it (kinesthetically). But alas, the man in the street hasn't a clue about function: all he thinks about is structure; when something hurts, it "has to be" due to a structural failure of some kind. Unfortunately his doctor may well think this way too, especially if he is a surgeon. One way to start to enlighten the structural purists is to liken pain to a shudderingly off-tune note on the violin: we are all agreed that the violin may be defective, but we all know that it is infinitely more probable that it is the violinist who is at fault and that he must learn to play in tune. And of course, quite often, the problem lies in both structure and function at the same time: what you do to correct it will depend on 1) how good you are at diagnosing the problem, 2) how good you are at treating what you have diagnosed, and 3) what particular mix of faulty structure and function exists in the case.

As with other therapies, there is no need to use Myotherapy exclusive of other approaches: for instance, in its use together with medication, one can complement the other; or its use postsurgery can facilitate return to function. In particular, in the common case in which pain is of both structural *and* functional origin, it may be vital to treat both causes either sequentially or simultaneously. It should be noted, however, that where it is a matter of trying (for want of objective precision) surgery first and Myotherapy second, or in the reverse order, it is a lot safer, cheaper, and less irreversible to try Myotherapy first!

Occasionally what seems structural may have a basis in function; for instance, surgical procedures exist to divide certain fibrous or muscular bands that are entrapping or otherwise mechanically interfering with nerve function. It is theoretically possible for Myotherapy, by releasing tension in said bands, to allow relaxation of function. In such cases, assuming success with both approaches (surgery and Myotherapy) it becomes a matter of patient-physician judgment as to which is the *simpler* approach: pressure is quick and easy for temporary erasure, but reeducation may be long and arduous for permanent control.

And occasionally what may at first *seem* an internal medical or surgical problem (such as pain in the gallbladder area or pain in the rectum) turns out to be an external problem in the surface musculature. Hence occasional control of unlikely diseases by Myotherapy—because the diagnosis was spurious!

With the exception of a small group of certified Bonnie Prudden Myotherapists personally trained and certified by Bonnie, all certified Bonnie Prudden Myotherapists are graduated from the Bonnie Prudden School of Physical Fitness and Myotherapy. Certified Bonnie Prudden Myotherapists are now certified by the International Myotherapy Association. One thousand three hundred hours of training are required for graduation, and forty-five hours of update every two years for recertification. They are competent in the uncovering and therapy of trigger points. They do not diagnose, which is why they will accept only patients referred by physicians or dentists. The requirement of the referring doctor is not so much that he *approve* the referral (for how can he approve the relatively unknown, and that untested by controlled trials?) but that he not *disapprove* the referral on grounds that more orthodox treatment is predictably, and more urgently, indicated.

August 1983
Lee, Massachusetts

Glossary of Terms

ABDUCT (L. *ab* + *ducere*). To draw away from the median plane.

ACRO'MION (Gr. *akromion*, from *akros*, extreme + *omion*, dim. of *omos*, shoulder). The lateral extension of the spine of the *scapula*, projecting over the shoulder joint and forming the highest point on the shoulder; called also the *acromial process* and the *acromion scapulae*.

AC'UPUNCTURE. The Chinese practice of piercing specific peripheral nerves with needles to relieve discomfort associated with painful disorders.

AD (L., to). A prefix expressing to or toward, addition to, nearness or intensification.

ADDUCT' (L. *adducere*, to draw toward). To draw toward the median plane.

ADRE'NAL (L. *ad*, to or toward or near to, + *renes*, kidneys). The adrenal glands, near the kidneys, play a large role in stress.

AG'ONIST (Gr. *agonistēs*, combatant). A muscle that contracts and is opposed by contraction in another muscle, the antagonist.

ALBEO, -ERE (L., to be white). Albumen, the white of an egg; *linea alba*, white line.

ALEXANDER TECHNIQUE. A technique, concerned with improving posture, devised by a Shakespearean actor, F. M. Alexander. The idea is that postural habits are learned and the uneconomical ones can be unlearned.

ALGESIS (Gr., pain). Algesireceptors are nerves that sense pain. An analgesic is the medication recommended for pain.

ALVEOLUS (L., dim. of *alveus*, hollow). Designates a small saclike dilation.

ANCO'NEUS (Gr. *ankon*, elbow). A muscle near the elbow.

ANGI- (Gr. *angeion*, vessel). Angiocarditis, inflammation of the heart and large blood vessel.

ANGI'NA (Gr. *ankonē*, a strangling, choking). Any disease with spasmodic or suffocating pain. Usually denoting chest pain associated with heart attack.

AN'KYL- (Gr., stiff). Ankylosis, the joining of one or more parts to form a single part, particularly a bone. Ankylosing of the spine.

ANOCOCCY'GEAL. Pertaining to the anus and the coccyx.

ANOM'- (Gr. *an*, not + *homalos*, even). Deviant. Deviation, or departure, from the normal or common order or rule; abnormality. Anomaly.

ANTA'GONIST (Gr. *antagonizesthai*, to struggle against). A muscle that opposes another muscle.

ANTE (L., before. *Ante* + *meridiem*, antemeridian, A.M.). Earlier, prior to, before; in front of. Anteroom.

ANTERIOR. To the front of or in the forward part of.

ANTI- (Gr., opposite). Antibiotic, against life *(bios)*. Antidote, given against.

ARTHR- (Gr., joint). Arthritis, an inflammation of the joints.

ARTICULATION. The place of union, or junction, between two bones.

APONEURO'SIS. A white flattened or ribbonlike tendinous expansion serving mainly to connect a muscle with the parts it moves.

ASTHMA. A condition marked by recurrent attacks of paroxysmal dyspnea (difficulty in breathing or labored breathing). It is accompanied by wheezing due to spasmodic contractions of the *bronchi*.

ATLAS (the Greek god who bears up the pillars of heaven). The first cervical vertebra, which articulates above with the occipital bone and below with the axis.

AUTOGE'NIC TRAINING. A kind of autohypnosis combining relaxation and affirmations (positive thinking) and guided by visualization; developed by Johannes H. Schultz, a German psychiatrist, in 1932.

AXIL'LA (L.) A small pyramidal space between the upper lateral part of the chest and the median side of the arm. Armpit. It houses many trigger points referring to distant parts.

AXIS (Gr. *axon*, axle). A line about which a revolving body turns or about which a structure would turn if it did revolve; a line around which specified parts of the body are arranged. The second cervical vertebra.

BEHAVIOR. Deportment, or conduct; any or all of a person's total activity, especially that which can be externally observed.

BEHAVIOR MODIFICATION. The modification of behavioral traits through psychological means, as reinforcement and aversion therapy.

BELL'S PALSY. A neuropathy of the facial nerve, resulting in paralysis, usually to one side. Responds to Myotherapy.

BI- (L., twice, two). Binocular, pertaining to both eyes.

BI'CEPS (L. *bi*, two + *ceps*, head). Any muscle having two heads.

BIO- (Gr. *bios*, life). Biochemistry, the chemistry of living things.

BIOENERGE'TICS. The study of energy transformations in living organisms.

BIOFEED'BACK. By amplifying biological signs with a variety of machines, biofeedback trains the individual to become aware of and control autonomic-nervous-system processes.

BRA'CHY (Gr., short). Brachycephalic, having a short head.

BRON'CHI (Gr. *bronkos*, windpipe). Any of the larger air passages to the lungs, having an interlacing network of smooth muscle.

BUR'SA (L., sac). A sac or saclike cavity filled with viscid fluid and situated at places in the tissues in which friction would otherwise develop.

BURSIT'IS (L. *bursa*, sac, + -itis, inflammation). An inflammation of a *bursa*, occasionally accompanied by a calcific deposit; the most common site is the subdeltoid *bursa*. Pain said to be caused by a *bursa* is often misdiagnosed and usually responds to Myotherapy.

CALCAR (L., spur). A spurlike process; calcarine, spurlike.

CALCIF'IC (Gr. *khalix*, pebble; L. *calx*, lime). Calcification: impregnation with calcium or calcium salts; hardening, as of tissue, by such impregnation.

CAPIT- (L. *cepit-*, *ceps*). Head.

CAPSULE (L. *capsula*, small box). General term for a cartilaginous, fatty, fibrous or membranous structure enveloping another structure or organ or part.

CAR'PAL. Pertaining to the *carpus*, or wrist, which is made up of eight bones, the *ossa carpi*.

CAR'PAL TUNNEL. The *osseofibrous* passage for the median nerve and the *flexor* tendons formed by the *flexor retinaculum* (a network of cells).

CAR'TILAGE (L. *cartilago*). A specialized fibrous connective tissue. There are several types, the most important of which are *hyaline cartilage*, elastic cartilage and fibrocartilage.

CAUDA (L., tail). The terminal portion of the spinal cord.

CE'CUM (L. *caecum*, blind, blind gut). The first part of the large intestine, forming a dilated pouch into which open the *ilium*, the *colon* and the *appendix vermiformis*.

CERVICAL (L. *cervix*, neck). Pertaining to the neck. The *cervix uteri*. Cervical vertebrae.

CERVICAL VERTEBRAE. The seven vertebrae that form the back of the neck.

CHIROPRAC'TIC. A system of therapeutics based on the claim that disease is caused by abnormal function of the nerve system. Manipulation and treatment of the structures of the body, especially of the spinal cord.

CHONDROMALA'CIA. A softening of the articular cartilage, most frequently in the *patella*. Often offered as the cause of knee pain. It sometimes is.

CLA'VICLE (Dim. of L. *clavis,* key, from its shape). The bone articulating with the *sternum* and the *scapula*. Curved like the letter *S,* it forms the anterior portion of the shoulder girdle on either side. Also called the collarbone.

COC'CYX (Gr. *kokkyx,* cuckoo, whose bill it is said to resemble). The small bone caudal to the *sacrum* in man. It is formed by the union of four, sometimes five or three, rudimentary vertebrae and forms the caudal extremity of the vertebral column.

CO'LON. That part of the large intestine which extends from the *cecum* to the *rectum.*

COLON'IC IRRIGATION. Enema irrigating the *colon*. Sometimes causes shock.

CONDYLE (Gr. *condylys,* knuckle). A rounded articulatory prominence at the end of a bone.

CONNECTIVE TISSUE. A highly vascular matrix that forms the supporting and connecting structure of the body.

COR'ACOID (Gr. *korakoeides,* like a raven's beak). The *coracoid process (processus coracoideus scapulae).*

CORNU. A hornlike excrescence or projection of bone.

CORONOID PROCESS (like a crow's beak). A projection from the upper part of the neck of the *scapula*. It overhangs the shoulder joint.

CORTISONE. A hydrocortisone medication used as an anti-inflammatory. To be used with great caution: side effects can be severe.

COS'TA (L., rib). One of the paired bones, twelve to a side, that extend from the thoracic vertebrae toward the median line on the ventral aspect of the trunk.

COS'TAL CARTILAGE (L. *costa* + *cartilago*). Part of a rib.

CREST (L. *crista*). A projection or projecting structure or ridge, especially one surmounting a bone or its border.

CUNE'IFORM (L. *cuneus,* wedge + -iform). The wedge-shaped bone of the wrist.

CUTA'NEUS. Cutaneous muscle, striated muscle that inserts into the skin.

DIAPHRAGM. The muscular membranous partition separating the abdominal and the thoracic cavities. It functions in respiration.

DISTAL. Located far from the origin or line of attachment, as a bone.

DORSAL. Pertains to the back or a portion nearer the back than some other object or structure.

DORSIFLEXION (L. *dorsum,* back, + flexion, bending). To bend back, as a hand or a foot.

EPICONDYLE. An eminence upon a bone, above its *condyle.*

ESTROGEN. The generic term for estrus-producing compounds; female sex hormones.

EXTENSION. The act of extending or being extended.

FASCIA. A sheet of fibrous tissue beneath the surface of the skin enveloping the body; encloses a muscle or muscle group and separating muscle layers.

FELDENKRAIS METHOD. A variant of the Alexander Technique of postural reconstruction. Its aim is a conscious reeducation of the central nervous system.

FIBROSI'TIS (L. *fibrosus,* fibrous, + -itis). Inflammatory hyperplasia of the white fibrous fascial layers of the locomotor system. According to Travell, it means too many things to too many people and should not be used. According to Kraus, it is the thickened tissue known as dimpled fat. Prudden accepts the latter as well as the idea that it is a by-product of stress.

FISSURES. Nonarticular depressions of bones.

FLEXION. The act of bending or being bent.

FORAMEN. A natural opening, or passage, especially into or through a bone.

FOR'CEPS. An instrument with two blades and a handle for compressing or grasping tissues. Used in childbirth to facilitate delivery of babies.

FOSSA (L., a trench or channel). A general term for a hollow or depressed area.

FRONTAL (L. *frontalis*). Pertaining to the forehead (*frons,* the front or forepart). The forehead region above the eyes. See *Glossary of Muscles.*

FUSION, SPINAL. A surgical creation of ankylosis between contiguous vertebrae. Spondylosyndesis.

GALEA APONEUROTICA. The *aponeurosis* connecting the *frontal* and *occipital* bellies of the *occipitofrontal* muscle.

GEST'ALT. Fritz Perls fathered the *Gestalt* (whole, in German) movement. Unlike the standard "talking it out" therapies, *Gestalt* aims for experiences that dissipate old, rigid patterns.

GLENOID CAVITY. A depression in the lateral angle of the *scapula* for articulation with the *humerus*.

GROOVES. Nonarticular depressions of bones.

HAIR ANALYSIS. To spot mineral deficiencies or poisonous levels of heavy metals in the body. A lock of hair is sent to a lab and a computer printout is returned detailing the mineral levels and usually a summary of the present research.

HEARTBURN. An *esophageal* symptom consisting of a *retrosternal sensation* of warmth or burning that rises in the chest. When severe it may include the neck and head and prevent lying down. Responds to Myotherapy to chest, arms and upper back.

HEMICRA'NIA (Gr. *hēmi-,* half, partial, partially + *kranion,* skull). Pain or aching on one side of the skull.

HERBO'LOGY. Uses herbal concentrates, extracts, infusions and poultices for nourishment and healing. Herbs provide the recipes for many modern-day medications. They, like the medications, *can* be dangerous.

HIA'TUS HERNIA. A protrusion of the stomach above the diaphragm. Often given as a diagnosis for abdominal and chest pain. It sometimes is the correct diagnosis. If the pain responds to Myotherapy it was probably wrong or there was more than one problem.

HOMEO'PATHY. The principle here is that like cures like. Attempts are made to build up the patient's resistance instead of attacking the disease itself. Homeopathic remedies are prepared and administered according to a carefully codified materia medica. If you suffered from insomnia you would be given diluted, homeopathically prepared caffeine.

HYSTERECTOMY. The surgical removal of the uterus.

IL'IUM. The expansive superior portion of the hipbone *(os coxae).* See *Glossary of Bones.*

INFERIOR. Situated below or directed downward. Used in referring to the lower surface of a structure or the lower of two or more similar structures.

INGUINAL. Pertaining to the groin.

INTEROSSEOUS MEMBRANE. A membrane between two bones.

IRIDO'LOGY. This is based on the principle that the iris is a miniature map of the body. The iridologist examines the iris for telltale specks, rings or cloudiness signaling disease elsewhere in the body.

ISTHMUS. A narrow connection between two larger bodies or parts.

JACOBSON TECHNIQUE. This uses a set of easy tensing and relaxing exercises, often as a prelude to autogenic training and other mind therapies.

JUICE FASTING, WATER FASTING or just FASTING. Means exactly that: fasting, not eating. Fasts of varying durations have been used down the centuries with varied results. Moderate fasting is often a good idea, especially in an overfed nation, but drastic diets or fasting can be dangerous and should not be undertaken without the help of professionals trained in the field.

KINE'SIOLOGY (Gr. *kinēsis,* from *kinein,* to move + -logy, a branch of learning). The study of muscles and their movements, especially as applied to physical conditioning.

KINE'SIOLOGY ACCORDING TO HOLISTIC APPROACHES. A do-it-yourself technique for ascertaining your body's reaction to food or any other stimulus—music, fluorescent lights—by testing the strength of your muscles before and during exposure.

KNEECAP. See PATELLA, in *Glossary of Bones.*

KYPHOSIS. An abnormally increased convexity in the curvature of the *thoracic spine* as viewed from the side. Hunchback.

LAMINECTOMY. A surgical excision of the posterior arch of a vertebra.

LATERAL. Pertains to the side.

LIGAMENT. A band of fibrous tissue, connecting bones or cartilages, serving to support and strengthen joints.

LINEA (L., line).

LINEA ALBA (L. *alba,* white). A tendinous raphe (a thick stratum of transversely directed nerve fibers) seen along the middle line of the abdominals extending from the ensiform cartilage *(xiphoid process)* to the *symphysis pubis,* to which it is attached.

LINEA ASPERA (L., rough). A prominent longitudinal ridge or crest on the middle third of the *femur* shaft. Provides attachments for the *gluteus maximus, vastus internus, vastus externus, adductor magnus,* short head of the *biceps, iliacus, pectineus* and *adductor brevis.*

LINE OF BONE. A rough, narrow elevation affording attachment for tissue.

LOIN. Part of the back between the *thorax* and the *pelvis.*

LORDOSIS. A forward curvature of the *lumbar spine.*

LUMBAR VERTEBRAE. The five largest movable vertebrae. Situated between the lowest ribs and the pelvis.

MALAR (L. *malaris,* from *mala,* cheekbone). See *Glossary of Bones.*

MASTOID PROCESS. The conical projection at the base of the mastoid portion of the temporal bone. See TEMPORAL BONES OF THE SKULL, in *Glossary of Bones.*

MEDIAL LINE. Pertaining to the middle. The midline of a body or structure.

MEDITATION. The act of reflecting upon or contemplating; an exercise in contemplation.

MEMBRANE. A thin layer of tissue that covers a surface, lines a cavity or divides a space or organ.

MYOFASCIAL TRIGGER POINT (Travell). A hyperirritable spot, usually within a taut band of skeletal muscle or the muscle's *fascia,* that is painful on compression and can give rise to characteristic referred pain, tenderness and autonomic phenomena.

NOTCHES. Nonarticular depressions of bones.

OLEC'RANON. A bony projection of the *ulna,* at the elbow.

ORBIT. The bony cavity containing the eyeball and its associated muscles, vessels and nerves.

ORTHOMOLECULAR PSYCHIATRY. This is sometimes called "clinical ecology," because it deals with heretofore undiagnosed allergies. Megavitamin therapy is commonly employed to treat phobias, nerves, even schizophrenia. It routinely uses hair analysis to check for vitamin and mineral deficiencies.

OSTEOP'ATHY. A respectable branch of Western medicine. It involves manipulation of the musculoskeletal system and confidence in the body's innate healing powers.

OSTEOPOROSIS. An abnormal rarefaction of bone. May be idiopathic or occur secondarily to other diseases.

PAROXYS'MAL. Pertaining to spasms.

PERINEUM. The pelvic floor and pelvic structures occupying the pelvic outlet.

PHA'LANX (pl. *phalanges;* Gr., "a line of soldiers"). A general term for any bone of a finger or toe. *Phalanges digitorum manus,* the fourteen bones composing the bones of the fingers. *Phalanges digitorum pedis,* the fourteen bones composing the skeleton of the toes. See *Glossary of Bones.*

PHYSIATRY. That branch of medicine using physical therapy in diagnosis, prevention and treatment of bodily disorders.

PITO'CIN. Solution of oxytocic hormone often used to induce labor.

PLANTAR FLEXION. Plantar pertains to the sole of the foot. Flexion means bending the foot toward the sole.

POLAR'ITY THERAPY. This was developed by Dr. Randolph Stone and is an amalgam of "right thinking," manipulation, exercise and diet. Its goal is to restore balance to the vital energy pictured by polarity therapists as flowing between positive (yang) and negative (yin) poles.

POPLITEAL. Pertaining to the back of the knee.

POSTERIOR. In back or on the back part of.

PRO'CESS (L. *processus,* advance). A prominence, or projection, as of bone.

PRODRO'MAL (Gr. *prodromos,* precursor, from *pro,* forward, and *dromos,* running). Indicating the onset of a disease or morbid state.

PROXIMAL. Nearest to a point of reference, as to a center, or median, line, or to the point of attachment or origin.

PSYCHOGENIC. Having an emotional, or psychological, origin.

RAMUS (L., a branch). A general term for a smaller structure.

REFLEXOLOGY. The foot is to a reflexologist what the eye is to an iridologist: a map of the human body through which improvements in health may be accomplished, by pressure.

REICHIAN THERAPY . . . BIOENERGETICS. Pioneer psychotherapist Wilhelm Reich (of orgone fame) believed that primal memories and emotions are locked into our musculature. Therapists use massage and manipulation to bring them to the surface.

RIDGE OF BONE. See LINE OF BONE.

ROLFING. A technique devised by Ida P. Rolf. It is called System of Structural Integration, and the purpose is said to be "verticality." It is a system of deep, painful massage of connective tissue.

SACRAL VERTEBRAE. Five fused vertebrae forming the posterior section of the *pelvis*.

SCA'PULA (L., shoulder blade). The flat triangular bone in the back of the shoulder. See *Glossary of Bones*.

SCIA'TICA. Pain radiating down the legs along the distribution of the *sciatic nerve;* may be more severe than back pain.

SCLEROMETER. A tool used in determining the relative resistance of measured tissue to outside pressure.

SHEATH. A tubular case or envelope.

SHIATSU. A gentle Japanese massage that works on the acupuncture system of meridians, applying finger pressure instead of needles.

SHIN SPLINTS. A strain of the long *flexor* muscles of the toes. Usually occurring in athletes and marked by pain along the shinbone.

SHOULDER BLADE. See SCAPULA.

SOMATIC. Pertaining to the characteristics of the body.

SPATIAL DISORIENTATION AND DIZZINESS. Disagreeable sensation which seems to come from within the head. Less often, called vertigo. The sensation of objects spinning around the patient. Often caused by trigger points in the sternocleidomastoid muscles.

SPHINCTER. A circular muscle that constricts a passage or closes a natural orifice.

SPINE (L. *spina,* thorn). A sharp, slender, pointed eminence.

SPONDYLOSIS. Ankylosis, or abnormal bone fusion, of a vertebral joint. A general term for degenerative changes in the spine.

SUBLUXATION. An incomplete or partial dislocation.

SUPERCILIARY. Pertains to the eyebrow.

SUPINATION (L. *supinatio*). The act of assuming the supine position, or the state of being supine. Applied to the hand, the act of turning the palm forward (anteriorly) or upward, performed by lateral rotation of the forearm.

SUPRA-. Prefix signifying above or over.

SUL'CUS. A narrow, deep fissure or groove, any of the narrow fissures separating adjacent cerebral convolutions. Another example: a rough, deep groove on the upper surface of the *calcaneus* (heel bone) between the medial and the posterior *articular surfaces* and giving attachment to the *interosseous talocalcaneal ligament*.

SWAYBACK. See LORDOSIS.

SYM'PHYSIS. A site or line of union. A type of joint in which the apposed bony surfaces are firmly united by a plate of fibrocartilage.

SYNO'VIAL MEMBRANE. The inner of two layers of the articular capsule of a synovial joint, having a free, smooth surface that lines the joint cavity.

TMJD. Temporomandi'bular joint dysfunction.

TEN'DON. A cord or band of strong, white fibrous tissue. It connects a muscle to a bone. When a muscle contracts, or shortens, it pulls on the tendon, which moves the bone.

THERAPEU'TIC TOUCH. Another way of saying "laying on of hands." A study in the early seventies is worth noting: Patients given "therapeutic touch" by nurses showed a significant change in hemoglobin (the oxygen carrier in the blood) compared with routinely treated patients.

THORA'CIC (Gr. *thōrakikos*). Pertaining to or affecting the chest.

TIC. Spasmodic twitching movement made involuntarily by muscles that are ordinarily under voluntary control.

TINNITUS. The perception of sound in the absence of acoustic stimulus; buzzing, ringing. It may be either intermittent or continuous.

TORTICOL'LIS (spasmodic). Intermittent spasm of the neck muscles, causing rotation and tilting of the head. Wry neck.

TRANSPERSONAL PSYCHOLOGY. From the personal (traumas, etc.), the individual voyages into the transpersonal realm of the "Self." It employs Eastern meditation, Jungian dream work and *Gestalt* methods. Psychosynthesis, another transpersonal therapy, fosters spiritual wholeness.

TRANSVERSE. Extending from side to side, situated at right angles to the long axis.

TRICEPS (L. *tri-*, three, + *ceps*, head). Any muscle having three heads.

TU'BERCLE (L. *tuberculum*, dim. of *tuber*, lump). A knoblike process on a bone.

TUBERO'SITY. An elevation, or protuberance, especially at one end of a bone for the attachment of a muscle or tendon.

UNGUAL (L. *unguis*, nail). Pertaining to the nails.

VENTER. The belly of a muscle.

VENTRAL. Pertains to the abdomen or a position nearer the abdominal surface than some other object or reference.

VERTEBRA (L., akin to *vertere*, to turn). Any of the bones of the spinal column, comprising *seven cervical, twelve thoracic, five lumbar, five sacral* and *four coccygeal.*

VISION IMPROVEMENT. The Bates method of sight improvement: mental relaxation techniques to train the individual out of the need for glasses.

WRY NECK. See TORTICOLLIS.

YOGA. The Indian system of postures and exercises. The one used most in the United States is Hatha-yoga. There are others, many using breathing techniques and meditation.

Glossary of Bones

ACETA'BULUM (L., vinegar cup, from *acetum*, vinegar). The cuplike cavity into which the head of the *femur* (thighbone) fits. It is a deep hemispherical depression formed internally by the *os pubis*, above by the *ilium* and behind and below by the *ischium*. It is also called the *cotyloid cavity*.

ACRO'MION PROCESS (Gr. *akrōmion*, from *akros*, extreme + *ōmion*, dim. of *ōmos*, shoulder). A large, somewhat triangular or oblong process flattened from behind forward, then curving forward and upward so as to overhang the *glenoid cavity*. Its upper surface gives attachment to some of the fibers of the *deltoid*. Its outer border presents three or four tubercles for the tendinous attachments of the *deltoid*. Its inner margin gives attachment to a portion of the *trapezius* muscle. Its apex is thin and attaches to the *coracoacromial ligament*. Articulation: the *humerus* and the *clavicle*.

ALVE'OLAR PROCESS. The thickest and most spongy part of the bone, excavated with deep cavities for the teeth. The *buccinator* muscle arises from the outer surface as far forward as the first molar tooth.

ASTRA'GALUS (Gr. *astragalos*, ankle bone). Situated in the middle and upper part of the *tarsus*, it supports the *tibia* above. It also articulates with the *malleoli* on either side, resting below on the *os calcis* and joined in front with the navicular. It articulates with the *tibia, fibula, os calcis* and *navicular*.

BONES. Bones are divided into four classes: long, short, flat and irregular. Long bones are found in the limbs and consist of a shaft and two extremities. Examples: the *humerus* and the *femur*. Damage to any part will leave trigger points in its wake. Short bones exist where a part of the skeleton is intended for strength and compactness. They are divided into a number of small segments held together by ligaments. Example: the *carpal bones* of the wrist. Flat bones appear where there is need for either extensive protection or broad surfaces for the attachment of muscles. Example: the *scapula*, or shoulder blade. Irregular, or mixed, bones have such peculiar shapes they do not fall into the foregoing categories. Example: the *vertebrae*.

BONES, their surfaces. The surfaces of bones have certain eminences and depressions that have distinctive names. There are two kinds: articular and nonarticular. An example of an articular eminence is the head of the *femur* (thighbone). An articular depression would be the *glenoid cavity* of the *acetabulum*. Nonarticular eminences are designated according to shape. A broad, rough, uneven elevation is called a *tuberosity;* a small rough prominence is a *tubercle;* a sharp, slender, pointed eminence, a *spine;* a rough, narrow elevation running along the surface, a *ridge*, or *line*. Nonarticular depressions differ in form and are known variously as *fossae, grooves, fissures, notches*, etc.

CALCA'NEUM, OS CALCIS (L. *os*, bone, *calx*, heel). The largest and strongest of the *tarsal* bones. It forms a strong lever for the calf muscles. It articulates with the *astragalus* and the *cuboid*. Eight attachments: *tibialis posticus, tendo Achilles, plantaris, abductor hallucis, abductor minimi digiti, flexor brevis digitorum, flexor accessorius* and *extensor brevis digitorum.*

CAR'PUS (Gr. *karpos*, wrist). These bones are eight in number and lie in two rows. In the top row are the *scaphoid, semilunar, cuneiform* and *pisiform* bones; in the lower row are the trapezium, trapezoid, *os magnum* and *unciform.*

CLA'VICLE (dim. of L. *clavis*, key). The collarbone forms the anterior portion of the shoulder girdle, linking the *sternum* and the *scapula.* It articulates by its upper extremity with the upper border of the *sternum* and by its outer extremity with the *acromion process* of the *scapula.* It affords attachments for six muscles: the *sternocleidomastoid, trapezius, pectoralis major,* deltoid, *subclavius* and sternohyoid.

COR'ONOID PROCESS (Gr. *koronē*, anything curved). A thin, flattened, triangular eminence of bone varying in shape and size. Serves chiefly as the attachment for the *temporalis* muscle. Its external surface affords attachment for the *temporal, masseter* and *buccinator* muscles.

COS'TAL CARTILAGES are bars of *hyaline cartilage* that serve to extend the ribs forward to the front of the chest. They give attachment to the *costoclavicular ligament* and the *subclavius* muscle, the *pectoralis major,* some of the great flat muscles of the abdomen, the *sternothyroid, triangularis sterni,* the *transversalis* muscle and the diaphragm. They also afford attachments to the *intercostal muscles.*

CU'BOID. It is situated on the outside of the foot, in front of the *os calcis* and behind the fourth and fifth *metatarsal bones.* It articulates with the *os calcis,* the *external cuneiform,* and the fourth and fifth *metatarsal* bones; occasionally with the *navicular.* It attaches to part of the *flexor brevis hallucis* and part of the *tibialis posticus* tendon.

CUNE'IFORM BONES (L. *cuneus,* wedge; *forma,* likeness). They are called first, second and third, counting from the inner to the outer sides of the foot . . . or internal, middle and external.

Internal cuneiform is the largest of the three. It articulates with four bones: *navicular, middle cuneiform* and the first and second *metatarsal bones.*

Muscle attachments: to three: *tibiales anticus* and *posticus* and *peroneus longus.*

Middle cuneiform—the smallest of the three. Articulates with four bones: *navicular, internal* and *external cuneiform* and the *second metatarsal* bone. Muscle attachments: a part of the *tibialis posticus.*

External cuneiform articulates with six bones: *navicular, middle cuneiform, cuboid* and second, third and fourth *metatarsal* bones.

FE'MUR. The longest and strongest bone in the skeleton. Its attachments are the *ligamentum teres* and the posterior part of the *capsular ligament* of the hip joint. The upper extremity presents a head, a neck and a *greater* and a *lesser trochanter.*

The head is globular in shape and is the ball that fits into the socket of the *acetabulum.* It provides attachment for the *ligamentum teres.*

The neck is a flattened pyramidal process of bone that connects the head with the shaft. It provides attachment for the posterior part of the *capsular ligament* of the hip joint.

Trochan'ters (Gr. *trekhein,* to run) are prominent processes of bone providing leverage to the muscles rotating the thigh on its axis. There are two, the greater and the lesser. The *greater trochanter* is a large, irregular eminence situated at the outer side of the neck at its juncture with the shaft. It provides attachments for tendons of the *gluteus medius* and *obturator externus* muscles, the *obturator internus* and the *gemelli.* It also provides attachments for the upper part of the *vastus externus* muscle and the *gluteus minimus.* The *lesser trochanter* is a conical eminence projecting from the lower and back part of the neck. Its summit gives attachment to the tendon of the *iliopsoas.* The *iliacus* attaches to the shaft just below the *lesser trochanter* between the *vastus internus* and the *pectineus.* There is a point projecting from the upper front part of the neck called the *tubercle of the femur,* which is the meeting point of five muscles: the *gluteus minimus, vastus externus, obturator internus* and the *gemelli*. The spiral line of the femur affords attachment for the *iliofemoral ligament* of the hip joint and to the *vastus internus*. The *linea quadrata*, descending along the back part of the shaft, affords attachment for the *quadratus femoris* and some fibers of the *adductor magnus* muscle.

LIN'EA AS'PERA (L. *asper*, rough). A prominent longitudinal ridge or crest on the middle third of the shaft of the *femur*. It is extended above by three ridges; one of them, the *gluteal ridge*, gives attachment to part of the *gluteus maximus*. Below, the *linea aspera* is extended by two ridges. The inner one terminates in the *adductor tubercle*, which provides attachment to the tendon of the *adductor magnus*.

To the inner lip of the *linea aspera* and its extensions are attached the *vastus internus*, the *vastus externus*, the *adductor magnus*, the *gluteus maximus*, the short head of the *biceps, iliacus, pectineus, adductor brevis* and *adductor longus*.

The anterior surface of the shaft of the *femur* affords attachment to the *crureus* muscle; the lower fourth affords attachment to the *subcrureus*. To the external surface is attached the outer portion of the *crureus* muscle.

The lower extremity of the *femur* is larger than the upper and is divided into two large eminences, the *condyles* (Gr. *condylos*, knuckle, a rounded articulatory prominence at the end of a bone). The outer *condyle* gives attachment to the external lateral ligaments of the knee. Immediately beneath it is a depression that gives attachment to the *popliteus* muscle. The inner surface of the outer *condyle* gives attachment to the anterior ligament. Just above and to the outer side is a depression for the tendon of the outer head of the *gastrocnemius*, above which is the attachment for the *plantaris*.

The inner *condyle* gives attachment to the posterior crucial ligament and the tendon of the inner head of the *gastrocnemius*.

FIB'ULA (L., clasp). The smaller of the two long bones situated on the outer side of the lower leg. It is the more slender of the two long bones. On the outer side of the *tibia*, it is connected above and below. It is connected below the level of the knee

joint and excluded from its formation. It articulates with two bones: the *tibia* and the *astragalus*.

Attachments: The head of the *biceps, soleus* and *peroneus longus, extensor longus digitorum, peroneus tertius, extensor proprius hallucis, tibialis posticus, flexor longus hallucis*, the *peroneus longus* and the *peroneus brevis*.

FOOT. The skeleton of the foot consists of three divisions: the *tarsus, metatarsus* and *phalanges*.

FOREARM is that portion of the upper extremity which is situated between the elbow and the wrist. The skeleton is composed of two bones: the *ulna* and the *radius*.

The lower extremity of the forearm articulates with the *carpus* and the *ulna*. It affords attachments for the anterior ligament of the wrist joint, the tendon of the *supinator longus* and the lateral and posterior ligaments of the wrist joint.

FRON'TAL BONE OF THE SKULL (forms the forehead). It resembles a cockleshell.

HAND. The hand is divided into three segments: *carpus*, or wrist bones; *metacarpus*, or bones of the palm and *phalanges*, the bones of the fingers.

HUM'ERUS (L., upper arm). The longest bone of the upper extremity, it affords attachments to twenty-four muscles: *supraspinatus, infraspinatus, teres minor, subscapularis, pectoralis major, teres major, latissimus dorsi, deltoid, coracobrachialis, brachialis anticus*, external and internal heads of the *triceps, pronator radii teres* and common tendon of the *flexor carpi radialis, palmaris longus, flexor sublimis digitorum* and *flexor carpi ulnaris, supinator longus, extensor carpi radialis longior*, the common tendon of the *extensor carpi radialis brevior, extensor communis digitorum, extensor minimi digiti, extensor ulnaris, supinator brevis* and *anconeus*.

ILIUM (L., groin or flank). So called from its support of the flank. It is the superior, broad and expanded portion of the pelvis, running upward from the *acetabulum* and forming the prominence of the hip.

Ilium attachments: *gluteus maximus, gluteus medius, gluteus minimus*, the reflected tendon of the *rectus femoris* muscle, the *iliacus*, the *obturator internus*, the posterior sacroiliac ligaments and the *erector* and *multifidus spinae*, the *tensor fasciae femoris*, *obliquus externus abdominis* and *latissimus dorsi*, the *fascia lata*, the internal oblique, *sartorius, iliofemoral ligament* and the *iliopsoas*.

IS'CHIUM (L., hip joint). The inferior and strongest portion of the bone, it proceeds downward from the *acetabulum*, expands into a large *tuberosity* and then, curving forward, forms, with the descending ramus of the *os pubis*, a large aperture, the *obturator foramen*.

Is'chium attachments: *obturator internus, gemellus inferior, gemellus superior, pyriformis, coccygeus, levator ani*, lesser sacroiliac ligament, *quadratus femoris, adductor magnus*, falciform prolongation of the great sacroiliac ligament, *transversi perinei, semimembranosus, semitendinosus, biceps, obturator externus*, and *erector penis* or *erector clitoridis*.

THE LEG. The skeleton of the leg consists of four bones: the *patella* (a large sesamoid bone in front of the knee), the *tibia*, the *fibula* and the femur.

LOWER EXTREMITIES. The bones of the lower extremities consist of those of the pelvic girdle, the leg and the foot.

MALAR. Pertaining to the cheekbone.

MAN'DIBLE, THE INFERIOR MAXILLARY BONE. The mandible (L. *mandere*, to chew) is the largest and strongest bone of the face. Serves to hold the lower teeth. It consists of a curved horizontal portion (body) and two perpendicular portions (the *rami*), which join the back part of the body nearly at right angles. Forms the chin. It affords attachments to the *levator menti* (or *levator labii inferioris*) and a portion of the *orbicularis oris*. On the internal surface is the attachment for the anterior *venter* (belly) of the digastric muscle.

MAXIL'LA, THE SUPERIOR MAXILLARY BONES. The *maxilla* (L., jawbone) is liable to many diseases. It is the largest bone in the face except for the mandible. The bone has a body and four processes: the *malar* (L. *mala*, cheekbone), the *nasal* (L. *nasus*, nose), the *alveolar* (L. *alveus*, hollow) and the *palatal* (L. *palatum*, taste, judgment) processes.

METACAR'PAL BONES. Five in number, they are long, cylindrical bones of the hand. The *metacarpal* bone of the thumb is shorter and wider than the others and provides attachments for the *flexor ossis metacarpi pollicis*, the *extensor ossis metacarpi pollicis*, the *flexor brevis pollicis* and the first dorsal interosseous. The metacarpal bone of the index finger is the longest. It attaches to six muscles: the *flexor carpi radialis*, the *extensor carpi radialis longior*, the *adductor obliquus pollicis*, the first and second *dorsal interosseous* and the first *palmar interosseous*. The *metacarpal* bone of the middle finger is a little smaller than that of the index finger. It attaches to the *extensor carpi radialis brevior*, the *flexor carpi radialis*, the *adductor transversus pollicis*, the *adductor obliquus pollicis* and the second and third *dorsal interosseous*. The *metacarpal* bone of the ring finger is shorter and smaller than the preceding. It attaches to the third and fourth *dorsal* and the second *palmar interosseous*. The *metacarpal* bone of the little finger attaches to the *extensor carpi ulnaris*, the *flexor carpi ulnaris*, the *flexor ossis metacarpi minimi digiti*, and the fourth *dorsal* and third *palmar interosseous*.

METATAR'SAL BONES. These are five in number and are numbered according to position from within outward. The first *metatarsal* attaches to three muscles: part of the *tibialis anticus*, the *peroneus longus*, and the first *dorsal interosseous*. The second *metatarsal* attaches to four muscles: the *adductor obliquus hallucis*, the first and second *dorsal interosseous* and a part of the tendon of the *tibialis posticus*; sometimes attached to the *peroneus longus*. The third *metatarsal* attaches to five muscles: the *adductor obliquus hallucis*, the second and third *dorsal*, and the first *plantar interosseous*. There are also some fibers from the *tibialis posticus* tendon. The fourth *metatarsal* affords attachments for five muscles: the *adductor obliquus hallucis*, the third and fourth *dorsal* and the second *plantar interosseous*. There are also some fibers from the *tibialis posticus* tendon. The fifth *metatarsal* attaches to six muscles: the *peroneus brevis*, the *peroneus tertius*, the *flexor brevis minimi digiti,* the *adductor transversus hallucis,* the fourth *dorsal* and the third *plantar.*

NA'SAL PROCESS. A strong triangular plate of bone projecting upward, inward and backward at the side of the nose. Gives attachment to the *levator labii superioris alaeque nasi, orbicularis palpebrarum* and *tendo oculi.*

NAVI'CULAR (or scaphoid) bone (L. *navicula,* dim. of *navis,* ship). Articulates with four bones: *astragalus* and three *cuneiform;* occasionally with the *cuboid.* Muscle attachments: part of the *tibialis posticus.*

OLE'CRANON PROCESS (Gr. *olekranon,* from *ōlenē,* elbow + *kranion,* head). The large point of the upper end of the *ulna* that projects behind the elbow and forms the point of the elbow. It affords attachments for the *triceps,* part of the posterior ligament of the elbow joint, the *flexor carpi ulnaris* and the *anconeus.*

OS INNOMINA'TUM (L. *in,* not + *nominatus,* named). A large, irregularly shaped, flat bone constricted in the center and expanded above and below. With its fellow on the opposite side it forms the two sides and anterior wall of the pelvic basin. The bone is divided into three parts: the *ilium,* the *ischium* and the *os pubis.*

OS MAG'NUM (L. *os,* bone + *magnus,* great). The largest bone of the *carpus,* it occupies the center of the wrist. It affords attachments for ligaments and part of the *adductor obliquus pollicis.*

OS PU'BIS (L., bone of the groin; *pubes,* groin). That portion of the pelvis which extends inward and downward from the *acetabulum* to articulate in the middle line with the bone of the opposite side. It supports the external organs of generation.

OS PUBIS ATTACHMENTS. *Adductor longus, obturator externus, levator ani, puboprostatic ligaments, Poupart's ligament,* the conjoined tendon of the *internal oblique* and *transversalis* muscles, *Gimbernat's ligament, rectus abdominis, pyramidalis,* internal pillar of the external abdominal ring, the *obturator membrane, pectineus,* the *psoas parvus, obturator internus, gracilis, obturator externus,*

adductores brevis and *magnus* and the *compressor urethrae.*

PA'LATE PROCESS. The partition separating the nasal and oral cavities.

PATEL'LA (L., small pan). A flat triangular bone situated at the anterior part of the knee joint, it serves to protect the front of the joint and increase the leverage of the *quadriceps extensor.* It provides attachments for four muscles: the *rectus femoris, vastus intermedius, vastus internus* and *vastus externus.*

PELVIC GIRDLE. Consists of a single bone, the *os innominatum,* by which the thigh is connected to the trunk.

PHALANGES (Gr. *phalanx*). The bones of the fingers are fourteen in number, three for each finger (index finger, middle finger, ring finger and little finger) and two for the thumb.

Thumb (two *phalanges*). Five attachments to the base of the first *phalanx: extensor brevis pollicis, flexor brevis pollicis, adductor pollicis, adductor transversus* and *obliquus pollicis.* To the second *phalanx,* two attachments: *flexor longus pollicis* and *extensor longus pollicis.*

Index finger (three *phalanges*). Two attachments to the first *phalanx:* first *dorsal* and first *palmar interosseous.*

Middle finger (three *phalanges*). Two attachments to the first *phalanx:* second and third *dorsal interosseous.*

Ring finger (three *phalanges*). Two attachments to the first *phalanx:* fourth *dorsal* and second *palmar interosseous.*

Little finger (three *phalanges*). Three attachments to the first *phalanx:* third *palmar interosseous, flexor brevis minimi digiti* and *abductor minimi digiti.*

To the second *phalanges* of all four: *flexor sublimis digitorum* and *extensor communis digitorum.* In addition, *extensor indicis* to the index finger and *extensor minimi digiti* to the little finger.

To the third *phalanges: flexor profundus digitorum* and *extensor communis digitorum.*

The *phalanges* of the foot, like those in the hand, number fourteen. In arrangement they are like the hand as well, two in the great toe and three each in the other four. The first row even resemble those in the hand. The bones in the second row are remarkably short, and they are broader than those in the first. The *ungual phalanges* resemble those of the fingers, having an expanded extremity for the support of the nail- and weight-bearing end of the toe.

Attachments to the first *phalanx:* the great toe, five muscles: the innermost tendon of the *extensor brevis digitorum, abductor hallucis, adductor obliquus hallucis, flexor brevis hallucis* and *adductor transversus hallucis.*

Second toe: three muscles: first and second *dorsal interosseous* and first *lumbrical.*

Third toe: three muscles: third *dorsal* and first *plantar interosseous* and second *lumbrical.*

Fourth toe: three muscles: fourth *dorsal* and second *plantar interosseous* and third *lumbrical.*

Fifth toe: four muscles: *flexor brevis minimi digiti, abductor minimi digiti, plantar interosseous* and *lumbrical.*

Attachments for the second *phalanx* of the great toe: *extensor longus hallucis* and *flexor longus hallucis.*

Other toes: *flexor brevis digitorum,* some fibers of the common tendon of the *extensores longus* and *brevis digitorum.*

Third phalanges: some fibers from the common tendon of the *extensores longus* and *brevis digitorum* and the *flexor longus digitorum.*

PISIFORM BONE (L. *pisum,* a pea). Small in size, it serves as attachment for the *anterior annular ligament,* the *flexi carpi ulnaris* and the *abductor minimi digiti.*

RADIUS (L., a ray or spoke of a wheel). A long bone situated on the outer side of the forearm parallel with the *ulna.* The upper end forms a small portion of the elbow joint. The lower end forms the chief part of the wrist. The upper extremity articulates with the radial head of the *humerus* and the *lesser sigmoid cavity* of the *ulna.* It provides attachments for the *supinator brevis* and the tendon of the *biceps* muscle. The shaft of the *radius* gives attachment to the *supinator brevis, flexor longus pollicis, flexor sublimis digitorum, rotator quadratus,* posterior *annular ligament* of the wrist and the tendon of the *supinator longus.* It also provides attachments for the *flexor lon-*

gus pollicis, pronator quadratus, extensor ossis metacarpi pollicis, supinator brevis, pronator radii, teres major and *teres minor.*

RIBS. Elastic arches of bone that form the chief part of the *thoracic* (chest) walls. They are twelve in number on each side. The first seven are connected behind with the *spine* and in front with the *sternum* through the intervention of the *costal* (L. *costa,* rib) *cartilages.* They are called *true* ribs. The remaining five are *false* ribs. The first three of the latter have their cartilages attached to the *cartilage* of the rib above. The last two are free at their anterior extremities (floating ribs). The ribs are situated one below the other, leaving spaces between called the intercostal spaces. The ribs serve as attachments for the *internal* and *external intercostals, scalenus anticus, scalenus medius, scalenus posticus, pectoralis minor, serratus magnus, obliquus externus, quadratus lumborum,* diaphragm, *latissimus dorsi, serratus posticus superior, serratus posticus inferior, iliocostalis, musculus accessorius ad iliocostalem, longissimus dorsi, cervicalis ascendens, levatores costarum* and *infracostales.*

SCAPHOID (Gr. *skaphoeidēs,* boatlike). Attaches to the anterior annular ligament of the wrist, a few fibers of the *adductor pollicis* and the *external lateral ligament* of the wrist.

SCAPULA (L., shoulder blade). Forms the back of the shoulder girdle. It is a large, flat bone, triangular in shape, situated at the posterior aspect and side of the *thorax* (chest) between the second and the seventh (sometimes the eighth) ribs. Its internal border, or base, is about an inch from and almost parallel with the *spinous processes* of the *vertebrae.*

The anterior surface presents a broad concavity, the *subscapular fossa.* Its oblique ridges give attachment to the tendinous intersections, and the surfaces between them to the *subscapularis* muscle.

The *scapula,* when judged by the number of attachments afforded, is one of the most important bones in the body, and when working on the surface one should not forget the underside. The *scapula* attaches to the *subscapularis* (posterior surface), *supraspinatus, infraspinatus* (spine), *trapezius,* deltoid (superior border), omohyoid (vertebral border), *serratus magnus, levator anguli scapulae, rhomboidei minor* and *major,* axillary *border,* triceps, *teres minor, teres major;* apex of *glenoid cavity,* long head of the *biceps; coracoid process, coracobrachialis, pectoralis minor* and *latissimus dorsi.*

Its margin affords attachment throughout its entire length to the *serratus magnus.* The summit of its arch serves to support its spine and the *acromion process.* The *posterior,* or *dorsum,* affords attachment for the *supraspinatus, infraspinatus, teres major* and *teres minor.* Sometimes the *latissimus dorsi* is attached by a few fibers.

The spine of the *scapula* is a prominent plate of bone. It commences at the *vertebral border* by a smooth, triangular surface over which the *trapezius* slides, terminating in the *acromion process,* which overhangs the shoulder joint. It affords attachments to part of the *infraspinatus* muscle. The *posterior,* or *crest,* of the *spine* is attached to the *trapezius* and the *deltoid.*

SPINE (L. *spina*). A flexuous and flexible column formed of a series of bones called *vertebrae* (L. *vertere,* to turn). There are thirty-three *vertebrae:* seven *cervical,* twelve *dorsal* (also called *thoracic*), five *lumbar,* five *sacral* and four *coccygeal.*

STERNUM (Gr. *sternon,* chest). A flat, narrow bone in the median line of the front of the chest, consisting of three portions. It is like a sword. The upper part, representing the handle, is the *presternum,* or *manubrium* (L. *manus,* hand, handle), triangular in form. Its anterior surface affords attachments on each side to the *pectoralis major* and the *sternal* end of the *sternocleidomastoid* muscle. Its posterior surface affords attachments on each side to the *sternohyoid* and *sternothyroid* muscles.

The middle and largest piece represents the blade, the *gladiolus* (L. dim. of *gladius,* sword). The inferior piece, the point of the sword, is the *ensiform* (L. *ensis,* sword + -form), or *xiphoid,* process (Gr.

xiphos, sword + *-oeidēs,* shape). The *gladiolus (mesosternum)* is longer, narrower and thinner than the first piece of the *sternum.* Its anterior surface affords attachments on each side to the *triangularis sterni* muscle. The *ensiform,* or *xiphoid process (metasternum)* is the smallest of the three pieces of the *sternum.* It is thin, elongated in form and *cartilaginous* in structure in youth but ossified at its upper part in adults. The anterior surface affords attachment to the *chondroxiphoid ligament,* and its posterior surface attachment to some of the fibers of the *diaphragm* and the *triangularis sterni.* Its pointed extremity gives attachment to the *linea alba.*

TARSUS (Gr. *tarsos,* ankle). There are seven bones of the *tarsus:* the *calcaneus,* or *os calcis; astragalus;* cuboid; navicular; and *internal, middle* and *external cuneiform* bones.

TEMPORAL BONES OF THE SKULL. Situated at the sides and base of the skull, they have *squamous* (L. *squama,* scale), *mastoid* (Gr. *mastos,* breast) and *petrous* (Gr. *petros,* stone) portions. The *squamous* portion affords attachment for the *temporal muscle.* The *mastoid* portion is set at the posterior part of the bone; its outer surface is rough and gives attachment to the *occipitofrontalis.* The *mastoid* portion is continued below into a conical projection, the *mastoid process.* Both size and form vary somewhat. This process serves for the attachment of the *sternocleidomastoid, splenius capitis* and *trachelomastoid* muscles. The *petrous* portion, a pyramidal process of bone wedged between the *sphenoid* and *occipital bones* at the base of the skull, contains in its interior the essential parts of the organs of hearing.

THIGH. That portion of the lower extremity which is situated between the pelvis and the knee, the thigh is the longest and strongest bone in the body. Attachments: *ligamentum teres* and the posterior part of the *capsular ligament* of the hip joint.

TIBIA (L., an ancient flute originally made from an animal's leg bone). The *tibia* is situated at the front and inner side of the leg and is the second-longest and second-largest bone in the body. The upper extremity, or head, has two lateral *tuberosities*, which articulate with the *condyles* of the *femur*. The lower extremity presents five surfaces. The *internal malleolus* attaches to a strong process of bone. The *inferior surface* articulates with the *astragalus*. The *anterior surface* of the lower extremity is covered by the tendons of the *extensor* muscles of the toes; the *posterior surface* presents a superficial groove for the passage of the tendon of the *flexor hallucis longus;* the *external surface* presents an attachment for the *inferior interosseous ligament*, connecting it with the *fibula*. This surface affords attachment to the *anterior* and *posterior tibiofibular ligaments*. The *internal surface* is extended downward to form a strong pyramidal process, the internal *malleolus*. The *inner surface* of this process articulates with the *astragalus;* its *anterior border* provides attachment of the anterior fibers of the *internal lateral* or *deltoid ligament;* its *posterior border* presents a deep groove that transmits the tendons of the *tibialis posticus* and *flexor longus digitorum* muscles. The summit of the internal *malleolus* provides the attachment for the *internal lateral ligament* of the ankle joint.

Attachments: *semimembranosus, tibialis anticus, extensor longus digitorum, biceps femoris, sartorius, gracilis, semitendinosus, popliteus, soleus, flexor longus digitorum, tibialis posticus, ligamentum patellae*, by which the *quadriceps extensor* is attached to the *tibia*. In addition, the *tensor fasciae femoris* is attached indirectly to the *tibia*, through the *iliotibial band* and the *peroneus longus*.

TRAPEZIUM (Gr. *trapezion*, small table, dim. of *trapeza*, table). Of very irregular form, the *trapezium* affords attachments for the *abductor pollicis, flexor ossis metacarpi pollicis, flexor brevis pollicis* and the *anterior annular ligament*.

TRAPEZOID. The smallest bone in the second row of the wrist. Affords attachments for ligaments.

ULNA (Gr. *olenē*, forearm). A long prismatic bone at the inner side of the forearm paralleling the *radius*, the *ulna* is a shaft with two extremities, the upper becoming the *olecranon process*, the *coronoid process* and two *concave articular cavities*, the greater and lesser *sigmoid cavities*. Articulates with wrist at lower (distal) end.

UNCIFORM (L. *uncus*, a hook + -form). Provides attachments for the *flexor brevis minimi digiti*, the *flexor ossis metacarpi minimi digiti* and the *flexor carpi ulnaris*.

UPPER EXTREMITY. The bones of the upper extremity consist of those of the shoulder girdle, arm, forearm and hand. The shoulder girdle is made up of the *clavicle* and the *scapula*.

VERTEBRAE, CERVICAL (L. *cervix*, neck). There are seven *cervical vertebrae* in the neck.

VERTEBRAE, COCCYGEAL (Gr. *kokkyx*, cuckoo, from its resemblance to the cuckoo's beak). There are four *coccygeal vertebrae*.

VERTEBRAE, DORSAL (L. *dorsum*, back). These are also called *thoracic vertebrae* (L. *thorax*, the chest). They are twelve in number.

VERTEBRAE, LUMBAR (L. *lumbus*, loin). There are five *lumbar vertebrae*, situated between the lowest ribs and the five *sacral vertebrae* of the pelvis.

VERTEBRAE, SACRAL (L. *os sacrum*, translated from Gr. *hieron osteon*, sacred bone). The five *sacral bones* are fused and form the posterior section of the *pelvis*.

Glossary of Muscles

ABDOMINALS: EXTER'NUS AB-DOM'INIS. The external oblique muscle of the abdomen. It attaches to the *lower eight ribs* at the *costal cartilages,* the crest of the *ilium* and the *linea alba* through the *rectus* sheath. It flexes and rotates the *vertebral column* and compresses the abdominal *viscera.*

ABDOMINALS: REC'TUS ABDOM'INIS. Attaches to the *pubis,* the *xiphoid process* and *cartilages* of the fifth, sixth and seventh ribs. It supports the abdomen.

ABDOMINALS: TRANSVER'SUS AB-DOM'INIS. The transverse muscle of the abdomen attaches to the *cartilages* of the six lower ribs, the *thoracolumbar fascia, iliac crest, inguinal ligament, linea alba* through the *rectus* sheath and conjoined tendon to the *pubis.* It compresses the abdominal *viscera.*

ABDUC'TOR HAL'LUCIS. The *abductor* muscle of the great toe. It attaches to the *medial tubercle* of the *calcaneus,* the *plantar fascia* and the medial surface of the *proximal phalanx* of the great toe.

ABDUC'TOR POL'LICIS BRE'VIS. The short *abductor* muscle of the thumb. It attaches to the *scaphoid ridge* of the *trapezium,* the *transverse carpal ligament* and the lateral surface of the base of the *proximal phalanx* of the thumb. Abducts the thumb.

ABDUC'TOR POL'LICIS LON'GUS. The long *abductor* muscle of the thumb. It attaches to the posterior surface of the *radius* and *ulna* and the radial side of the base of the first *metacarpal bone.* Extends thumb.

ACHILLES TENDON. A fibrous cord of connective tissue. An alternative term for the *calcaneal tendon:* a powerful tendon at the back of the heel which attaches the *triceps surae* muscle to the tuberosity of the *calcaneus.*

ADDUC'TOR BRE'VIS. The *short adductor* muscle. It attaches to the outer surface of the *inferior ramus* of the *pubis* and the upper part of the *linea aspera* of the *femur.* It rotates and flexes the thigh.

ADDUC'TOR HAL'LUCIS. The *adductor* muscle of the great toe, it has two heads. Attaches to the bases of the second, third and fourth metatarsals and the sheath of the *peroneus longus,* capsules of the metatarsophalangeal joints of the three outside toes and the outside of the base of the proximal *phalanx* of the great toe. It adducts the great toe.

ADDUC'TOR LON'GUS. The *long adductor* muscle attaches to the crest of the *symphysis pubis* and the *linea aspera* of the *femur.* It flexes the thigh.

ADDUC'TOR MAG'NUS. The *great adductor* muscle has two parts. The deep part attaches to the *inferior ramus* of the *pubis,* the *ramus* of the *ischium* and the *linea aspera* of the *femur.* The superficial part attaches to the *ischial tuberosity* and the *adductor tubercle* of the *femur.* The deep part adducts the thigh, and the superficial part extends the thigh.

ADDUC'TOR MIN'IMUS. The smallest *adductor* muscle. This is the name given to a portion of the *adductor magnus.* It attaches to the *ischium* and the body and *ramus* of the *pubis.* It adducts the thigh.

ADDUC'TOR POL'LICIS. The *adductor* muscle of the thumb, it has two heads. Attaches to the sheath of the *flexor carpi radialis*, the *anterior carpal ligament*, the *capitate bone*, the bases of the second and third *metacarpals*, the lower two-thirds of the anterior surface of the third *metacarpal* and the medial surface of the base of the *phalanx* of the thumb. It adducts and apposes the thumb.

ANCONE'US. The *anconeus* muscle attaches back of the *lateral epicondyle* of the *humerus*, to the *olecranon* and to the posterior surface of the *ulna*. It extends the forearm.

ARTICULA'RIS CU'BITI. The *articular* muscle of the elbow attaches to the deep surface of the *brachii* and the *posterior ligament* of the *synovial membrane* of the elbow joint.

ARTICULA'RIS GE'NUS. The *articular* muscle of the knee attaches to the shaft of the *femur* and the *synovial membrane* of the knee joint. It lifts the capsule of the knee joint.

AURICULA'RIS ANTE'RIOR. The *anterior auricular* muscle attaches to the *superficial temporal fascia* and the *cartilage* of the ear. It draws the auricle (ear) forward.

AURICULA'RIS POSTE'RIOR. *Posterior* means in back of or in the back part of. *Auricular* pertains to the ear. The *posterior auricular* muscle attaches to the *mastoid process* and to the *cartilage* of the ear. It draws the ear backward.

AURICULA'RIS SUPE'RIOR. The *superior* muscle of the *auricle* attaches to the *galea aponeurotica* and the *cartilage* of the ear. It raises the auricle (ear).

BI'CEPS BRA'CHII. A *biceps* is a muscle with two heads. The *biceps brachii* is a muscle in the upper arm attaching to the upper border of the *glenoid cavity*, the *apex of the coracoid process* and the *radial tuberosity* and *fascia* of the forearm. It flexes the forearm and supinates the hand.

BI'CEPS FEM'ORIS. The *biceps* muscle in the thigh. It attaches to the *ischial tuberosity*, the *linea aspera* of the *femur*, the head of the *fibula* and the *lateral condyle* of the *tibia*. It flexes the leg and extends the thigh.

BRACHIA'LIS. The *brachial* muscle attaches to the anterior (situated to the front of or in the forward part of) surface of the *humerus* and the *coracoid process* of the *ulna*. It flexes the forearm.

BRACHIORADIA'LIS. Attaches to the *supracondylar ridge* of the *humerus* (*supra*- is a prefix signifying above or over). It also attaches to the lower end of the *radius*. It flexes the forearm.

BUCCINA'TOR. The *buccinator* muscle attaches to the *buccinator ridge* of the *mandible*, the *alveolar process* of the *maxilla*, the *pterygomandibular ligament* and the *orbicularis oris*, at the angle of the mouth. It compresses the cheek and retracts the angle of the mouth.

COCCYG'EI. The *coccygeal* muscles. These are the muscles acting upon the *coccyx*, including the *coccygeal* and the *dorsal* and *ventral sacrococcygeal* muscles. (*Dorsal* pertains to the back and *ventral* pertains to the belly or a position nearer the belly surface than some other object of reference.)

COCCYG'EUS. The *coccygeal* muscle attaches to the *ischial spine* and lateral border of the lower part of the *sacrum* and *upper coccyx*. It supports and raises the coccyx.

COL'LI. Muscles of the neck, including the *sternocleidomastoid*, the *longus colli*, the *suprahyoid*, the *infrahyoid* and the *scalene* muscles.

CORACOBRACHIA'LIS. Attaches to the *coracoid process* of the *scapula* and the medial surface of the shaft of the *humerus*. It flexes and adducts the arm.

CORRUGA'TOR SUPERCIL'II. (*Superciliary* pertains to the eyebrow.) This muscle attaches to the medial end of the *superciliary arch* (medial pertains to the middle) and the skin of the eyebrow. It draws the brow downward and medially.

DELTOI'DEUS. The *deltoid* attaches to the *clavicle*, the *acromion*, and the spine of the *scapula*. It abducts, flexes and extends the arm.

EREC'TOR SPI'NAE. The *erector* muscle of the spine: a name given the fibers of the deep muscles of the back, originating from the *sacrum*, spines of the *lumbar* and the eleventh and twelfth *thoracic* vertebrae and the *iliac crest*, which split and insert as the *iliocostalis, longissimus* and *spinalis* muscles.

EXTEN'SOR CAR'PI RADIA'LIS BRE'VIS. The short *radial extensor* muscle of the wrist. Attaches to the *lateral epicondyle* of the *humerus* and the third *metacarpal* bone. It extends and abducts the wrist joint.

EXTEN'SOR CAR'PI RADIA'LIS LON'GUS. The long, *radial extensor* muscle of the wrist attaches to the *lateral supracondylar ridge* of the *humerus* and base of the *metacarpal bone* and extends and abducts the wrist.

EXTEN'SOR CAR'PI ULNA'RIS. The *ulnar extensor* muscle of the wrist (two heads) attaches to the *lateral epicondyle* of the *humerus,* the *dorsal border* of the *ulna* and the base of the *fifth metatarsal bone.* It extends and adducts the wrist joint.

EXTEN'SOR DIGITO'RUM. The *extensor muscle* of the fingers. Attaches to the *lateral epicondyle* of the *humerus* and the *common tendon* of each finger. Extends the wrist joint and the fingers.

EXTEN'SOR DIGITO'RUM BRE'VIS. The *short extensor muscle* of the toes attaches to the *dorsal surface* of the *calcaneus* and the *extensor tendons* of the first, second, third and fourth toes. It extends the toes.

EXTEN'SOR DIGITO'RUM LON'GUS. The *long extensor muscle* of the toes attaches to the *anterior surface* of the *fibula, lateral condyle* of the *tibia,* the *interosseus membrane* and the common *extensor tendon* of the four outside toes. Extends toes.

EXTEN'SOR HAL'LUCIS BRE'VIS. The *short extensor* muscle of the great toe. A name given to the portion of the *extensor digitorum brevis* muscle that goes to the great toe.

EXTEN'SOR HAL'LUCIS LON'GUS. The *long extensor muscle* of the great toe attaches to the front of the *fibula,* the *interosseous membrane* and the *dorsal surface* of the base of the *distal phalanx* of the great toe. Dorsiflexes the ankle joint and extends the great toe.

EXTEN'SOR IN'DICIS. The *extensor muscle* of the index finger attaches to the *dorsal surface* of the body of the *ulna,* the *interosseous membrane* and the *common tendon* of the index finger. It extends the index finger.

EXTEN'SOR POL'LICIS BRE'VIS. The *short extensor muscle* of the thumb attaches to the *dorsal surface* of the *radius* and the *interosseous membrane* and the *dorsal surface* of the *proximal phalanx* of the thumb. It extends the thumb.

EXTEN'SOR POL'LICIS LON'GUS. The *long extensor muscle* of the thumb attaches to the *dorsal surface* of the *ulna,* the *interosseous membrane* and the *dorsal surface* of the *distal phalanx* of the thumb. Extends and abducts the thumb.

FLEX'OR CAR'PI RADIA'LIS. The *radial flexor* muscle of the wrist attaches to the *medial epicondyle* of the *humerus* and the base of the *second metacarpal.* It flexes and abducts the wrist.

FLEX'OR CAR'PI ULNA'RIS. The *ulnar flexor* of the wrist (two heads) attaches to the *medial epicondyle* of the *humerus,* the *pisiform,* the *hook of the hamate* and the *proximal* end of the *fifth metacarpal* bone. It flexes and adducts the wrist.

FLEX'OR DIGITO'RUM BRE'VIS. The *short flexor muscle* of the toes attaches to the *medial tuberosity* of the *calcaneus, plantar fascia* and the *middle phalanges* of the four outside toes. It flexes the toes.

FLEX'OR DIGITO'RUM LON'GUS. The *long flexor muscle* of the toes attaches to the *posterior shaft* of the *tibia* and *distal phalanges* of the four outside toes. It flexes the toes and extends the foot.

FLEX'OR DIGITO'RUM PROFUN'DUS. The deep *flexor muscle* of the fingers attaches to the *shaft of the ulna,* the *coronoid process* and the *distal phalanges* of the fingers. It flexes the *distal phalanges.*

FLEX'OR DIGITO'RUM SUPERFI'CIA'LIS. The *superficial flexor muscle* of the fingers (two heads) attaches to the *medial condyle* of the *humerus,* the *coronoid process* of the *ulna,* the *oblique* line of the *radius,* the *anterior border* and the *middle phalanges* of the fingers. It flexes the *middle phalanges.*

FLEX'OR HAL'LUCIS BRE'VIS. The *short flexor muscle* of the great toe attaches to the under surface of the *cuboid,* the *lateral cuneiform* and the base of the *proximal phalanx* of the great toe. It flexes the great toe.

FLEX'OR HAL'LUCIS LON'GUS. The *long flexor muscle* of the great toe attaches to the *posterior surface* of the *fibula* and the base of the *distal phalanx* of the great toe. It flexes the toe.

FLEX'OR POL'LICIS BRE'VIS. The *short flexor muscle* of the thumb attaches to the *transverse carpal ligament*, the ridge of the *trapezium* and the base of the *proximal phalanx* of the thumb.

FLEX'OR POL'LICIS LON'GUS. The *long flexor muscle* of the thumb attaches to the *anterior surface* of the *radius*, the *coracoid process* of the *ulna* and the base of the *distal phalanx* of the thumb.

FRONTA'LIS. See OCCIPITOFRONTALIS.

GASTROCNE'MIUS. The calf muscle (two heads) attaches to the *popliteal surface* of the *femur*, the upper part of the *medial condyle* and *capsule* of the knee; also, the *lateral condyle* and *capsule* of the knee. The *aponeurosis* unites with the tendon of the *soleus* to form the *calcaneal tendon* (Achilles tendon).

GEMEL'LUS INFE'RIOR. The *inferior gemellus* muscle attaches to the *tuberosity* of the *ischium* and the *greater trochanter* of the *femur*. It rotates the thigh laterally.

GEMEL'LUS SUPE'RIOR. The *superior gemellus* muscle attaches to the *spine* of the *ischium* and the *greater trochanter* of the *femur*. It rotates the thigh laterally.

GLU'TEUS MAX'IMUS. The greatest *gluteal muscle* attaches to the *lateral surface* of the *ilium*, the *dorsal surface* of the *sacrum* and *coccyx* and the *gluteal tuberosity* of the *femur*. It extends, abducts and rotates the thigh laterally.

GLU'TEUS ME'DIUS. The *middle gluteal muscle* attaches to the *lateral surface* of the *ilium* between the *anterior* and *posterior gluteal lines* and to the *greater trochanter* of the *femur*.

GLU'TEUS MIN'IMUS. The least of the *gluteal muscles* attaches to the *lateral surface* of the *ilium* between the *anterior* and *inferior lines* of the *gluteals* and to the *greater trochanter* of the *femur*. It abducts and rotates the thigh medially.

GRA'CILIS. This muscle attaches to the *inferior ramus* of the *pubis* and the *medial surface* of the shaft of the *tibia*. It adducts the thigh and flexes the knee joint.

HYOGLOS'SUS. The *hyoglossal muscle* attaches to the body of the greater *cornu*

of the *hyoid bone* and the side of the tongue. It depresses and retracts the tongue.

ILI'ACUS. Attaches to the *iliac fossa* and the base of the *sacrum* and the *lesser trochanter* of the *femur*. It flexes thigh, trunk on limb.

ILIOCOCCYG'EUS. The *iliococcygeal* muscle, a name given to the posterior portion of the *levator ani*, which attaches as far forward as the *obturator canal* and attaches also on the side of the *coccyx* and the *anococcygeal body*. It helps support the pelvic *viscera* and resist increases in intra-abdominal pressure.

ILIOCOSTA'LIS. The *iliocostal muscle:* the lateral division of the *erector spinae*, which includes the *iliocostalis cervicis*, *iliocostalis thoracis* and the *iliocostalis lumborum*.

ILIOCOSTA'LIS CER'VICIS. The *iliocostalis* of the neck attaches to the third, fourth, fifth and sixth *ribs* and the *transverse processes* of the fourth, fifth and sixth *cervical vertebrae*. It extends the cervical spine.

ILIOCOSTA'LIS LUMBO'RUM. The *iliocostal muscle* of the loins attaches to the crests and angles of the lower six or seven *ribs* and extends the lumbar spine.

ILIOCOSTA'LIS THORA'CIS. The *iliocostal muscle* of the *thorax* attaches at the upper borders of the angles of the six lower *ribs*, the six upper *ribs* and the *transverse process* of the seventh *cervical vertebra*. It keeps the spine erect.

ILIOPSO'AS. The *iliopsoas* muscle is a compound muscle consisting of the *iliacus* and the *psoas major*.

INFRASPINA'TUS. This muscle attaches to the *infraspinous fossa* of the *scapula* and the *tubercle* of the *humerus*. It rotates the *humerus* laterally.

INTERCOSTA'LES EXTER'NI. The *external intercostal muscles* (eleven on each side) attach to the inferior borders of the *ribs* and *intercostals* and draw the *ribs* together in respiration and expulsive movements.

INTERCOSTA'LES INTER'NI. The *internal intercostal muscles* (eleven on each side) attach to the inferior borders of the *ribs* and *costal cartilage*, and to the superior borders of the *ribs* and the *costal carti-*

lage below, and draw the *ribs* together in respiration and expulsive movements.

ISCHIOCAVERNO'SUS. The *ischiocavernosus* muscle attaches to the *ramus* of the *ischium*, and the *crus penis (crus clitoridis)*. It maintains erection of the penis (clitoris).

LATIS'SIMUS DOR'SI. Attaches to the spines of the *thoracic* and *lumbar vertebrae*, the *thoracolumbar fascia, iliac crest*, lower *ribs*, the inferior angle of the *scapula* and the crest of the *intertubercular sulcus* of the *humerus*. It adducts, extends and rotates the *humerus* medially.

LEVA'TOR A'NI. The name applied collectively to important muscular components of the *pelvic diaphragm*, including the *pubococcygeus (levator prostatae* and *pubovaginalis)*, the *puborectalis* and the *iliococcygeus* muscles.

LEVA'TOR GLAN'DULAE THYROI'DAE. The *levator muscle* of the *thyroid gland* is an inconstant muscle attaching to the *isthmus* or *pyramid* of the *thyroid gland* and the body of the *hyoid bone*.

LEVA'TOR PROSTA'TAE. The *levator* muscle of the *prostate* is a name applied to a part of the anterior portion of the *pubococcygeus* muscle, which attaches to the *prostate* and the tendinous center of the *perineum*. It supports and compresses the prostate and is involved in micturation (passage of urine).

LEVA'TOR SCAP'ULAE. The *levator muscle* of the *scapula* attaches to the *transverse process* of the upper four *cervical vertebrae* and the medial border of the *scapula*. It raises the *scapula*.

LONGIS'SIMUS. The *longissimus* is the longest element of the *erector spinae*, which includes the *longissimus capitis*, the *longissimus cervicis* and the *longissimus thoracis*.

LONGIS'SIMUS CAP'ITIS. The *longissimus* of the head attaches to the *transverse processes* of four or five upper *thoracic vertebrae* and the *mastoid process* of the *temporal* bone. It draws the head backward and rotates the head.

LONGIS'SIMUS CER'VICIS. The *longissimus* of the neck attaches to the *transverse processes* of four or five of the upper *thoracic vertebrae* and the *transverse processes* of the second to sixth *cervical vertebrae*. It extends the *cervical vertebrae*.

LONGIS'SIMUS THORA'CIS. The *longissimus* of the *thorax* attaches to the *transverse* and *articular processes* of the *lumbar vertebrae*, the *thoracolumbar fascia*, *transverse processes* of all the *thoracic vertebrae* and nine or ten lower *ribs*. It extends the *thoracic vertebrae*.

LON'GUS CAP'ITIS. The long muscle of the head attaches to the *transverse processes* of the third to the sixth *cervical vertebrae* and the basal portion of the *occipital bone*.

LON'GUS COL'LI. The long muscle of the neck attaches to the *transverse processes* of the third to fifth *cervical vertebrae*, the bodies of the first to third *thoracic vertebrae*, the bodies of three *upper-thoracic* and three *lower-cervical vertebrae*, the *tubercle* of the anterior arch of the *atlas*, the *transverse processes* of the fifth and sixth *cervical vertebrae* and the bodies of the second to fourth *cervical vertebrae*. It flexes and supports the *cervical vertebrae*.

MASSE'TER. The *masseter* muscle. Attachments: *pars superficialis:* the *zygomatic process* of the *maxilla* and the lower border of the *zygomatic arch; pars profunda:* the lower border and medial surface of the *zygomatic arch; pars superficialis:* the angle and *ramus* of the *mandible; pars profunda:* the upper half of the *ramus* and lateral surface of the *coronoid process* of the *mandible*. Closes the jaws.

OBLI'QUUS CAP'ITIS INFE'RIOR. The *inferior oblique muscle* of the head attaches to the *spinous process* of the *axis* and the *transverse process* of the *atlas*. Rotates the *atlas* and the head.

OBLI'QUUS CAP'ITIS SUPE'RIOR. The *superior oblique* muscle of the head attaches to the *transverse process* of the *atlas* and the *occipital* bone. Extends and moves the head laterally.

OBLI'QUUS EXTER'NUS ABDOM'INIS. The *external oblique* muscle of the abdomen attaches to the lower eight *ribs* at the *costal cartilages*, the crest of the *ilium* and the *linea alba* through the *rectus* sheath. Compresses abdominal *viscera*.

OBLI'QUUS INTER'NUS ABDOM'INIS.
The *internal oblique* muscle of the abdomen attaches to the *inguinal ligament,*
the *iliac crest,* the *lumbar aponeurosis,*
the lower three or four *costal cartilages,*
the *linea alba* and the conjoined tendon
to the *pubis.* It flexes and rotates the vertebral column and compresses the *viscera.*

OBTURATOR'IUS EXTER'NUS. The *external obturator* muscle attaches to the
pubis, the *ischium,* the superficial surface
of the *obturator membrane* and the *tro-
chantic fossa* of the *femur.* It rotates the
leg laterally.

OBTURATO'RIUS INTER'NUS. The *internal obturator* muscle attaches to the pelvic surface of the hipbone, the margin of
the *obturator foramen,* the *ramus* of the
ischium, the inferior *ramus* of the *pubis,*
the internal surface of the *obturator
membrane* and the *greater trochanter* of
the *femur.* It rotates the thigh laterally.

OCCIPITA'LIS. *Venter occipitalis musculi
occipitofrontalis.* See OCCIPITOFRON-
TA LIS.)

OCCIPITOFRONTA'LIS. The *occipitofrontalis* muscle attaches to the *venter occipitalis* (the highest point on the *nuchal line*
of the *occipital bone*), and the *venter
frontalis* (the skin of the eyebrows and
the root of the nose). The *venter frontalis*
raises the eyebrows, and the *venter occipitalis* draws the scalp backward. Note:
Venter means belly of a muscle. The two
bellies here are connected from the frontal bone (forehead) to the occipital bone
at the back of the head by the *galea aponeurotica* over the top of the head. Trigger points in one muscle, usually the *occipitalis,* can refer pain to the other.
(Important in headaches.)

ORBICULA'RIS. A muscle that encircles a
body such as the mouth or the eye.

ORBICULA'RIS OC'ULI. The *orbicular*
muscle of the eye. The oval *sphincter*
muscle surrounding the eyelids consists
of three parts: *Pars orbitalis, pars pal-
pebralis,* and *pars lacrimalis.*

ORBICULA'RIS O'RIS. The *orbicular* muscle of the mouth, comprising a *pars la-
bialis,* fibers restricted to the lips, and a
pars marginalis, fibers blending with
those of adjacent muscles. It closes and
protrudes the lips.

PALMA'RIS BRE'VIS. The *short palmar
muscle* attaches to the *palmar aponeurosis* and the skin of the medial border
of the hand. It tenses the palm of the
hand.

PALMA'RIS LON'GUS. The *long palmar
muscle* attaches to the *transverse carpal
ligament* and the *palmar aponeurosis.* It
flexes the wrist joint.

PECTIN'EUS. The *pectineal muscle* attaches
to the *iliopectineal* line, the *spine* of the
pubis and the *femur* distal to the *lesser
trochanter.* It flexes and adducts the
thigh.

PECTORA'LIS MA'JOR. The *greater pectoral muscle* is attached to the *clavicle,*
the *sternum,* six upper *ribs* and the *aponeurosis* of the *obliquus externus abdominis* (external oblique). These are reflected in the subdivision of the muscle
into clavicular, sternocostal and abdominal parts. It is also attached to the *crest*
of the *intertubercular groove* of the *humerus.* It adducts, flexes and rotates the
arm medially.

PECTORA'LIS MI'NOR. The *smaller pectoral* muscle attaches to the third, fourth
and fifth *ribs* and the *coracoid process* of
the *scapula.* It draws the shoulder forward and downward.

PERONE'US BRE'VIS. The *short peroneal
muscle* attaches to the lateral surface of
the *fibula* and the base of the fifth *metatarsal bone.*

PERONE'US LON'GUS. The *long peroneal
muscle* attaches to the *lateral condyle* of
the *tibia,* the lateral surface of the *fibula,*
the *medial cuneiform* and the first *metatarsal.* It abducts, everts and plantar-
flexes the foot.

PERONE'US TER'TIUS. The *third peroneus
muscle* attaches to the medial surface of
the *fibula* and the fifth *metatarsal.* It
everts and dorsiflexes the foot. It is also
called the *fibularis tertius,* or third fibular,
muscle.

PIRIFOR'MIS. The *piriform muscle* attaches
to the *ilium,* the second to fourth *sacral
vertebrae* and the upper border of the
greater trochanter. It rotates the thigh
laterally.

PLANTA'RIS. The *plantaris muscle* attaches
to the *lateral condyle* of the *femur* and
the posterior part of the *calcaneus.* It
plantar-flexes the foot.

PLATYS'MA. A plate-like muscle that attaches to the *fascia* of the *cervical region*, the *mandible* and the skin around the mouth. Wrinkles the skin of the neck and depresses the jaw.

POPLITE'US. The *popliteal muscle* attaches to the *lateral condyle* of the *femur* and the posterior surface of the *tibia*. It flexes and rotates the leg medially.

PROCE'RUS. The *procerus muscle* attaches to the skin of the nose and the skin of the forehead. It draws the brows together.

PRONA'TOR TE'RES. Attaches to the *medial epicondyle* of the *humerus*, the *coronoid process* of the *ulna* and the lateral surface of the *radius*. It pronates the hand.

PRONA'TOR QUADRA'TUS. Attaches to the anterior border of the distal third or fourth of the *ulna* and the distal fourth of the shaft of the *radius*. Pronates the hand.

PSO'AS MA'JOR. The greater *psoas* muscle attaches to the *lumbar vertebrae* and *fascia* and the *lesser trochanter* of the *femur*. It flexes the trunk and flexes and rotates the thigh medially.

PSO'AS MI'NOR. The smaller *psoas* muscle attaches to the last *thoracic* and first *lumbar vertebrae* and the *iliopectineal eminence*. It flexes the trunk on the pelvis.

PTERYGOI'DEUS LATERA'LIS. The *lateral pterygoid* muscle has two heads. It attaches to the lateral surface of the greater wing of the *sphenoid* and *infratemporal crest*, the lateral surface of the *lateral pterygoid plate*, the neck of the *condyle* of the *mandible* and the *temporomandibular joint capsule*. It protrudes the mandible, opens the jaws and moves the mandible from side to side.

PTERYGOI'DEUS MEDIA'LIS. The *medial pterygoid* muscle attaches to the *lateral pterygoid plate*, the *tuberosity* of the *maxilla* and the medial surface of the *ramus* and angle of the mandible. It closes the jaws.

PUBOCOCCYG'EUS. The *pubococcygeal muscle*. This is a name applied to the anterior portion of the *levator ani* and originating in front of the *obturator canal*. It is attached to the *anococcygeal ligament* and the side of the *coccyx*. It helps support the pelvic *viscera* and resist increases in intra-abdominal pressure.

PUBORECTA'LIS. *Puborectal muscle* is a name applied to a portion of the *levator ani*. It helps support the pelvic *viscera* and resists increases in intra-abdominal pressure.

PUBOVAGINA'LIS. *Pubovaginal muscle* is a name applied to the part of the anterior portion of the *pubococcygeal muscle* that is inserted into the *urethra* and *vagina*. It is involved in the control of micturition (the passage of urine).

PUBOVESICA'LIS. *Pubovesical muscle* is a name applied to smooth muscle fibers extending from the neck of the *urinary bladder* to the *pubis*.

PYRAMIDA'LIS. The *pyramidal muscle* attaches to the front of the *pubis*, the anterior *pubic ligament* and the *linea alba*. It tenses the abdominal wall.

QUADRA'TUS FEM'ORIS. The *quadrate muscle* of the thigh attaches to the upper part of the lateral border of the *tuberosity* of the *ischium* and the *quadrate tubercle* of the *femur*. It adducts and rotates the thigh.

QUADRA'TUS LUMBO'RUM. Attaches at the crest of the *ilium*, the *thoracolumbar fascia*, the *lumbar vertebrae*, the twelfth *rib* and the *transverse processes* of the four upper *lumbar vertebrae*. Flexes the *lumbar vertebrae* laterally.

QUADRA'TUS PLAN'TAE. The *quadrate muscle* of the sole attaches to the *calcaneus* and *plantar fascia* and the *lateral plantar*. It aids in flexing the toes.

QUAD'RICEPS FEM'ORIS. The *quadriceps muscle* of the thigh. This is a name applied collectively to the *rectus femoris*, the *vastus intermedius*, the *vastus lateralis* and the *vastus medialis*. They are attached by a *common tendon* that surrounds the *patella* and ends on the *tuberosity* of the *tibia*, acting to extend the leg upon the thigh. See individual components.

RECTOCOCCYG'EUS. The *rectococcygeal muscle* consists of smooth muscle fibers originating on the anterior surface of the second and third *coccygeal vertebrae* and attaching to the posterior surface of the *rectum*. It retracts and elevates the *rectum*.

REC'TUS ABDOM'INIS. The *abdominal muscle* attaches to the *pubis*, the *xiphoid process* and the *cartilages* of the fifth, sixth and seventh *ribs*. It flexes the *lumbar vertebrae* and supports the abdomen.

REC'TUS FEM'ORIS. The *thigh muscle* that attaches to the *anterior inferior iliac spine*, the rim of the *acetabulum*, the *patella* and a *tubercle* of the *tibia*. It extends the leg and flexes the thigh.

RHOMBOI'DEUS MA'JOR. The *greater rhomboid muscle* attaches to the *spinous processes* of the second, third, fourth and fifth *thoracic vertebrae* and the medial margin of the *scapula*. It retracts and elevates the *scapula*.

RHOMBOI'DEUS MI'NOR. The *lesser rhomboid muscle* attaches to the *spinous processes* of the seventh *cervical* to the first *thoracic vertebrae*, the lower part of the *ligamentum nuchae* and the medial margin of the *scapula* at the root of the *spine*. It adducts and elevates the *scapula*.

SARTO'RIUS. Attaches to the *anterior superior iliac spine* and the medial side of the proximal end of the *tibia*. It flexes the thigh and leg.

SCALE'NUS ANTE'RIOR. The *anterior scalene muscle* attaches to the *transverse process* of the third to sixth *cervical vertebrae* and the *tubercle* of the first *rib*. It raises the first *rib*.

SCALE'NUS ME'DIUS. The *middle scalene muscle* attaches to the *transverse process* of the second to the sixth *cervical vertebrae* and the first rib.

SCALE'NUS MIN'IMUS. The *smallest scalene muscle:* a band *occasionally* found between the *scalenus anterior* and the *scalenus medius*.

SCALE'NUS POSTE'RIOR. The *posterior scalene muscle* attaches to *all* the *tubercles* of the fourth to sixth *cervical vertebrae* and the second *rib*. Raises the first and second *ribs*.

SEMIMEMBRANO'SUS. The *semimembranosus* muscle attaches to the *tuberosity* of the *ischium* and the *medial condyle* of the *tibia*. It flexes the leg and extends the thigh.

SEMISPINA'LIS. A muscle composed of fibers extending obliquely from the *transverse processes* of the *vertebrae* to the *spines* (pointed projection on each vertebra), *except* for the *semispinalis capitis;* it includes the *semispinalis cervicis* and the *semispinalis thoracis*.

SEMISPINA'LIS CAP'ITIS. Attaches to the *transverse processes* of five or six upper *thoracic* and four lower *cervical vertebrae* and the *occipital bone*. It extends the head.

SEMISPINA'LIS CER'VICIS. Attaches to the *transverse process* of the five or six *upper thoracic vertebrae* and the *spinous processes* of the second to fifth *cervical vertebrae*. It extends and rotates the vertebral column.

SEMITENDINO'SUS. This muscle attaches to the *tuberosity* of the *ischium* and the upper part of the medial surface of the *tibia*. Flexes the leg and extends the thigh.

SERRA'TUS ANTE'RIOR. Attaches to eight or nine *upper ribs* and the *medial border* of the *scapula*. It raises the shoulder in abduction of the arm.

SO'LEUS. The *soleus* muscle attaches to the *fibula*, the *popliteal fascia*, the *tibia* and the *calcaneus* by the *tendo calcaneus*. It plantar-flexes the ankle joint.

SPHINC'TER. A sphincter muscle is a ring-like muscle that closes a natural orifice.

SPINA'LIS. The medial division of the *erector spinae*, including the *spinalis capitis*, *spinalis cervicis* and *spinalis thoracis*.

SPINA'LIS CAP'ITIS. Attaches to the *upper thoracic* and *lower cervical vertebrae* and the *occipital bone*. It extends the head.

SPINA'LIS CER'VICIS. Attaches to the *spinous processes* of the fifth, sixth and seventh *cervical* and the two upper *thoracic vertebrae*, the *spinous process* of the *axis* and sometimes of the second to fourth *cervical vertebrae*. It extends the vertebral column.

SPINA'LIS THORA'CIS. Attaches to the *spinous processes* of the two *upper lumbar* and the two *lower thoracic vertebrae* and the *spines* of the *upper thoracic vertebrae*. Extends the vertebral column.

SPLE'NIUS CAP'ITIS. This all-important muscle for headaches attaches to the lower half of the *ligamentum nuchae*, the *spines* of the seventh *cervical* and three *upper thoracic vertebrae* and the *occipital bone*. It extends and rotates the head.

SPLE'NIUS CER'VICIS. Attaches to the *spinous processes* of the third to sixth *thoracic vertebrae* and the *transverse processes* of two or three *upper cervical vertebrae.* It extends the neck and the head.

STERNOCLEIDOMASTOI'DEUS. The *sternocleidomastoid muscle* (two heads) attaches to the *sternum,* the *clavicle,* the *mastoid process* and the *superior nuchal line* of the *occipital bone.* It flexes the vertebral column and rotates the head.

SUBCLA'VIUS. The *subclavius muscle* attaches to the first *rib* and its *cartilage* and the lower surface of the *clavicle.* Depresses the lateral end of the *clavicle.*

SUBSCAPULA'RIS. The *subscapular muscle* attaches to the *subscapular fossa* of the *scapula* and the *lesser tubercle* of the *humerus.* It rotates the *humerus* medially.

SUPINA'TOR. The *supinator muscle* attaches to the latter *epicondyle* of the *humerus,* the *ulna* and the elbow-joint *fascia.* It supinates the hand.

SUPRASPINA'TUS. The *supraspinatus muscle* attaches to the *supraspinous fossa* of the *scapula* and the *greater tubercle* of the *humerus.* It abducts the *humerus.*

TEMPORA'LIS. The *temporal muscle* attaches to the *temporal fossa* and *fascia* and the *coronoid process* of the *mandible.* It closes the jaws.

TEN'SOR FAS'CIAE LA'TAE. The *tensor muscle* of the *fascia lata.* It attaches to the *iliac crest* and the *iliotibial band* of the *fascia lata.* It flexes and rotates the thigh medially.

TE'RES MA'JOR. Attaches to the inferior angle of the *scapula* and the crest of the *intertubercular sulcus* of the *humerus.* It adducts, extends and rotates the arm medially.

TE'RES MI'NOR. Attaches to the lateral margin of the *scapula* and the *greater tuberosity* of the *humerus.* It rotates the arm laterally.

TIBIA'LIS ANTE'RIOR. The *anterior tibialis muscle* attaches to the *tibia,* the *interosseous membrane,* the *medial cuneiform* and the *first metatarsal.* It dorsiflexes and inverts the foot.

TIBIA'LIS POSTE'RIOR. The *posterior tibial muscle.* It attaches to the *tibia,* the *fibula,* the *interosseous membrane* and the bases of the *metatarsals* except the talus. It plantar-flexes and inverts the foot.

TRAPE'ZIUS. The *trapezius muscle* attaches to the *occipital bone,* the *ligamentum nuchae,* the *spinous process* of the seventh *cervical* and *all* the *thoracic vertebrae,* the *clavicle,* the *acromion* and the *spine* of the *scapula.* It rotates the *scapula* to raise the shoulder in abduction of the arm and also draws the *scapula* backward.

TRI'CEPS BRA'CHII. The *triceps muscle* of the arm has three heads. It attaches to the *infraglenoid tubercle* of the *scapula,* the *posterior* surface of the *humerus,* the *lateral border* of the *humerus,* the *lateral intermuscular septum,* the *posterior surface* of the *humerus* below the radial groove, the medial border of the *humerus,* the *medial intermuscular septa* and the *olecranon* of the *ulna.* It extends the forearm and adducts and extends the arm.

TRI'CEPS SU'RAE (L. *sura,* calf). Name used when the *gastrocnemius* and *soleus* are considered together. (For Myotherapy, highly important.)

ZYGOMAT'ICUS MA'JOR. The *greater zygomaticus* muscle attaches to the *zygomatic bone* in front of the *temporal process* and the angle of the mouth. It draws the angle of the mouth backward and upward.

ZYGOMAT'ICUS MI'NOR. The *lesser zygomaticus* muscle attaches to the *zygomatic bone* near the *maxillary suture,* the *orbicularis oris* and the *levator labii superioris.* It draws the upper lip upward and laterally.

Bibliography

Books

How to Keep Slender and Fit After Thirty. Rev. ed. New York: Pocket Books, Inc., 1980.

A complete exercise program plus the philosophy needed to implement it after the age of thirty. Useful at any age.

How to Keep Your Child Fit from Birth to Six. New York: Harper & Row, Publishers, 1964. Rev. ed. New York: The Dial Press, 1983.

Exercise should begin at birth, and the foundation for a strong, healthy body is laid down between birth and six. The major damage caused by sedentary living is visited on children *before* school days . . . and parents can prevent it.

Fitness from Six to Twelve. New York: Harper & Row, Publishers, 1972. Rev. ed. New York: The Dial Press, 1983.

American schools are not equipped to repair the physical and emotional damage resulting from years of sedentary living, TV viewing and confinement to strollers, car seats, high chairs, playpens and preschools lacking in physical preparation for life. The second six years of life are literally the last chance for building a child's body to anywhere near its potential. This book is a complete guide for parents and teachers who want to provide their children with even a modest degree of fitness.

Teenage Fitness. New York: Harper & Row, Publishers, 1965. Rev. ed. New York: The Dial Press, 1983.

Teenagers are the victims of the American way of life. Provided with "things," rather than strong, healthy bodies and training in physical fitness, they lack the physical outlets needed to compensate for rising levels of emotional stress. Results are both obvious and ominous. This is an excellent coed program of physical activity for young people as well as the philosophy needed to keep it going. Presport and how-to exercises.

Teach Your Baby to Swim. New York: The Dial Press, 1983.

If you want your baby to become water wise, enjoy the water and come to know you better, this is a thoroughly delightful book that will show you how. If you are a swim teacher, this is the program that put the hundreds of Y Baby Swim and Gym programs into being.

How to Keep Your Family Fit and Healthy. Stockbridge, Mass.: Bonnie Prudden Press, 1975.

Families want to and *should* exercise together, but what programs appeal to every age and can be adapted for each generation? This book provides the information.

Exer-Sex. Stockbridge, Mass.: Bonnie Prudden Press, 1979.

A gentle book about feelings and sex, with exercises that improve both as well as the quality of life. A different, better way of imparting information about sex, sensuality and loving.

Physical Fitness for You (a talking book for the blind). New York: The American Foundation for the Blind, 1964.

The complete book of exercise for the blind, partially blind and for older people who may be limited in what they can do for their level of fitness by handicaps. It can be ordered from

The American Foundation for the Blind, 15 West 16th Street, New York, N.Y. 10011.

Pain Erasure: The Bonnie Prudden Way. New York: M. Evans & Co., Inc., 1980, hardcover. New York: Ballantine Books, Inc., 1982, paperback.

This was the first book ever written about Myotherapy, a revolutionary method of relieving pain. It would be useful as an adjunct to *Bonnie Prudden's Guide to Pain-Free Living*. The more you know about a subject, the better you understand the world around you.

Records

Keep Fit—Be Happy, Volume I. Los Angeles: Warner Brothers, 1959.

An excellent program of exercise with delightful music. A special band for running at home *and off the road*. Two bands on progressive relaxation. Recommended as a beginning program and as an aid in recovering from injuries caused by many fitness programs today.

Keep Fit—Be Happy, Volume II. Los Angeles, Warner Brothers, 1961.

Advanced exercise plus floor progressions, weight lifting and tumbling routine.

Film

Your Baby Can Swim. 15mm, color, sound, 12 minutes. Stockbridge, Mass.

Bodos

The bodos shown in this book are handmade wooden tools used for erasing muscle pain by extinguishing trigger points. Their chief value is they can be used by people who live or travel alone and who must depend on their own hands for help. Available only from the Bonnie Prudden Institute for Physical Fitness and Myotherapy, Stockbridge, Mass. 01262.

An annual brochure providing places and dates of Pain-Erasure Seminars and workshops is sent on request and to those on the center's mailing list. Include a stamped business envelope.

WARNING:

Recently, several unauthorized persons have been calling themselves "Myotherapists." Bonnie Prudden-certified Myotherapists spend two years learning the art at the Bonnie Prudden School for Physical Fitness and Myotherapy. This requires thirteen hundred hours. They graduate as certified Bonnie Prudden Myotherapists and Certified Exercise Therapists or both . . . and they have the papers to prove it. Certified Bonnie Prudden Myotherapists are required to update their training every two years with forty-five hours of work leading to recertification. *They do not accept patients without a doctor's referral.* When offered Myotherapy by *anyone*, ask for proof of training.

For further information, contact the Bonnie Prudden School for Physical Fitness and Myotherapy.^SM

Books Mentioned

Stress Without Distress, by Hans Selye
 1974 (hardcover) by Lippincott
 1975 (paperback) by New American Library
The Virtue of Selfishness, by Ayn Rand
 1964 (original edition) by New American Library
 no date (paper) by New American Library
The Cinderella Complex, by Colette Dowling
 1981 (hardcover) by Summit Books
 1982 (paperback) by Summit Books
Immaculate Deception—A New Look at Women and Childbirth in America, by Suzanne Arms
 1975 (paperback) by Bantam Books
Poisons in Your Food, by William Longgood
 out of print

YOU DESERVE A PAIN-FREE LIFE

Pain-Free Living. A one-hour video cassette. The audio-visual aid for this book. Read it, see it, hear it, *do it yourself*.

A program designed for both group and individual instruction, featuring a new, non-invasive, drug-free method for getting at the cause of pain.
The Bonnie Prudden Approach to Pain Erasure/Myotherapy^{SM}

Easy-to-follow instructions for erasing the pain of backache, headache, leg cramps, shin splints, groin pain, menstrual cramps, shoulder and neck pain, tired feet and other assorted aches and pains including many of those attributed to arthritis.

Demonstrations of *safe*, effective, exciting exercises for everyone and every age. Improve your posture and increase your strength, flexibility, coordination and endurance. Exercises for warm-up before sports, dance or *any* demanding physical activity.

Exercises for children, prevention of sports injuries, help for the sidelined athlete . . . even pain erasure for your pets.

Baby exercises to be begun at once and proceeding through every age. Exercises for the executive. Exercises and pain erasure to prevent aging.

No special equipment or setting necessary. Use what's around the house right there in the house.

HAVEN'T YOU SUFFERED ENOUGH? Order now. Available in VHS and BETA. Write to: Bonnie Prudden, Inc., P. O. Box 625, Stockbridge, Mass. 01262.

Index